Fourth Edition

Research Design and Evaluation in Speech-Language Pathology and Audiology

Franklin H. Silverman
Marquette University
Medical College of Wisconsin

Allyn and Bacon
Boston • London • Toronto • Sydney • Tokyo • Singapore

To those who use the information in this book, in the words of Socrates, "to kindle a flame, not fill a vessel."

Executive Editor: Stephen D. Dragin
Editorial Assistant: Elizabeth McGuire
Editorial-Production Administrator: Joe Sweeney
Editorial-Production Service: Walsh & Associates, Inc.
Composition Buyer: Linda Cox
Manufacturing Buyer: Megan Cochran
Cover Administrator: Suzanne Harbison

Library of Congress Cataloging-in-Publication Data

Silverman, Franklin H., 1933–
    Research design and evaluation in speech-language pathology and
audiology / Franklin H. Silverman.—4th ed.
        p.   cm.
    Includes bibliographical references and index.
    ISBN 0-205-19799-X
    1. Speech disorders—Research—Methodology.   2. Language
disorders—Research—Methodology.   3. Audiology—Research—
Methodology.   I. Title.
    [DNLM: 1. Communicative Disorders.   2. Research—methods.   3. Data
Collection.   4. Speech-Language Pathology—methods.   WM 475 S587r
1997]
RC423.S519   1997
616.85'5'0072—dc21
DNLM/DLC
for Library of Congress   97-6601
                                                                           CIP

Printed in the United States of America

10 9 8 7 6 5 4 3 2 1   00 99 98 97

Contents

Preface

During the twenty years since this book was first published, I have received comments from a number of clinicians and instructors of research methodology courses about my position that clinicians should be producers as well as consumers of research. While most of these comments indicated agreement with my position, some have expressed reservations about it. The gist of the most frequent one I have received is that while in an "ideal" world clinicians would do clinical research, in the real world very few are likely to do it. Consequently, it is not essential that they know how to do research—they just have to know how to evaluate it. While it is true that relatively few masters-level speech-language pathologists and audiologists publish research in professional journals and present it at professional meetings, nevertheless, they all do it and publish it. That is, they assess the impacts of their intervention (management) strategies on clients and "publish" their findings about such impacts in reports to clients, employers, insurance companies, and government agencies. Such dissemination of information is recognized as publication by U.S. copyright law. Dissemination (publication) by report, incidentally, is the method used by corporations for disseminating research that they regard as proprietary and by agencies of the U.S. government for disseminating "classified" research.

The process clinicians should use for answering questions to document therapy outcome to maximize the likelihood of a correct answer is identical to the one they should use for answering other research questions. The same is true for the process they should use for answering questions during an evaluation (diagnostic) session. Consequently, clinicians not only need a knowledge of research methodology that is adequate for evaluating the validity, reliability, and generality of the answers to questions posed by others, but also one that is adequate for answering clinical and other research questions that they pose. Clinical documentation is single-subject research!

In this fourth edition of *Research Design and Evaluation in Speech-Language Pathology and Audiology* I have sought not only to bring the text up to date but to strengthen it in several ways. The material on single-subject research methodology—particularly as it pertains to clinical documentation—has been expanded considerably. A chapter has been added on the use of inferential statistical techniques for estimating the reliability and generality of data yielded by single-subject designs.

The material on inferential statistical techniques for group designs has been expanded. Sections have been added to Chapter 10 on multivariate analysis of variance (MANOVAS) and multivariate analysis of covariance (MANCOVAS).

There is a second new chapter in this edition that deals with cultural considerations in designing and interpreting clinical research (Chapter 17). This is a topic to which practitioners and researchers in our field have become particularly sensitive in recent years. My own sensitivity to it comes in part from reading relevant literature and in part from training Palestinians in the Gaza Strip to do clinical research.

The protection of human subjects in clinical research continues to be of concern to all health professionals—both those who do and don't engage in it. The wording of the World Health Association statement on their protection in Appendix D has been modified slightly to increase its relevancy as a guideline for speech-language pathologists and audiologists.

There is a greater emphasis on the use of computers for measurement and data analysis in this edition than in previous ones. The material on instrumentation measurement schemes in Chapter 8 has been revised extensively to reflect the use of microcomputers for simulating such schemes. Also, the commands for doing *all* of the exercises in Appendix A with MINITAB statistical software are now included. This program, which was developed in 1972 at Pennsylvania State University to help teach introductory courses in statistics, has been updated frequently and is utilized in such courses at more than 1500 colleges and universities. It is available for almost all mainframe and minicomputers as well as for Macintosh and Windows-compatible microcomputers. These exercises, of course, can also be done with other statistical software packages.

It is impossible to give credit to all of the sources from which the concepts presented in this book have been drawn. The book is the result of years of reading and thousands of hours of conversation with students and colleagues in the areas of communicative disorders and research methodology. Thus, I often cannot credit this or that concept to a specific person, but I can say "thank you" to all who have helped, particularly my students at Marquette University and in the Gaza Strip whose questions and criticisms through the years have helped me to clarify my own ideas.

I am pleased by reports that the first three editions of the text have helped a little to break down the dichotomy in the minds of many speech-language pathologists and audiologists between clinical work and clinical research. I am also pleased by reports that it has provided many with information needed to become informed consumers and producers of clinical research. Hopefully, the information they gain from functioning as a clinician-investigator will help them fulfill the A.S.H.A. ethical injunction "to hold paramount the welfare of persons served professionally."

I would also like to thank the followintg reviewers: Michael W. Casby, Michigan State University, and Paxton E. Oliver, Northeast Louisiana University.

Part *I*

Introduction

Chapter 1

Utilization of Research Methodology in Speech-Language Pathology and Audiology

The intent of this chapter is to demonstrate the relevance of pure (or basic) and applied research to evaluation and therapy (clinical process) in speech-language pathology and audiology. *Pure research* is intended to increase our understanding of the etiology (that is, the predisposing, precipitating, and maintaining causes) of communicative disorders. *Applied research* is intended to increase our understanding of how to prevent the development of, or modify behaviors contributing to, communicative disorders. Some research serves both functions: It provides data relevant to the etiology of communicative disorders as well as to their diagnosis, prevention, or treatment.

The term *research* in this book refers to the processes underlying the *asking and answering* of questions as well as to the "answers" that can be abstracted from the observations provided by such processes. In a sense, the overall objective of this book is to clarify and elaborate upon this definition of research as it applies to clinical process in speech-language pathology and audiology.

You, the reader of this book, have to make some assumption(s) about the relevance of research to your activities before deciding how much to invest in acquiring a knowledge of research methodology. The amount you are willing to invest to attain a goal is at least partially a function of the return you anticipate. If you expect a substantial return, you usually will be willing to invest more than if you anticipate little, if any, return. The stronger your belief that learning certain material will directly benefit you, the more time and energy you are likely to invest in doing so. Also, the stronger your belief that learning certain material will benefit you, the more willing you are likely to be to tackle material you expect to be difficult, such as statistical and research design concepts. And the more willing you are to tackle such material and the more time and energy you devote to doing so, the more likely you are to master it. Some persons who have difficulty understanding statistical and research design concepts do *not* appear to experience it because of a lack of ability, but because they are not convinced that learning such concepts will be helpful to them in the "real world" and, hence, they do not invest the time and energy necessary to grasp them. One of my goals in this chapter and the one that follows is to strengthen your belief in the relevance of research and research design concepts to your functioning as a clinician.

Questioning and Clinical Effectiveness

We will begin our discussion of the relevance of research to clinical process in speech-language pathology and audiology with the following premise: To be even minimally effective, a clinician must be able to at least partially answer certain questions. These questions include:

1. Is the communicative behavior of the child or adult whom I am evaluating "within normal limits"?
2. If his or her communicative behavior is not "within normal limits," what is the reason?
3. How can his or her communicative behavior be modified to bring it "within normal limits," or as close as possible to this goal?

If we are not aware of "normal limits" for the various attributes of speech, language, and hearing, we will be unable to determine with an acceptable degree of accuracy whether a child or adult (particularly a child) has a communicative disorder. We will tend to make one or both of the following errors more often than we should: (1) classifying a person whose communicative behavior is "within normal limits" as having a communicative disorder, or (2) classifying a person who has a communicative disorder as having communicative behavior "within normal limits." We may, for example, classify a 3-year-old who has an IQ of approximately 100 and consistently substitutes /w/ for /r/ as not being "within normal limits." Also, we might classify a 3-year-old who is "effortlessly" repeating some syllables as beginning to stutter. To answer questions concerning the normality of a 3-year-old's communicative behavior, we must have information concerning the communicative behavior of "normal" 3-year-olds. That is, we must have access to relevant normative data.

If the answer to the first question is no (that is, if we do not judge the person's communicative behavior to be "within normal limits"), we then attempt to answer the second, or "why," question. To answer this question, we have to be able to specify the possible causes for the deviation or deviations we have observed. We need this information to perform a differential diagnosis—to rule in and rule out possible causes systematically. We also need this information to plan therapy. For a therapy strategy to have maximum probability of success, it should be based upon, or derived from, our assumption or assumptions about why a client's communicative behavior is not "within normal limits" (Williams, 1968).

Once we have at least partially established the reason or reasons for a client's communicative behavior not being "within normal limits," we then develop an intervention strategy that will hopefully either bring it "within normal limits" or as close as possible to the goal. To develop such a strategy, or to answer the "how" question, we need information concerning the relative effectiveness of the various strategies that could be used. For each possible strategy, we also need related information, including negative side effects and susceptibility to relapse. Such information provides guidelines for answering the "how" question and thereby helps to maximize the probability of achieving the therapy goal or goals.

Need for Systematic Observation in Answering Questions

How do we go about answering questions such as the three previously discussed so that the probability of a correct answer is maximized? Answering questions in this manner requires the type of data that results from systematic observation. The term *data* as used here refers to numerical and verbal descriptions of attributes of events. Attributes of the event "speech," for example, would include "voice quality" and "amount of syllable repetition." And attributes of the event "listening" would include "sound discrimination ability" and "level of comprehension." Numerical descriptions of attributes of events are referred to as *quantitative* and verbal as *qualitative*.

Systematic observation is a process that permits us to describe individual attributes of events. We decide in advance which attributes of which events we wish to describe and then for each attribute devise a "filter" that will permit us to make the desired observations. The filter makes each target attribute—each attribute we seek to describe—stand out sufficiently from the others so that it can be described reliably. The filter, then, enhances the figure-background relationship (the target attribute being the figure and the other attributes the background). The filter may include instrumentation to enhance our ability to restrict our observational processes, or it may consist solely of a "set" we give ourselves to do so. Speech-language pathologists usually give themselves such a set during the administration of a picture articulation test, since they pay most attention to the particular speech sound each picture was included to elicit. This sound would be the figure (i.e., the target attribute), the other sounds in the word would be the background. Instrumentation used by speech-language pathologists and audiologists for this purpose is described in Chapter 8.

Systematic observation maximizes the probability that the data used to answer questions will yield correct answers by maximizing the probability that they will possess adequate validity and reliability for the purpose. By adequate *validity* in this context, we mean that the filter used to observe and describe a particular attribute of a particular event actually permits us to observe and describe that attribute of that event. If we wished, for example, to determine how frequently a child produced a lateral /s/ (attribute) during conversational speech (event), having observers listen to tape recordings of the child's conversational speech and identifying instances of lateral /s/ on typescripts of the recordings should yield data that possess adequate validity for this purpose.

By maximizing the probability that the data used to answer a question will possess adequate *reliability*, we mean that the filter used to observe and describe an attribute of an event permits this to be done with a *sufficient level of accuracy*—that is, a level that permits the minimum desired degree of confidence in the correctness of the answer. The less distortion (or error) introduced by the filter, the more reliable will be the resulting data. As indicated in the previous paragraph, a valid method for estimating how frequently a child produced a lateral /s/ probably would be to tape record his conversational speech and have trained listeners indicate instances of lateral /s/ on a typescript of the recording. For this methodology to be adequately reliable as well as valid, the tape recordings would have to be of sufficiently high quality that instances of lateral /s/ could be identified from them with minimal error.

Systematic observation, in addition to maximizing the probability that the data used to answer a question will possess adequate levels of validity and reliability for the purpose, also provides a methodology for determining whether this goal has been achieved. In fact, this methodology permits us to estimate the validity and reliability levels of a set of data. These constructs will be discussed further in Chapter 12.

Satisfying the Need for Systematic Observation

The preceding section discussed why systematic observation could be expected to yield the type of data that maximizes the probability of correct answers to questions. We will now consider how pure and applied research can satisfy, at least partially, the need for systematic observation.

Systematic observation is used in both pure and applied research. It is, in fact, a component (as will be shown in Chapter 3) of the scientific method that underlies almost all research. For this reason, data yielded by both types of research can be used by speech-language pathologists and audiologists to answer questions of professional interest, including those on clinical process.

The previous section discussed three questions that a clinician needs to be able to answer to function effectively. How can data from pure and applied research help to maximize the probability of a correct answer to each question?

The first of these questions was: Is the communicative behavior of the child or adult whom I am evaluating "within normal limits"? To maximize the probability of a correct answer, a clinician needs *normative data*—data that help to define "normal limits" for each attribute of communicative behavior being evaluated. Such data have been reported for a number of attributes of communicative behavior in research papers appearing in such journals as the *American Journal of Audiology*, the *American Journal of Speech-Language Pathology*, the *Journal of Speech and Hearing Research*, and *Language, Speech, and Hearing Services in Schools*.

The second question was: If the client's communicative behavior is not "within normal limits," what is the reason? To answer this question, we need to know the possible causes for each deviation from "normal limits" a client exhibits. Considerable relevant research-based information has appeared in the *American Journal of Audiology*, the *American Journal of Speech-Language Pathology*, the *Journal of Speech and Hearing Research*, and *Language, Speech, and Hearing Services in Schools*. Such research-based information, incidentally, is the source of lists of possible causes of articulation disorders, voice disorders, fluency disorders, children's language disorders, hearing loss, and other communicative disorders that appear in speech-language pathology and audiology textbooks.

The final question was: How can the client's communicative behavior be modified to bring it "within normal limits," or as close as possible to this goal? To answer this question, we need information concerning the possible impacts of each intervention strategy we are considering on the client in general and his or her communicative behavior in particular. We are not only interested in information about the possible positive effects of an intervention strategy on a client's communicative disorder, but also in information about possible negative side effects and the permanence of changes in a client's communicative behavior resulting from its use. Relevant data for some therapy approaches used to treat communicative disorders have been reported in such journals as the *American Journal of Audiology*, the *American Journal of Speech-Language Pathology*, and *Language, Speech, and Hearing Services in Schools*. There is a need for considerably more therapy outcome research. This need is explored further in Chapters 2 and 14.

Questions and Answers

To demonstrate the relevance of research to clinical decision making in speech-language pathology and audiology, we have argued that a clinician has to be able to answer certain questions to be even minimally effective. In this section we will indicate more specifically how research can provide the data needed to maximize the probability of correct answers to questions concerning evaluation and therapy. We will pose five questions a clinician might need to answer and indicate how data published in several *randomly* selected issues of the *Journal of Speech and Hearing Research* could provide at least a partial answer to each question. The format used for each question will be: (1) a statement of the question, (2) a reference for the data, (3) a description of the observational procedures, (4) a summary of the observations made (i.e., data) that are relevant to answering the question, and (5) a tentative answer to the question. In addition to demonstrating the relevance of research to clinical decision making, this presentation is also intended as an informal introduction to the structure of a research report.

1. ARE THE EARPHONES I USE FOR MY CLINICAL AUDIOLOGICAL EVALUATION LIKELY ENOUGH TO BECOME CONTAMINATED TO WARRANT THE EXPENSE OF ROUTINE DECONTAMINATION?
  Data Source. Talbott, R.E. (1969). Bacteriology of earphone contamination. *Journal of Speech and Hearing Research*, 12, 326–329.
  Observational Procedure. Bacterial samples of earphone earcushions used for clinical audiological evaluations in a hospital setting were examined for the presence of three pathogenic microorganisms that have been associated with otitis media and otitis externa.
  Observations Made. Staphylococcus aureus, a pathogenic microorganism, was recovered "in great quantities" from all earcushions sampled.
  Tentative Answer to Question. Earphones used for clinical audiological evaluations appear likely enough to become contaminated by pathogenic microorganisms to warrant the expense of routine decontamination.
  Remarks. A clinician also could obtain data to answer this question through systematic observations of his or her own earphones.

2. CAN SAMPLES OF CONVERSATIONAL SPEECH THAT ARE SUFFICIENTLY REPRESENTATIVE TO BE USEFUL FOR ASSESSING A 4-YEAR-OLD CHILD'S PRAGMATIC ABILITY BE ELICITED IN A PRESCHOOL PLAYROOM ENVIRONMENT?

Data Source. Schober-Peterson, D., & Johnson, C.J. (1989). Conversational topics of four-year-olds. *Journal of Speech and Hearing Research*, 32, 857–870.

Observational Procedure. Ten dyads (pairs) of 4-year-old children were videotaped during play in a typical preschool playroom environment. Ten-minute samples were analyzed according to a number of topic-dependent measures.

Observations Made. All dyads evidenced some lengthy topics (13-91 utterances). Longer topics were characterized by three text-level functions: enacting scenarios, describing, and problem solving.

Tentative Answer to Question. Samples of conversation that are likely to have adequate generality for revealing a 4-year-old's pragmatic ability can be obtained by recording him or her during play in a preschool playroom setting.

3. HOW TRANSPARENT ("GUESSABLE") ARE 91 ONE-HANDED AMERICAN INDIAN HAND-TALK (AMER-IND) SIGNS?

Data Source. Campbell, C.R., & Jackson, S.T. (1995). Transparency of one-handed Amer-Ind hand signals to nonfamiliar viewers. *Journal of Speech and Hearing Research*, 38, 1284–1289.

Observational Procedure. Each of 30 subjects after viewing each of the 91 hand signals twice in succession on videotape wrote at least one word for the signal's meaning. The percentage of correct guesses for each hand signal was determined.

Observations Made. The percentage of correct guesses for the hand signals ranged from 0% to 100%.

Tentative Answer to Question. The correct-guess percentages for 91 hand signals are reported in a table.

4. WHAT FACTORS SHOULD I CONSIDER WHEN MAKING A PROGNOSIS FOR LANGUAGE RECOVERY FOLLOWING A STROKE?

Data Source. Holland, A.L., Greenhouse, J.B., Fromm, D., & Swingell, C.S. (1989). Predictors of language restitution following stroke: A multivariate analysis. *Journal of Speech and Hearing Research*, 32, 332–338.

Observational Procedure. A consecutive sample of 50 language impaired patients was evaluated prospectively during the first three to four months following a unilateral left- or right-hemisphere stroke with regard to the relative importance of eight variables on the likelihood of language recovery.

Observations Made. The variables that were found to be most strongly associated with language recovery were age (favoring younger patients) and length of hospital stay (favoring shorter stays). Gender (favoring males), type of stroke (favoring hemorrhages), and site of lesion (favoring right) also appeared to influence language recovery, but not as strongly as age and length of hospital stay. Neither race nor history of previous stroke appeared to influence language recovery.

Tentative Answer to Question. These data suggest that the age of the patient is probably the best single predictor of language recovery following stroke. If the length of the patient's hospital stay was not influenced by financial (insurance) considerations, this also could be a good predictor.

5. CAN A COCHLEAR IMPLANT INTERFACED WITH A WEARABLE SPEECH PROCESSING DEVICE ASSIST A DEAF PERSON IN UNDERSTANDING SPEECH?

Data Source. Dowell, R.C., Martin, L.F.A., Tong, Y.C., Clark, G.M., Seligman, P.M., & Patrick, J.F. (1982). A 12-consonant confusion study of a multiple-channel cochlear implant patient. *Journal of Speech and Hearing Research, 25,* 509–516.

Observational Procedure. A 49-year-old man with total bilateral deafness who had been fitted with a cochlear implant and a wearable speech processing device was asked to identify 12 consonant sounds (in a VCV context) spoken by a male and a female speaker. He could not see the speakers' faces. The percentage of the consonants that were correctly identified was determined.

Observations Made. The subject correctly identified 48 percent of the consonants.

Tentative Answer to Question. Judging by the fact that this subject was able to understand almost half of the consonant sounds, it would appear that a cochlear implant interfaced with a wearable speech processing device can significantly assist *some* deaf persons in understanding speech. More subjects, of course, would have to be tested before a reliable estimate could be made of the percentage of deaf persons who would be likely to benefit significantly from such an approach.

Has the Need Been Met?

This chapter stressed the fact that existing research can provide data helpful in answering questions concerning clinical process. This was not meant to imply that the need for such data has been met. To the contrary, more such data are needed. This need is, incidentally, one of the main reasons for my arguing in the next chapter that clinicians should be producers as well as consumers of research.

Exercises and Discussion Topics

1. Select any single issue of the *Journal of Speech and Hearing Research*. Formulate three questions a clinician might want to answer that could be at least partially answered using data reported in this issue. For each indicate the data source (i.e., the title of the paper) and summarize the observational procedures used and the observations made. Then indicate the tentative answer to each question. Five examples of this type of analysis are included in the chapter.

2. The need for systematic observation in answering research questions is explored in this chapter. Discuss why systematic observation also is needed for answering *clinical* questions, particularly those that clinicians attempt to answer when evaluating clients.

3. Suppose that there will be no further research on communicative disorders. What impacts would this have on clinical practice in speech-language pathology and audiology?

4. Select a paper from the *Journal of Speech and Hearing Research*, the *American Journal of Audiology*, the *American Journal of Speech-Language Pathology*, or *Language, Speech, and Hearing Services in Schools* in which a therapy approach is described. Show how pure and applied research contributed to the development of the approach, using the studies cited in the paper.

5. You are a research audiologist working for a hearing aid manufacturer. Your employer has developed a new type of hearing aid and wants you to do research to evaluate its impacts on hard-of-hearing persons. What research questions might you attempt to answer to accomplish this objective?

Chapter 2

Research, Research Methodology, and the Clinician

The previous chapter dealt with the need for research in speech-language pathology and audiology to answer questions relating to clinical practice. This chapter will present the need for clinicians to be able *both* to evaluate answers to such questions and to answer them through research. Specifically, we will argue that it is important for clinicians to function as both consumers and producers of research. Both roles require a knowledge of research methodology. It is used in the first for *evaluating* research and in the second for both *evaluating and designing* research.

The Consumer Role

All speech-language pathologists and audiologists are consumers of research. They read research reports in professional journals and utilize information presented in them in their clinical practice. They need to understand research methodology (particularly that aspect dealing with descriptive and inferential statistics) to *evaluate* the information presented in them. Specifically, they need it to determine whether the data reported possess levels of validity, reliability, and generality that are adequate for them to be utilized clinically. Data reported in professional journals may not possess levels of one or more of these that would be adequate for this purpose. The reasons are discussed in Chapter 12.

The Producer, or Clinician-Investigator, Role

The term *clinician-investigator* will be used in this book to designate a speech-language pathologist or audiologist who functions both as a clinician and a clinical investigator, or researcher. A hyphen was inserted between "clinician" and "investigator" to indicate that the two roles are not independent but interdependent. Thus, being a clinician would probably influence the kinds of research questions an investigator would ask, and being an investigator would probably influence a clinician's approach to problem solving in diagnosis and therapy. Also, a speech-language pathologist or audiologist might perform both functions simultaneously. That is, he or she might gather clinical research data while performing clinical functions (diagnosis and therapy). The individual clinical case study that utilizes data gathered as part of diagnosis or therapy, or both, illustrates this combined function (Bromley, 1986). The term *clinician-investigator*, incidentally, was derived from *teacher-investigator*, a term used in some colleges and universities to designate the dual interrelated roles of a professor—teaching and research.

Why should a clinician be a clinician-investigator? One of the most compelling reasons is to function in a manner that is consistent with the Code of Ethics of the American Speech-Language-Hearing Association. The current (1996) version of the Code states that "individuals shall evaluate services rendered to determine effectiveness." Thus, for clinicians to function ethically they *must* systematically evaluate the impacts of the services they render. And to be able to do so they must acquire a knowledge of clinical research methodology.

There are a number of benefits in addition to satisfying the requirements of the ASHA Ethical Code that a clinician can derive from functioning as a clinician-investigator. The following discussion suggests several of them. The order in which they are discussed is not intended to reflect their relative importance.

First of all, functioning as a clinician-investigator would probably make one's job more stimulating, less routine, and would probably increase the possibilities for positive reinforcement. In addition to feeling successful at clinical activities, the clinician-investigator would have a second potential source of reinforcement—his or her research activities. This reinforcement could arise from any of the following factors: the feeling of accomplishment that comes from formulating a research question (or questions) and making the necessary observations to answer it (or them) at least partially; reporting the results of research to professional colleagues informally, on the program of a professional meeting (for example, a state speech and hearing association or the American Speech-Language-Hearing Association), or in a professional journal; and knowing that your professional efforts can help not only your own clients but also those of other practitioners. Thus, communicating your clinical knowledge and experience of the communicatively handicapped can spread the benefits to others.

Functioning as a clinician-investigator also would help you to satisfy your employer's requirements for *accountability* (Olswang, 1990). Almost all speech-language pathologists and audiologists are required by their employers to document the impacts of their therapy programs on their clients. Incidentally, for speech-language pathologists employed in the public schools such documentation is mandated by Public Law 94-142. And for those employed in medical settings, such documentation is also essential because it is required for managed care (Vekovius, 1995) and other insurance purposes.

Next, functioning as a clinician-investigator could probably help you become a more effective clinician, for several reasons. First, the dual role could provide answers to questions relevant to managing your own caseload. For example, it could help you to determine whether a therapy approach you are using is effective and whether, therefore, you should continue to use it. Or it could help you to determine whether a newer therapy approach is more effective than one you are currently using and, therefore, whether you should adopt the newer approach. It could also help you to establish whether your diagnostic procedures are adequately reliable and to provide normative data for diagnostic procedures you use that are not standardized on the specific populations in your caseload (see Chapter 17). Finally, it could provide documentation for the efficacy of new clinical services offered by your facility that would be helpful when seeking funding to continue them.

Functioning as a clinician-investigator could improve your effectiveness by helping you to develop a more "scientific" approach to clinical decision making. The problem-solving approach based on the scientific method that is essential for functioning as an investigator is also desirable for functioning as a clinician. This approach has several aspects, including: (1) stating goals, or objectives, clearly; (2) asking questions that are "answerable" and stating hypotheses that are "testable"; (3) being systematic in making observations to answer questions and test hypotheses; and (4) being aware of the *tentative* nature of answers and hypotheses.

The need for clinical goals and objectives to be stated clearly has been discussed by a number of authors (e.g., Johnson, 1946; Silverman, 1984, 1995b; Williams, 1968). Obviously, if a clinical objective or goal were not clearly stated, a clinician could never be reasonably certain whether it had been achieved. This situation probably would not be positively reinforcing for either client or clinician.

Another clinically relevant aspect of this approach is asking questions that are "answerable" and stating hypotheses that are "testable." Rather than asking, for example, whether a given therapy approach has been effective, you would ask whether it resulted in certain behavioral changes. (The reason why the second question would be more "answerable" than the first will be discussed in Chapter 5.) Also, rather than hypothesizing that a child is slow in learning to talk because he is "emotionally disturbed," you would define operationally what you meant by being emotionally disturbed. This definition would suggest the diagnostic procedures you would need to test your hypothesis.

A third aspect is being systematic in making observations to answer questions and test hypotheses. The considerations described in Chapter 14 for designing research to evaluate the effects of therapies, for example, are relevant *clinically* for making observations to evaluate the effects of therapies you are using with clients. That is, the approaches used to answer systematically clinical questions for both clinical and research purposes are identical. The approaches used for both for making observations to "test" clinically relevant hypotheses are also identical. There should be no difference, therefore, in the way you would go about answering clinically relevant questions or testing clinically relevant hypotheses for clinical and research purposes. This similarity in approach is not surprising, since no sharp line of demarcation exists between clinical work and clinical research. Overlap is particularly evident with regard to the individual case study and other clinical research that utilizes a single subject design (e.g., Barlow & Hersen, 1984; Connell & Thompson, 1986; Kazdin, 1982a, 1982b; Kearns, 1986; McReynolds & Kearns, 1983; McReynolds & Thompson, 1986; Tawney & Gast, 1984).

The final aspect of the scientific approach, being aware of the *tentative* nature of answers and hypotheses, is one of the most important, because it indicates that no answer to a question or test of a hypothesis is *final*. As new information becomes available, hypotheses that appeared viable may no longer appear so. The answer to every question and the viability of every hypothesis must therefore be regarded as tentative. Both have implicit qualifiers attached. For answers to questions, the implicit qualifier would be: "With the information I currently have available, the answer to the question is . . ." And for statements concerning the viability of hypotheses, the implicit qualifier would be: "Judging by the information I currently have available, the hypothesis seems viable." These implicit qualifiers, of course, should be attached to clinical question answers and hypotheses, not just research ones.

The tentative nature of answers and hypotheses is due at least partially to the fact that observations are never complete. In other words, "the data are never all in." It is more appropriate to conclude, therefore, that available research *suggest* a therapy is effective, rather than available data *prove* a therapy is effective. This concept is discussed further in Chapter 3.

If clinicians functioned as clinician-investigators, furthermore, they would provide data needed for answering questions on diagnosis and therapy. The answers to many questions sought by clinicians require observations that can be made at least as validly and efficiently in the clinic as in the laboratory. If you wished to evaluate, for example, a therapy approach intended for use in a school setting, it probably would make most sense for you to evaluate it in a school setting. One reason is that the setting in which therapy is done may place constraints upon what can be done. Thus, a therapy approach that is effective but requires a child to be seen five days a week for an hour a day would not be practical in a typical school setting. Also, data on the long-term effects of therapies probably can be gathered as validly, and more efficiently, in a clinical setting as it can in a laboratory setting. Additionally, the populations that must be observed to answer certain clinical questions may be more available to an investigator who works in a setting where such cases are seen for therapy than to one who is not employed in such a setting.

Finally, the data necessary to answer many clinically relevant questions can be gathered over a period of time as a part of diagnosis and therapy. Some of the best data we have on the symptomatology, etiology, diagnosis, and treatment of communicative disorders have come from this source. One example is the data on psychogenic stuttering of adult onset reported by Roth, Aronson, and Davis, Jr. (1989).

A clinician often is in a better position to make the observation needed to answer questions of clinical interest than is an investigator not actively engaged in clinical work. As previously mentioned, a clinician sometimes can make and record such observations within the context of his or her clinical work. In fact, the observations a clinician makes and records during diagnosis and therapy may be used to answer clinically relevant questions. It is necessary, though, that these observations be made in such a way that they possess relatively high levels of validity and reliability. This, incidentally, would also be a requirement for making such observations for clinical purposes. Observations that are not adequately reliable and valid would not be particularly useful for these purposes, either.

A clinician may also be able to make the observations needed to answer certain questions more reliably than an investigator not actively engaged in clinical work because of his or her clinical background and experience. This would be especially likely, for example, if the observations were of performance on clinical diagnostic tests. An experienced administrator's and interpreter's observations of performance on a diagnostic test probably would be more reliable than those of an investigator who is not experienced with the test, particularly one who did not administer or interpret it prior to doing so for a research project.

A clinician-investigator would also probably be better able both to evaluate therapies and to design research for this purpose than would an investigator not actively engaged in clinical work. This is especially likely to be true if the research involves experimental therapy and the design calls for the investigator to serve as clinician. An experienced clinician probably would do a better job administering an experimental therapy than an inexperienced one would. Additionally, an experienced clinician would probably be more aware of the "reality" factors that have to be considered when designing clinical research, particularly those introduced by the environment in which the data are being gathered. It may not be realistic, for example, to expect a classroom teacher to consistently reinforce "target" behaviors in a specified manner.

Thus far we have argued that: (1) many questions to which clinicians seek answers require observations that are at least as validly made in the clinic as in the laboratory, and (2) a clinician may be in a better position to make the observations necessary to answer such questions than an investigator not actively engaged in clinical work. Hopefully, we have demonstrated why a speech-language pathologist or audiologist would have the *possibility* of functioning as a clinician-investigator. Is there a *need*, however, for speech-language pathologists and audiologists to function in this manner? We believe such a need exists for several reasons, including the following:

1. He or she may be in the best position to make the observations necessary to answer clinically relevant questions, particularly those related to diagnosis and therapy. There are several reasons why the clinician-investigator might be in an advantageous position to answer such questions, including: (a) the setting in which he or she works, (b) the populations in his or her caseload, (c) his or her background and experience, (d) the availability of equipment and facilities for making the necessary observations, (e) the availability of collaborators from other disciplines, (f) the availability of an existing research program as a part of which the desired observations could be made, and (g) the availability of consultants and other supportive research personnel. The first three reasons were discussed earlier in the chapter; let us briefly examine the others here.

A speech-language pathologist or audiologist may be in an excellent position to make the observations necessary to answer certain questions of clinical interest because of available facilities that are unique or not generally available. An audiologist, for example, may have testing instrumentation or facilities that are unavailable in most audiological settings because of their cost or relatively limited usefulness. A speech-language pathologist may have one or more instruments for behavior modification, augmentative communication, or diagnostic testing that are not available in most clinics. If a speech-language pathologist or audiologist is able to exploit such facilities or instrumentation, he or she may be in a unique position to gather data necessary to answer questions of clinical importance.

A speech-language pathologist or audiologist may also have the opportunity to collaborate with investigators in other disciplines. A speech-language pathologist might collaborate with an otolaryngologist to assess the effects of a therapy on vocal nodules, or with a reading specialist to determine the effect of phonological errors on reading ability. An audiologist might collaborate with a microbiologist to determine if audiometer earphones are likely to contain pathogenic microorganisms. Again, if a speech-language pathologist or audiologist "exploits" opportunities for interdisciplinary research, he or she may be able to make observations necessary for answering questions that are significant clinically.

Another opportunity for a speech-language pathologist or audiologist to gather clinically relevant data is to become involved with an ongoing research program, especially an interdisciplinary one. If a clinician is working in a setting where research is being conducted in a related area such as psychology, learning disabilities, physical therapy, occupational therapy, rehabilitation counseling, social work, medicine, or dentistry, he or she may be able to gather clinically relevant data on communicative disorders by participating in the research program. In fact, by becoming involved when such a program is being planned, the clinician may be able to arrange for relevant data on communicative disorders to be gathered at the same time subjects are being seen by the other discipline or disciplines involved. To illustrate how this combining of interests can be accomplished, in the late 1950s a group of audiologists at a Veterans' Administration Outpatient Center were able to gather data on the hearing of men well past the age of 70 by arranging to do an audiometric evaluation on each of a group of Spanish-American War veterans being seen at the Center for other reasons. In this way speech pathologists and audiologists can take advantage of available opportunities to gather the data they need to answer clinically relevant questions.

The final factor to consider is the availability of consultants and supportive research personnel. Included here would be persons with expertise in statistics and electronics. When such persons are available, a clinician with clinically relevant questions to answer that require expertise in these areas can utilize the opportunity.

2. Much of the needed clinical research probably will not be done unless more clinicians are willing to function as clinician-investigators. In the first place, investigators who are not actively involved in clinical work are unlikely to be as *aware* as those who are of at least some clinically relevant questions that need to be answered. This is particularly true for practical questions concerning clinical program procedure. Such questions might deal with the effectiveness of paraprofessionals in various roles in speech, language, and hearing habilitation and rehabilitation, or with the efficacy of pediatrician referral for identifying children younger than three years who have or are "at risk" of developing a communicative disorder.

Second, investigators who are not clinicians are unlikely to be as *interested* as those who are in answering some questions of clinical interest, particularly those on clinical program procedure and therapy outcome. Such investigators may view questions on clinical program procedure as having limited theoretical significance. They may also be less interested in questions on therapy outcome for one or more of the following reasons: (1) The effects of extraneous variables are more difficult to control than in much laboratory research;

(2) the time it takes to collect data may be longer than for many types of laboratory research; and (3) the likelihood of a publishable result may not be as high in outcome research as in many types of laboratory research.

Third, investigators who are not clinicians might lack the *opportunity* to make the observations needed to answer many clinically relevant questions even if they were interested in doing so. Possible reasons for this lack of opportunity have already been discussed.

3. More clinicians functioning as clinician-investigators would probably help break down the clinician-researcher dichotomy that exists to some extent in speech-language pathology and audiology (Attanasio, 1986; Costello, 1979; Hamre, 1972; Jerger, 1963a, 1963b, 1964a; Ringel, 1972; Schultz, Roberts, & Yairi, 1972; Siegel & Spradlin, 1985). While this is certainly not the primary reason speech-language pathologists and audiologists should function as clinician-investigators, it nevertheless is an important one, since (for reasons previously discussed) it seems reasonable to conclude that clinical research and clinical practice are interdependent activities.

Who Can Be a Clinician-Investigator?

The previous section attempted partially to answer the question, "What benefits would a clinician derive from functioning as a clinician-investigator?" The word *partially* was inserted here to indicate that the reasons discussed are not the only possible ones. As general semanticists (e.g., Johnson, 1946) and others have pointed out, it is quite doubtful that any question can be completely answered or, for that matter, that everything can be said about anything.

This section will attempt partially to answer the question: "What attributes and competencies are necessary for a clinician to function successfully as a clinician-investigator, and how do these differ from those necessary to function solely as a clinician?" It will also attempt to answer the related question: "What attitudes and competencies are not essential for a clinician to function successfully as a clinician-investigator that might be regarded as necessary for him or her to function successfully in this role?" Its objective is to help the reader develop a more objective attitude toward research.

Why is it necessary for you to be concerned about developing a more objective attitude toward research? The term *objective attitude* is used here to indicate that your attitude toward research and your ability to function as a researcher should be as rational, or reality-oriented, as possible. If you were to view research as an activity possible for Ph.D.'s in universities but not for clinicians who have master's degrees and work as practitioners in educational and medical settings, your attitude would not be objective. Speech-language pathologists and audiologists employed in these settings who are not Ph.D.'s both have done and continue to do research.

Viewing research as an activity that requires extensive training in statistics and research methodology or a considerable expenditure of time is likewise not an objective attitude, because neither is absolutely essential for at least some clinical research.

The more objective your attitude toward research, the higher the probability you will consider functioning as a clinician-investigator. That is, the more certain you are that it is possible for you to function in this role, the more likely you are to attempt to do it. Some clinicians do not function as clinician-investigators because their attitudes toward research are not objective—not because their interest is lacking. They may assume, for example, that to do clinical research, a speech-language pathologist or audiologist must have a doctoral degree, advanced training in statistics or research design, considerable time available, or certain personal attributes that are not generally regarded as essential for clinicians. While these are not the only such assumptions made by clinicians, they appear to be among the most frequent, judging by the results of a national survey of ASHA members certified in speech-language pathology (Kelly & McReynolds, 1987). For this reason, the validity of each assumption will be considered here.

Neither a Ph.D. degree nor extensive training in statistics is essential for a speech-language pathologist or audiologist to make many (but not necessarily all) of the observations needed to answer clinical questions and report the answers in oral convention presentations or journal articles. While training at the doctoral level is desirable for an investigator because it is usually in large part research training, it is not a prerequisite. The investigator responsible for the scientific exhibit that won First Prize for Scientific Excellence at the 1972 Annual Convention of the American Speech-Language-Hearing Association was a high school student. His competition consisted of nineteen exhibits by speech-language pathologists, audiologists, and speech and hearing scientists with doctoral degrees (including the author). Perhaps the strongest evidence that a Ph.D. is not a prerequisite for at least some clinical research is the fact that clinical research done by speech-language pathologists and audiologists with master's degrees has been reported at annual conventions of the American Speech-Language-Hearing Association, those of state speech and hearing associations, as well as in clinical journals including those that are (or were) published by the American Speech-Language-Hearing Association.

Extensive knowledge of statistics and research methodology, like doctoral level training, though desirable for a speech-language pathologist or audiologist who wishes to function as a clinician-investigator, is not essential. The information presented in this book will suffice to formulate a plan for making the observations needed to answer some clinical questions. To answer others, the clinician-investigator may have to consult with persons who are knowledgeable in statistics and research design. Such consultants are available in many school systems, hospitals, rehabilitation centers, and other clinical settings. In addition, there may be faculty members at nearby colleges and universities who would be willing to consult with you about research design problems.

Another potentially unobjective attitude is that doing clinical research requires more time than a speech-language pathologist or audiologist would have available for the purpose. This reason was one of the most frequently mentioned for not doing research in the survey of certified speech clinicians cited previously. The objectivity of this attitude is a function of the question, or questions, the clinician seeks to answer. If these questions require observations that *the clinician has to make as part of his or her routine clinical responsibilities* (or observations he or she would not routinely make but could make within the context of his or her clinical responsibilities), this attitude would probably not be objective. Such questions might deal with the effectiveness of therapies being used with clients in the clinician's caseload. It seems reasonable to assume that the clinician would make some observations to evaluate the effectiveness of the therapies being used, if for no other reason than to satisfy his or her employers' demands for accountability. If these observations were reasonably reliable and valid (which also would be necessary for them to be useful clinically), they could be used for answering clinical research questions concerning therapy outcome. Gathering research data in this manner should not be particularly time-consuming.

Other research likely to place minimal demands upon a clinician's time is that which utilizes client folder data—that is, the diagnostic and therapy data recorded in clients' folders or in computer database equivalents. For such data to be usable for this purpose, they must be easily retrievable: that is, the files must be organized so that the folders of clients in the "population" to be studied can be located fairly easily. A variety of clinically relevant questions can be answered, at least partially, through the use of such data. These would include ones pertaining to: (1) factors influencing the prognosis for various communicative disorders, (2) interrelationships between test results (e.g., audiometric test results) for specific clinical "populations," (3) negative side effects of specific therapies, (4) positive effects of specific therapies upon specific communicative disorders, and (5) factors that influence the probability a client will terminate therapy before the clinician feels he or she is ready.

A final misconceived attitude is that clinicians, to do research, need more of certain personal attributes than is necessary for them to function well clinically. One attribute most frequently mentioned by speech-language pathologists is "intelligence." Many clinicians surveyed indicate that they did not consider themselves sufficiently intelligent to do clinical research. Several assumptions appear to underlie this attitude. One is that clinical research is relatively homogeneous in the demands it places on an investigator's intelligence—that is, the level of intelligence required to answer most questions of clinical interest is approximately the same. A second, related assumption implicit here is that the level of intelligence required to answer clinically relevant questions for research purposes exceeds that required to answer such questions for clinical purposes. (We are assuming here that a clinician would regard his or her level of intelligence as adequate for answering clinically relevant questions for clinical purposes.)

While clinical research may possibly be relatively homogeneous in the demands it places on an investigator's intelligence, this still seems quite unlikely, for several reasons. First, this assumption would violate the principle posited by general semanticists (e.g., Johnson, 1946) and others that the members of a "class of events" (clinical research studies would constitute such a class) are not identical in any attribute. In other words, events do not replicate themselves. Second, it would be necessary to assume that the observations required to answer clinically relevant questions place approximately equal demands on an investigator's intelligence. Such an assumption would be counterintuitive, since some observational procedures appear to place greater demands on an investigator's intelligence and ingenuity than others do. Questions that, to be answered, required an observational procedure that was well developed and standardized (such as a standardized test) would not intuitively appear to place as great a demand on an investigator's intelligence as would those requiring an observational procedure that the investigator has to devise and standardize.

The second assumption (probably the more important of the two with reference to the ability of a clinician to function as an investigator) is that the level of intelligence required to answer clinically relevant questions for research purposes exceeds that required to answer such questions for clinical purposes. If a clinician feels sufficiently intelligent to answer certain clinically relevant questions for clinical purposes, he or she should rationally also feel sufficiently intelligent to answer the same questions for research purposes. It is no less important for a clinical question to be answered correctly than it is for a research one.

Thus far, this section has dealt with attributes and competencies that do *not* appear to be essential for a speech-language pathologist or audiologist to function successfully as a clinician-investigator. What attributes and competencies *do* appear to be necessary for him or her to have a reasonable chance for success as a clinician-investigator? Since few relevant research data have been reported, the answer to this question that is given here should be regarded as speculative.

The personal attributes that appear necessary for a speech-language pathologist or audiologist to have a reasonable chance of functioning successfully as a clinician-investigator also appear, for the most part, necessary for him or her to have a reasonable chance of functioning successfully as a clinician. Partial support for this conclusion is provided by the findings of a study (Silverman, Halbach, & Palmer, unpublished data) in which a national random sample of speech-language pathologists ascribed essentially the same attributes to "a speech-language pathologist who does clinical work" as a second such random sample ascribed to "a speech-language pathologist who does clinical work and clinical research." While these data generally support the conclusion that the attributes of a successful clinician-investigator are essentially the same as those of a successful clinician, they obviously do not constitute a direct test of this hypothesis. A direct test would require comparing a number of personal attributes of a group of clinician-investigators with those of a group of clinicians who do not function as investigators.

What competencies are essential for speech-language pathologists or audiologists to function successfully as clinician-investigators? A general answer to this question would be that they must know how to: (1) formulate "answerable" questions and make the observations necessary to answer them with adequate levels of validity and reliability, (2) relate their answers to existing theories and knowledge, and (3) communicate questions, answers, and relations. The information in this book, hopefully, will assist in developing these competencies.

Exercises and Discussion Topics

1. Why might you resist functioning as a clinician-investigator? How might your resistance to doing so be modified?

2. Indicate for each of the following statements whether you agree or disagree and why:

   a. "Diagnosis, therapy, and clinical research are interrelated activities."

   b. "I can visualize myself doing a research project and reporting the results in a professional journal."

   c. "I can visualize one or more of my classmates doing a research project and reporting the results in a professional journal."

   d. "Having a knowledge of clinical research methodology tends to make one a better clinician."

   e. "It is unethical for clinicians to use their clients for clinical research."

   f. "Male clinicians tend to be better suited for doing research than female ones."

   g. "I feel that I am smart enough to be a good clinician, but I do not feel that I am smart enough to do clinical research."

   h. "Clinicians usually do not have time available for doing therapy outcome research."

Asking/Answering Questions and the Scientific Method

In the first two chapters I attempted to demonstrate why it is essential for you, as a clinician, to be knowledgeable about research methodology. This chapter discusses the *scientific method*—the set of rules from which this methodology was derived. My primary objective will be to demonstrate that the scientific method, as applied to research, can be viewed as a set of rules for asking and answering questions and for evaluating answers to questions.

It is desirable for you to have an intuitive understanding of the scientific method from the frame of reference of the history of science (how it has functioned) as well as that of the philosophy of science (how it is supposed to function). The methods that have been used by investigators to answer questions (and to arrive at "correct" answers) have not always been those that philosophers of science would regard as being consistent with the scientific method (Bush, 1974; Kuhn, 1962). That is, what the philosopher of science regards as being the method of science is not always what the historian of science has found to have been used. Consequently, the scientific method will be considered in this chapter from both points of view. Several examples relevant to speech-language pathology and audiology will be presented to illustrate the difference between them, including Franz Joseph Gall's discovery of the importance of the anterior portion of the brain for motor speech.

In addition to understanding the set of rules used for formulating and answering questions based on the scientific method, it is also desirable that you understand the assumptions (or presuppositions) on which the scientific method—and hence these rules—are based. It is desirable that you understand what you are required to accept on "faith" when you interpret research findings. Science, like religion, requires you to accept some things on faith!

The scientific method can be viewed as a game. Like any game, it has objectives and strategies for maximizing the probability of achieving them. In fact, as Agnew and Pyke (1975) pointed out in their provocative and entertaining description of "the science game,"

*The ingredients of any great game can be found in science—massive effort, goals,
great plays, mediocre plays, lousy plays; umpires making clear calls, judgment
calls, biased calls, and of course, mistaken calls. There are prizes and penalties.
You will find integrity, dignity, and deals, along with good luck and bad luck—but
above all you will find commitment. (Agnew & Pyke, 1975, pp. vii–viii)*

To learn the rules of the "science game," you should study them from the frame of reference of both the philosophy of science and the history of science. The philosophy of science provides information on strategies that, theoretically, should lead to success at it; the history of science provides information on strategies that have led to success at it in the past.

A knowledge of the scientific method can also be helpful to you in your role as a clinician. All else being equal, you probably will be a more effective diagnostician and behavior manager if you know something about the scientific method. Diagnosis, particularly differential diagnosis, consists in large part of asking "answerable" questions (or forming "testable" hypotheses) and making the observations needed to answer (or test) them. The scientific method offers a set of rules for maximizing the probability of "correct" answers to such questions (or of reliable and valid tests of such hypotheses). As such, it is relevant for your functioning as a diagnostician. It also is relevant for your functioning as a behavior manager. Rules associated with the scientific method are applicable to both decision making in intervention and documentation of the impacts of intervention strategies on clients.

There is disagreement about the amount of impact that "rules" derived from the scientific method both do and should have on research and clinical practice in speech-language pathology and audiology. For lively discussions of relevant issues, see Bench (1989), Bloodstein (1988), Ingham and Siegel (1989), Panush (1989), Perkins (1986), Prutting, Mentis, and Nelson (1989), Ringel, Tachtman, and Prutting (1984), Siegel (1988), and Siegel and Ingham (1987).

What Is the Scientific Method?

Now that we have briefly considered the "why" question (Why is knowledge of the scientific method relevant for speech-language pathologists or audiologists?), we are ready to deal with the "what" question: What is the scientific method? As a partial answer, some of its objectives, characteristics, and underlying assumptions will be discussed. These are not the only ones that have been attributed to the scientific method, nor is there universal agreement that they are a necessary part of it. However, they are among those that tend to be mentioned most frequently by philosophers and historians of science.

Objectives

The scientific method is a set of rules that can be used for *describing* events, *explaining* events, and *predicting* events. The term *event*, as used here, includes anything that is observable and consequently includes phenomena usually classified as objects. Objects are classified as events because their configuration (e.g., appearance) is not constant. It changes as a function of time. An automobile that is five years old, for example, is likely to differ in both appearance and function from what it was like when it was new. Consequently, a detailed description of an object at one point in time is likely to differ—at least a little—from that at another, particularly if the two points are fairly widely separated.

Description

Describing events means partially answering questions beginning with "who," "what," "when," "where," "how," and "which," questions concerning events. The following are examples:

- *Who* is likely to benefit from a particular approach to dysphagia therapy?
- *Who* should be encouraged to use a telecommunication relay service?
- *What* factors have caused a particular client to begin to stutter?
- *What* is the attitude of a particular client toward wearing a hearing aid?
- *When* did the child first produce sounds that her parents interpreted as a meaningful word?
- *When* is a hearing loss educationally significant?
- *Where* can a client purchase the software needed for using a Macintosh PowerBook computer as a direct selection, speech-generating augmentative communication device?
- *Where* in a particular factory should ear protectors be worn?
- *How* does a client produce /s/?
- *How* does pacing speech with a metronome affect a client's speech fluency?
- *Which* of three symbol systems—English, Blissymbols, or photographs/drawings—comes closest to enabling a severely communicatively impaired client who has cerebral palsy meet her communication needs?
- *Which* of two hearing aids yields the highest speech discrimination score for a client?

Questions that when answered describe events can, of course, begin with other words.

Explanation

Explaining events means dealing with the "why" question—that is, specifying the reason(s) for events occurring. After you describe an event, you may be interested in explaining why it occurred. If your management approach resulted in a reduction in the severity of a client's communicative disorder, you probably would have some interest in being able to specify the reason or reasons why it did so. If, for example, you could identify the aspect, or aspects, of the therapy that were responsible for the observed change, you might be able to "simplify" the therapy and thereby make it more efficient. Or if you could identify and isolate the active ingredient in the therapy, you might be able to incorporate it into a new therapy approach that would be more effective than the one you used originally. Also, if you could determine why the frequency, duration, and complexity of behaviors that contribute to communicative disorders vary in predictable ways under specified laboratory conditions, you might be able to incorporate the active components of such conditions into programs of therapy for communicative disorders. If, for example, you could explain why the frequency of stuttering decreases under certain laboratory conditions (e.g., reading in chorus), you might be able to incorporate the active components of such conditions into programs of therapy for stuttering.

The scientific method sheds some light on the degree of confidence you can have in answers to "why" questions—questions of causality. These questions are particularly difficult to answer in the biological and behavioral sciences, which, of course, are the ones to which most of the questions asked by speech-language pathologists and audiologists relate. Philosophers of science have pointed out several reasons why questions of causality are difficult to answer with a high degree of confidence, including the following.

First, *more than one explanation for an event may be possible from descriptions of it*. Even if the existing data support only one explanation that has been posited for an event, they could conceivably support as well—or possibly even better—an explanation for it that has not yet been suggested. Also, while existing data may support one explanation for an event more than others, new data may become available that would make one of the other explanations appear more viable. Under these circumstances, no explanation of an event can be accepted as absolutely certain. All we can conclude based on the scientific method is that judging by what we know about an event, the most plausible explanation for it appears to be. As the amount of information we have about an event increases, our judgment about the most plausible explanation for it may change. One of the most important rules, or principles, of the scientific method is that explanations for events must be regarded as *tentative* and subject to change when new information becomes available.

Second, *because two events are highly correlated does not necessarily mean that one is causally related to the other*. Even though receptive language development is fairly highly related to articulation proficiency in preschool-age children, this does not necessarily mean that a deficit in receptive language development is a cause of articulation disorders. The two may appear to be related because they are both related to a *third variable*, such as mental age. If a child were developing mentally at a slower-than-normal rate, both receptive language and articulation proficiency would be developing slowly. The possibility that two variables that appear closely related are actually both causally related to a third variable is another reason why explanations for events must be regarded as tentative and, consequently, subject to change whenever new information—descriptions of attributes of the events—becomes available.

Third, *all events in a system are interrelated*. Causation, therefore, is apt to be complex. A system, for example, could be "centered" around a client and could include all events in both the client's internal and external environments that affect him or her. Because of the existence of such systems, if a client improves following a period of therapy, we can never be certain that the improvement was due solely to the therapy he or she received. Even if we isolate one aspect of therapy (event associated with therapy) that always seems to be present when improvement occurs, we cannot conclude this is the only event that has to be present for it to occur. In fact, we could not even be certain that the event isolated was related to the observed improvement. There could be events we have not abstracted, or identified, that were wholly or partially responsible for it.

Another possibility that needs to be considered here is that an aspect of therapy might be more likely to result in improvement if it is combined with a particular value of another variable, or variables. Organismic and therapist variables would be relevant here. A given therapy, for example, may be more effective with clients who have one cultural background than with those who have another (Anderson, 1991, 1992; Hammer, 1994; Maestas & Erickson, 1992; Terrell & Hale, 1992; van Kleeck, 1994). Also, this same therapy might be more effective if it were administered by a clinician who expected it to be effective (positive placebo effect) than if it were administered by one who did not expect it to be effective (negative placebo effect).

For a discussion both of problems that are likely to be encountered when attempting to establish causal relationships in communication disorders and of a strategy (path analysis) that can be helpful for doing so, see Duffy, Watt, and Duffy (1981).

We can conclude our discussion of the role of the scientific method in explanation with this generalization: Answers to "why" questions should be regarded as tentative and subject to change when new information becomes available.

Prediction

Predicting events means making probability statements about the likelihood of their future occurrence—that is, estimating the odds that a specific event will occur during a specific period of time. Once an event has been described and information becomes available concerning the conditions under which it occurs, its future occurrence may be predicted with "greater than chance" accuracy. The degree of accuracy with which such predictions can be made is at least partially a function of the amount of information available about the conditions under which the event occurs. The greater the available information about these conditions, the more accurately an event usually can be predicted.

Weather forecasting illustrates the application of the scientific method to predicting events. Weather forecasters estimate the odds a specific event (rain) will occur during a specific time period (e.g., next 24 hours). They base their predictions on available information about: (1) the conditions under which specific weather events occur, and (2) the conditions that are likely to be present during the period for which they are making their prediction. For each event they predict, they usually make a probability statement (20 percent chance of rain) about the likelihood of its occurrence.

What kinds of events do speech-language pathologists and audiologists attempt to predict? One is the probable outcome of therapy. This prediction is incorporated into the statement of prognosis. In this statement a speech-language pathologist or audiologist attempts to predict the probable impact of a specific program of therapy on a specific client's communicative disorder (possibly within a specific period of time). To make this statement, he or she consciously or unconsciously uses: (1) information about the conditions that have to be present for improvement to occur in persons who have a particular communicative disorder and (2) his or her judgment concerning the likelihood that these conditions will be operative for the client. The statement of prognosis could have a statement of either verbal (little chance for further improvement) or numerical (less than a 10 percent chance for further improvement) probability attached to it.

Characteristics

We will now consider some of the characteristics of the scientific method, particularly as they relate to clinical research and practice in speech-language pathology and audiology. This discussion can be viewed as a partial *operational definition* (Bridgman, 1927) of the scientific method, because it describes aspects of how you would have to behave—both clinically and otherwise—to function in a manner consistent with it. The terms used for the characteristics and the definitions of them are those of Feigl (1953), a philosopher of science. There is a discussion of the relevance of each characteristic to our field following Feigl's definition of it.

Intersubjective Testability

This term refers to "the requirement that the knowledge claims of science be in principle capable of test (confirmation or disconfirmation, at least indirectly and to some degree) on the part of any person properly equipped with intelligence and the technical devices of observation or experimentation" (Feigl, 1953, p. 11). If, for example, you develop a program that you claim is effective for modifying an aspect of a communicative disorder, you must describe your program in sufficient detail that it can be tested by someone else. Before any claim can be accepted, it must be confirmed (*replicated*) by others. A claim cannot be accepted simply because a person regarded as an authority makes it and/or the claim appears in print. Claims concerning the effectiveness of clinical management programs have appeared in our literature that could not be confirmed by those who tested them. The claims of one management program that had this status when this chapter was written was facilitated communication (Janzen-Wilde, Duchan, & Higginbotham, 1995).

Reliability

The "knowledge-claims" of science are required to have "a sufficient degree of confirmation. This second criterion of scientific knowledge enables us to distinguish what is generally called 'mere opinion' (or worse still, 'superstition') from knowledge (well-sustained belief)" (Feigl, 1953, p. 12). Degree of confirmation can vary from none to considerable. Obviously, the weight you give a claim should be at least partially a function of the degree to which it has been confirmed. The greater the degree to which a claim has been confirmed, the more confidence you can place in it and consequently, the more weight it would be reasonable for you to give it in decision making.

The claims, or observations, that speech-language pathologists and audiologists utilize in clinical decision making have been confirmed to varying degrees. Some have been confirmed beyond reasonable doubt while others are no more than hunches. Examples of claims relevant to speech-language pathology and audiology that appear to have received enough degree of confirmation to be regarded as well-substantiated belief include:

- Anticipation of stuttering somehow contributes to precipitating moments of stuttering.
- Damage to the anterior portion of the left cerebral cortex in right-handed persons is more likely to result in expressive aphasia than damage to the corresponding portion of the right cerebral cortex.
- Vocal abuse is a cause of vocal nodules.
- A characteristic of at least some types of noise-induced hearing loss is a greater degree of loss by air conduction at 4000 Hz than at 2000 Hz and 8000 Hz.

Definiteness and Precision

It is necessary that "the concepts used in the formulation of scientific knowledge-claims be as definitely delimited as possible. On the level of the qualitative-classificatory sciences this amounts to the attempt to reduce all border-zone vagueness to a minimum. On the level of quantitative science the exactitude of the concepts is enormously enhanced through the application of the techniques of measurement" (Feigl, 1953, p. 12). Communicative disorder specialists utilize both qualitative-classificatory and quantitative concepts. An example of a qualitative-classificatory concept that they utilize is *beginning stuttering*. The objective of much research during the past fifty years has been to define it with sufficient "definiteness and precision" to differentiate it from normal childhood disfluency (Silverman, 1996). And an example of a quantitative concept that they utilize is *threshold for pure tones* in decibels.

Why is it crucial that the concepts dealt with by science be as definitely delimited as possible? An attribute of an event referred to by a concept cannot be investigated unless it can be defined with enough precision that it is likely to be identified both when it does and does not occur. Before we can assess the impact of intervention on a client's "lateralized" /s/ (concept) we must be able to detect with precision both when his or her /s/ is and is not being lateralized. The meaning of precision in this context is illustrated by Figure 3-1. If precision is high, /s/ will be identified as lateralized when it is lateralized and will not be identified when it is not lateralized. Almost all of the judgments will fall into one of the two cells marked with Xs. The more frequently /s/ is judged to be lateralized when it is not lateralized and judged not to be lateralized when it is lateralized, the lower the precision of the judgments—that is, the lower the percentage of judgments that will fall into one of the two cells marked with Xs. To maximize the precision of such judgments, it would be necessary to define as precisely as possible what is meant by a lateralized /s/.

The borderline vagueness between categories sometimes can be reduced by supplementing verbal definitions with extensional ones. A category, or term, can be *defined extensionally* "by pointing to or exhibiting somehow the actual objects, phenomena, etc., to which the term refers" (Johnson, 1946, p. 507). Thus, the borderline vagueness between the categories "lateralized" and "nonlateralized" /s/ probably could be reduced by preparing an

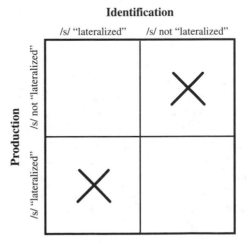

FIGURE 3-1   A four-cell bivariate table for assessing accuracy of judgments of /s/ lateralization. If accuracy is perfect, all judgments will fall into one of the two cells marked with Xs.

audiotape recording on which there are both labeled examples of /s/ that the definer considers lateralized and labeled examples of /s/ that he or she does not consider to be so.

Thus far, we have considered why it is necessary for qualitative-classificatory concepts to be defined as precisely as possible. You also deal with quantitative concepts. The attributes of events referred to by them are *measured*—that is, they are described by numerals (rather than words). (Measurement, which can be defined as the assignment of numerals to events according to rules, is discussed in depth in Chapter 8.) Quantitative concepts with which you may have to deal professionally include degree of hearing loss (in decibels), language age (in years), and frequency of stuttering (in percentage of words stuttered).

The amount of borderline vagueness that can be tolerated is dependent upon the purpose for which a conceptual scheme is being used. To answer some questions, the conceptual scheme must be highly precise—have little borderline vagueness. To answer others, a conceptual scheme could have considerable borderline vagueness and still be adequate for the purpose. As Feigl has indicated "there is no point in sharpening precision to a higher degree than the problem in hand requires. (You need no razor to cut butter.)" (Feigl, 1953, p. 12).

Coherence or Systematic Structure

In science we seek "not a mere collection of miscellaneous items of information, but a well-connected account of the facts." (Feigl, 1953, p. 12). This is true on both descriptive and explanatory levels.

On the *descriptive level*, the need for coherence or systematic structure "results, for example, in systems of classification—in diagrams, statistical charts and the like" (Feigl, 1953, pp. 12–13). An articulation test response form can be viewed as a chart for organizing qualitative information about the types of articulatory errors (i.e., substitutions, omissions, distortions, additions) a child produces. And an audiogram can be viewed as a diagram for organizing certain quantitative information about a person's hearing.

Items of information about a phenomenon can be viewed as pieces of a puzzle. New ones "fill in holes" and improve our ability to describe the phenomenon.

To satisfy the need for coherence or systematic structure on the *explanatory level*, "sets of laws, or theoretical assumptions, are utilized. The laws, theories, or hypotheses form the premises from which we derive logically, or logico-mathematically, the observed, or observable facts" (Feigl, 1953, p. 13). The interpretation of pure tone audiograms can be used to illustrate this process. After a person's hearing acuity for pure tones in the left ear has been plotted by air and bone conduction on an audiogram form (see Figure 3-2), we can attempt to explain the pathology responsible for the air-bone threshold differences that we observe on the form. We could hypothesize several pathologies that could account for the observed threshold differences and then attempt to determine how well each hypothesis could explain them. Two explanations (hypotheses) we undoubtedly would consider are outer/middle ear pathology and inner ear pathology. We would consider by reasoning deductively from each hypothesis what we would expect the configuration of air- and bone-conduction curves (thresholds) to be if it were the mechanism responsible. If the pathology were in the outer or middle ear, we would expect the air conduction curve to be relatively flat and the bone conduction curve to indicate essentially normal hearing. On the other hand, if the pathology were in the inner ear, we would expect the configuration of the air conduction curve to indicate greater loss in the high frequencies than in the low frequencies;

we would also expect the bone conduction curve to indicate approximately the same amount of loss as the air conduction curve. Since the configurations of the curves in Figure 3-2 more closely approximate what we would expect if the pathology were in the outer or middle ear pathology than in the inner ear pathology, we would conclude that outer or middle ear pathology appears to be the more viable explanation. In other words, we would conclude that the data plotted in Figure 3-2 are *consistent with the hypothesis* that the person has outer or middle ear pathology in his or her left ear.

Because a hypothesis is consistent with the data that we have on a phenomenon does not necessarily mean that it explains the phenomenon. There could be other hypotheses that are as consistent or even more consistent with the data. This dilemma was aptly described by Einstein and Infeld in *The Evolution of Physics*:

> *In our endeavor to understand reality we are somewhat like a man trying to understand the mechanism of a closed watch. He sees the face and the moving hands, even hears it ticking, but he has no way of opening the case. If he is ingenious he may form some picture of a mechanism that could be responsible for all the things he observes, but he may never be quite sure his picture is the only one which could explain his observations. He will never be able to compare his picture with the real mechanism and he cannot even imagine the possibility or the meaning of such a comparison. (Einstein & Infeld, 1938)*

This statement reinforces the conclusion we reached earlier in this chapter that explanations for phenomena must be regarded as tentative and subject to change whenever new information becomes available (which is the topic of the next characteristic of the scientific method we will consider).

FIGURE 3-2   Pure-tone audiogram indicating degree of hearing in left ear by air conduction (x) and bone conduction (<).

Comprehensiveness or Scope of Knowledge

According to Feigl (1953, p. 13), "Instead of presenting a finished account of the world, the genuine scientist keeps his unifying hypotheses open to revision and is always ready to modify or abandon them if evidence should render them doubtful. This *self-corrective aspect* [italics added] of science has rightly been stressed as its most important characteristic. . . . It is a sign of one's maturity to be able to live with an unfinished world view."

You have to be able to tolerate living professionally with an "unfinished world view." The "facts" you know about communicative disorders are not really facts but hypotheses subject to revision. Such facts (or beliefs) include those about their symptomatology, incidence, etiology, prognosis, evaluation, prevention, and treatment. You will have to modify your beliefs about their etiology, for example, if new evidence renders them doubtful. Many speech-language pathologists who believed during the 1930s that stuttering resulted from a lack of unilateral cerebral dominance eventually abandoned this belief when new data rendered it doubtful (Silverman, 1996). The abandonment of this belief took a number of years, which is not unusual. People tend to resist changing their beliefs until the evidence supporting competing ones is overwhelming.

How can you determine whether the evidence is sufficiently compelling to necessitate your modifying or abandoning a belief? There is no simple answer to this question. A number of factors are likely to influence your decision, including the following: (1) your internal standard for what constitutes compelling evidence, (2) the evidence itself, and (3) your ego-involvement with the belief.

People's internal standards for what constitutes compelling evidence differ. Evidence that you would regard as being compelling someone else may not consider to be so.

Another relevant factor is the evidence itself. Some data will almost universally be regarded as more compelling than others.

A third factor that influences the probability that you will consider evidence to be compelling is your ego-involvement with the belief to which it relates. The greater your ego-involvement, the stronger the evidence would have to be before you would be likely to regard it as sufficiently compelling to necessitate your modifying or abandoning your belief. Some persons become quite ego-involved with their beliefs and for this reason have difficulty evaluating them objectively. They tend to filter out evidence that might require them to modify or abandon their beliefs. In extreme cases, the filtering is so complete that they communicate (verbally, nonverbally, or both) to those who challenge their beliefs *that their minds are already made up and they don't wish to be confused by the facts.*

Underlying Assumptions

Thus far in our discussion of the scientific method we have dealt with its objectives and characteristics. We now will consider its underlying assumptions, or presuppositions. These beliefs—like some of those of all religions—must be accepted *on faith* because they have not been, and presumably cannot be, proven to be true empirically. They are being discussed here not only to help you develop an intuitive understanding of the method, but also to help you develop an objective attitude toward it. That is, you must realize that while the method is extremely useful because it provides a "set of rules" for asking and answering questions that appear to maximize the probability of correct answers, it is based on assumptions that are not empirically verifiable. Three of them are discussed here: (1) the principle of causality, (2) the principle of uniformity, and (3) the principle of the finitude of relevant factors. The terminology and definitions used are those of Pap, a philosopher of science.

Principle of Causality

One assumption, or presupposition, of the scientific method is that "every event has a cause" (Pap, 1949, p. 403). Without this assumption, two objectives of the scientific method—explanation and prediction—could not be achieved. To explain an event, we must assume it has a cause; otherwise, it would make no sense to try to explain it. Also, predicting an event requires a knowledge of its cause or causes. If events cannot be assumed to have causes, then attempting to predict their future occurrence with greater than chance accuracy makes no sense.

You implicitly or explicitly make this assumption every day while functioning professionally. It underlies, for example, such a statement as "The cause of your disorder is."

Is it reasonable to assume that all events have causes? The success of the scientific method in explaining and predicting events during the past 300 years offers some support for the reasonableness of this assumption. If events did not have causes, then predicting their occurrence with greater than chance accuracy would be impossible. However, it cannot be established that *every* event has a cause until every event has been studied. This, of course, is an impossible condition to satisfy since new events are constantly occurring. The assumption is worth making because it has *heuristic value*. That is, by making it we are more likely to be able to explain and predict events than we are by not making it.

Principle of Uniformity

Another presupposition of the scientific method related to causality is the "so-called principle of uniformity—i.e., '*same cause, same effect*' [italics added]" (Pap, 1949, p. 405). Without making this assumption, you could not predict the effects that your intervention strategies would be likely to have on clients with *greater than chance accuracy* because they could not be counted on to produce the same effect. (The role of "chance" in prediction is discussed in Chapter 10.)

Principle of the Finitude of Relevant Factors

The third and final presupposition of the scientific method we will consider—the principle of the finitude of relevant factors—states that "only a small, and in fact enumerable, set of circumstances is causally related to the observed effect" (Pap, 1953, p. 27). If you didn't make this assumption when evaluating a client, you probably would be unable to specify the etiology of his or her communicative disorder because you could not conclude with confidence that it had only a small number of causes.

Is this assumption viable? Some theoreticians in several disciplines—including general semantics (Korzybski, 1958), general systems theory (Buckley, 1968), and chaos theory (Briggs & Peat, 1989)—have suggested that it might be more reasonable to assume the set of circumstances that are causally related to an observed effect is relatively complex. That is, it might be reasonable to assume that all parts of a system are interrelated—that all events within a system are, to some extent, causally related to all other events in that system. The value of such an assumption has been demonstrated in several fields including ecology and economics. The causes of such events as "environmental pollution" and "inflation" apparently are quite complex.

How crucial is this assumption to the scientific method? If causation could not be assumed to be relatively simple, would this invalidate the method? The assumption does not appear crucial to the validity of the method. However, substituting the opposite assumption—that causality tends to be complex—would probably necessitate some revision in the methodology used to answer "why" questions and make predictions. Greater emphasis would be placed, for example, on the use of multivariate statistical techniques—techniques that permit us to assess the combined, or composite, effects of a number of variables—particularly nonlinear ones (Briggs & Peat, 1989). (The rationale for, and application of, such techniques is discussed in Chapter 10.)

Historical Perspective

Thus far, we have considered research primarily from the frame of reference of the philosophy of science. There is a second frame of reference through which it may be viewed—that of the history of science. The first is concerned with how research is *supposed* to be done; the second, with how it has been done. The two, in fact, are sometimes not synonymous (Bush, 1974; Kuhn, 1962). Scientists have made the observations needed to answer questions accurately and to develop and test hypotheses by methods that deviated to some extent from the scientific method. For example, Gall in 1818 was apparently the first to hypothesize that the "faculty of speech" is located in the anterior portion of the brain. His hypothesis appears to have arisen from the following observations:

> . . . he was sent in his ninth year to an uncle who was a cure in the Black Forest. Here he was educated with another boy of his own age who excelled him in learning his lessons. The two youths passed on to school at Baden, and Gall discovered that, when it was a question of learning by heart, he was beaten by those who were greatly inferior to him in written composition. Two of his new schoolfellows surpassed even his first companion in the ease with which they learnt by heart, and because they had large and prominent eyes [italics added] . . . they received the nickname of "Ox eyes." Three years later at Bruchsal and again at the University of Strasbourg he continued to notice that those who learnt easily by heart had the same sort of eyes. He began to associate this conformation with a good verbal memory, and so arrived at the conclusion that this faculty was situated in that part of the brain which lay behind the orbits. From such fantastic beginnings sprang the idea that memory for words was situated in the frontal lobes. (Head, 1963, p. 9)

Here we have a classic example of a person answering a question correctly for the wrong reason(s). Historians of science have reported a number of such cases (Bush, 1974; Kuhn, 1962).

If you can answer questions correctly by using procedures that are not compatible with the scientific method, why is it important for you to use procedures that are compatible with it? The use of such procedures *maximizes the probability* that the answers to your questions will be correct. While it does not guarantee that they will be correct, they are more likely to be if such procedures are used than they would be otherwise.

The Scientific Method as a Set of Rules for Asking and Answering Questions

My objective in this final section is to illustrate how the rules that make up the scientific method—particularly those that are implied by its characteristics—can be applied to asking and answering questions, particularly clinical ones.

The characteristics of the scientific method that are discussed in this chapter implicitly or explicitly suggest rules or criteria for formulating questions, making observations to answer them, and relating the answers to the existing body of knowledge. The criterion we referred to as "intersubjective testability" suggests that the observational procedures used to answer questions should be described in sufficient detail that they can be repeated by others. That is, the methodology used to arrive at an answer should be described in sufficient detail that someone else could attempt to replicate the answer—that is, arrive at the same answer. The tasks that you use during an evaluation, for example, should be described in sufficient detail in the report to enable another clinician to redo them to determine whether the client has changed and if so, in what ways.

The second criterion of the scientific method that we discussed, "reliability," in this context suggests that a sufficient number of observations should be made before we attempt to answer a question to enable us to have a reasonable degree of confidence in the accuracy of the answer. Furthermore, it suggests that we should provide an estimate of the reliability of the observations that we use to answer a question so that consumers of our "answers" can judge the maximum degree of confidence they can have in their accuracy. Clinically, this means that before you attach a diagnostic label to a client (assuming that you feel obliged to do so), you should observe him or her enough to be reasonably certain that the label is accurate and furthermore, you should communicate clearly in the report how confident you are that the label is accurate and why you are so.

The characteristic of the scientific method that we referred to as "definiteness and precision" suggests that the concepts that you refer to in questions should be as definitely delimited (unambiguous) as possible. If they are not clearly defined, questions that contain them probably will not be answerable. (What makes a question answerable will be discussed in Chapter 5.) It also suggests that the language you use to answer questions (e.g., to communicate your observations in evaluation reports) should be as unambiguous as possible.

The characteristic we referred to as "coherence or systematic structure" also has relevance here. Before you attempt to answer a question, you should organize the pieces of relevant information resulting from the observational process to make them coherent. This increases the probability of a correct answer. (Strategies for organizing qualitative and quantitative information to answer questions are discussed in Chapters 9, 10, and 11.)

The final characteristic of the scientific method we will consider here is "comprehensiveness or scope of knowledge." It indicates that answers to questions should be regarded as *tentative* and subject to change when new information becomes available. It's acceptable for you to change your diagnoses, management approaches, prognoses, and other clinical decisions when new information becomes available. In fact, it's not only acceptable, it's essential if you want to be in compliance with the ASHA Ethical Code injunction "to hold paramount the welfare of persons served professionally"!

I have attempted to indicate in this chapter why the scientific method can be conceptualized as being a set of rules for asking and answering questions that maximizes the likelihood of answers being correct. For our purposes, we will conceptualize research as a process for asking and answering questions that is governed by the rules of the scientific method.

Exercises and Discussion Topics

1. You are an audiologist who fits hearing aids. Indicate how each of the following assumptions that underlie the scientific method would be relevant when performing this task.
    a. The principle of causality
    b. The principle of uniformity
    c. The principle of the finitude of relevant factors
2. You are asked to evaluate Mary, a 6-year-old who is reported by her parents to be saying some speech sounds incorrectly. You, therefore, have to make the observations necessary for answering the question: "What articulation errors is Mary making?" How might each of the following characteristics of the scientific method influence the manner in which you would make the observations needed to answer this question?
    a. Intersubjective testability
    b. Reliability
    c. Definiteness and precision

d. Coherence or systematic structure
e. Comprehensiveness or scope of knowledge
3. In what ways is the scientific method applicable when making statements of prognosis?
4. Research is viewed in this chapter as a process that consists mainly of asking and answering questions. To what extent can the clinical evaluation (diagnosis) process also be conceptualized in this way?
5. A speech-language pathologist determined the level of phonological development of 100 children between the ages of 6 months and 12 years. He also measured the length of each child's foot. The correlation between the measures of foot length and phonological development was very high (over 0.85). Based on the strength of this correlation he concluded that foot length is a valid measure of phonological development. Do you agree or disagree that the correlation he obtained warrants this conclusion? Why?

Chapter 4

Literature Searching

Whether you are functioning as a consumer or producer of research, you have to be able to locate information efficiently. As a consumer of research, you have to be able to do so to keep up-to-date on the disorders you treat and to maximize the effectiveness of your intervention strategies for them. And as a producer of research, you have to do a systematic search for relevant literature whenever you begin (or contemplate beginning) a research project. Since the literature on most communicative disorders is relatively large and widely scattered, information usually cannot be located efficiently without using an *index*. Trying to do so would be as inefficient as trying to locate certain information in a book by thumbing through the pages. Several types of indexes to *portions* of the communicative disorder literature are described in this chapter. Unfortunately, there isn't a single index to all of it, and those that are available are unlikely to identify all relevant papers. They are particularly unlikely to identify all older ones and ones that were convention presentations. Nevertheless, if you use these indexes, you are likely to locate the information you want more quickly than you would otherwise.

There are two main types of indexes that can be used for accessing the literature in a particular field (e.g., communicative disorders): abstracts journals and online, interactive computer-based information retrieval systems. Abstracts journals contain abstracts of papers that have been published in other journals rather than original papers. Each of them abstract papers that are likely to be of interest to persons in a particular field—for example, *Psychological Abstracts* abstracts papers that are likely to be of interest to psychologists, and *Index Medicus* abstracts ones that are likely to be of interest to physicians. Papers that they abstract, of course, could also be of interest to persons in other fields—for example, speech-language pathology and audiology. In the final issue of each volume (usually the last issue for the year), there is an index to all of the abstracts in that volume. You can use this index for identifying papers that are likely to contain the information you are seeking.

Online, interactive computer-based information retrieval systems are "tools" for retrieving information from computer databases (Borgman, Moghdam, & Corbett, 1984). They are referred to as being *online* because the user is in direct communication with the computer containing the database through a terminal or a microcomputer that has been programmed to function as one. The computer on which they are located can be at the user's institution or on a computer network, such as the Internet. And they are referred to as being *interactive* because the user and computer engage in a "conversation" in which the computer responds quickly. The databases they access contain information similar to that in abstracts journals. In some cases, the information in an abstracts journal is essentially the same as that in a database. For example, the information in the Medline database (Albright, 1988; *PlusNet2 Medline System: End-user Introduction*, 1990; Reiner & Ludlow, 1979a, 1979b, 1981) is essentially the same as that in the abstracts journal *Index Medicus*, and that in the PsycLIT one (Gosling, Knight, & McKenney, 1989) is essentially the same as that in the abstracts journal *Psychological Abstracts*. However, the contents of these abstracts journals and databases are not identical (Pfaffenberger, 1990).

The "index" used for identifying relevant papers with a computer database is accessed by entering one or more terms in it into the computer via its keyboard or a terminal. Printouts of the terms that the index for a particular database will recognize have been published for most of them, including the Medline and PsycLIT ones. Partial printouts of this index for the Medline database have been published for specialists in communicative disorders (Reiner & Ludlow, 1979a, 1979b, 1981).

While abstracts journals and online, interactive computer-based information retrieval systems are the most frequently used "tools" for doing literature searches, they are not the only ones. Three others that can be used for supplementing them are published and unpublished bibliographies, reference lists in books and papers (particularly review papers), and convention abstracts. Bibliographies have been compiled for a number of topics relevant to communicative disorders, including the following: augmentative communication (Silverman, 1977a, 1989, 1995b; Villarruel, Mathy-Laikko, Ratcliff, & Yoder, 1987), microcomputer applications (Silverman, 1987, 1997), and stuttering (Silverman, 1996). Bibliographies and reference lists can be particularly helpful when searching for information in books, convention (and other unpublished) papers, and "older" published papers and monographs.

Published abstracts of papers presented at national conventions can be a valuable source for locating information on some topics—e.g., microcomputer applications in communicative disorders (see the reference/bibliography listing in Silverman, 1997). I have found the abstracts for the ASHA Convention to be particularly valuable in this regard. Extended abstracts, handouts, and/or copies of papers can often be obtained from presenters by writing to them.

Literature Searching with Online, Interactive Computer-Based Information Retrieval Systems

There are several computer databases that can be used with online, interactive information retrieval software for searching portions of the international communicative disorders literature. The one that probably has been used most often for this purpose by speech-language pathologists and audiologists is Medline. This database indexes papers in more than 3000 journals (including some of those published by the American Speech-Language-Hearing Association) dealing with medicine and related subjects from 1966 to the present. It is available in two forms: one that is stored on tape and requires the use of a mini- or mainframe computer to access and one that is stored on compact disks (CDs) and can be accessed with a microcomputer. A single compact disk can store as many as 275,000 pages of typed information (Pfaffenberger, 1990). One CD-based database—CD+Medline—stored the entire Medline database on eight CDs when this chapter was written. While the 3000+ journals indexed by this database include most that publish papers on communicative disorders, it does not include them all. The *Journal of Fluency Disorders*, for example, was not indexed when this chapter was written.

Another computer database that indexes a portion of the communicative disorders literature and is available on CDs is PsycLIT (Gosling, Knight, & McKenney, 1989). This database, which is produced by the American Psychological Association, indexes papers on psychology and related subjects in more than 1300 journals from 1974 to the present. Among the journals indexed are some of the ones published by the American Speech-Language-Hearing Association. Since some journals that publish papers on communicative disorders are indexed by PsycLIT but not by Medline and vice versa, using both is likely to result in a more complete search than using only one.

There are a number of other computer databases available in one or both of these forms that index portions of the communicative disorders literature. Three that speech-language pathologists and audiologists are likely to find particularly helpful are the following:

- *ERIC* (Educational Resources Information Center) indexes papers in 700+ educational journals from 1966 to present.
- *Dissertation Abstracts* indexes titles and abstracts in dissertations from 1980 to the present and titles only prior to that.
- *PsycINFO*, which like PsycLIT is produced by the American Psychological Association, indexes papers dealing with psychology and related areas from 1967 to the present. It differs from PsycLIT in that it is not available on CDs, includes both dissertations and published papers, and is updated monthly rather than quarterly (Gosling, Knight, & McKenney, 1989).

Most college and university libraries employ at least one research librarian who is knowledgeable about such databases and can recommend ones that would be worth searching for particular topics.

Deciding When to Use

It may be possible to do a literature search for a particular topic using either an abstracts journal or a computerized database. The same information may be in both. Topics with one or more of the following characteristics are likely to utilize the capabilities of computerized literature searching to their fullest (Borgman, Moghdam, & Corbett, 1984, pp. 21–22):

1. Searches that require the coordination of two or more distinct concepts; for example, "the effect of vitamin C on the common cold." The two concepts are "vitamin C" and "the common cold."
2. Searches on topics so new or obscure that they may not yet appear as subject headings in printed indexes.

3. Searches for information that is known to be more recent than the printed index, and it is known that the online database is current.
4. Searches on topics that may be stated in so many synonymous terms that manual searching of indexes would be unreasonably time-consuming.
5. Searches that are relatively narrow in scope and are likely to result in rather small retrieval.
6. Topics covered in databases that do not have a corresponding printed index. While many databases include information that duplicates printed indexes [abstracts journals], some databases have no printed counterpart.

Literature searching using online, interactive computer-based information retrieval systems tends to be faster than doing so using abstracts journals because a number of years can be searched simultaneously. For example, with the PlusNet2 Medline database relevant papers published between 1986 and 1991 can be identified from a single search. On the other hand, it usually is not possible to search as far back using a database as it is using an abstracts journal. With the PsycLIT database, for example, it is only possible to search from 1974 to the present (Gosling, Knight, & McKenney, 1989). However, with the journal *Psychological Abstracts* it is possible to do so as far back as 1927.

Planning the Search

Before performing a search using a computerized database, it is necessary to decide the following:

- The keywords that will be included in the search and the manner in which they will be "linked." Ways in which they can be linked are discussed in the next section.
- The database(s) that will be searched.
- The range of years that will be included in the search.
- Whether the search should be limited in any way(s), e.g., English language only, children only, females only, human subjects only, or review articles only.
- Whether abstracts, if available, will be printed.

After these have been decided, the search can be performed by either a research librarian or the enduser (You!). If a database to be searched is on CDs or tape at one of the college's or university's computer facilities, it should be possible for the enduser to do the search himself or herself. However, if the database is on a mini- or mainframe computer that does not belong to the institution and is accessed via a terminal and modem over telephone lines, the institution may require that searches be performed by a librarian. This is particularly likely to be the case if there is a charge for using the database. If a search cannot be performed by the enduser, then information defining the search usually will be communicated to the librarian on a special form (see Figure 4-1).

Doing the Search

Search Strategies
Most computer databases are searched in a similar fashion—through the use of keywords and the Boolean logic connectors AND, OR, and NOT (Berkman, 1990). (Boolean logic

COMPUTER SEARCH REQUEST—MARQUETTE UNIVERSITY LIBRARIES

DATE _____   FACULTY _____ STAFF _____ GRADUATE _____

Name_____   UNDERGRAD _____ ID NUMBER _____

School or Dept _____

Address _____   _____ Dissertation/thesis

Phone   Day _____ Night_____   _____ Coursework

   (In case further information is needed)   _____ University research

                         _____ Other (specify)

SEARCH TOPIC   Please explain in sentences exactly what you want covered. Be specific! Define terms that have special meanings. Feel free to attach another page.

SUGGESTED KEYWORDS/DESCRIPTORS	Which indexes or abstracts have you searched? Which subject headings were useful?
Please list a few recent relevant articles or books (authors, titles, journals, dates).	How many citations do you need? _____ A few relevant articles (under 25) _____ An exhaustive search that may retrieve a substantial number of irrelevant citations _____ Something in-between Time period to be covered _____ Current (last 2–3 years) _____ All years possible _____ Other time period (specify) _____ English _____ All languages _____ Other languages (specify) _____
Can you think of an ideal journal article title on the subject?	

FIGURE 4-1   A representative search request form.

FIGURE 4-2   A single keyword search strategy.

was named after the mathematician who invented it, George Boole.) The manner in which this is done is illustrated in Figures 4-2 through 4-9. Let's represent the keywords "hearing loss," "otitis media," and "children" by A, B, and C respectively. The strategy diagrammed in Figure 4-2 is one in which we are searching for all references containing a particular keyword (which can consist of more than one word). We would use this strategy, for example, if we were interested in retrieving from a database all references containing the keyword "hearing loss."

The strategy diagrammed in Figure 4-3 is one in which we are searching for all references containing two keywords. We could use this strategy, for example, if we were interested in retrieving from a database all references containing the keywords "hearing loss" AND "otitis media." That is, we would use it if we were only interested in retrieving references dealing with hearing loss resulting from otitis media.

The strategy diagrammed in Figure 4-4 is referred to as the *inclusive* OR strategy because it not only will retrieve references containing one of two keywords, but also those containing both of them. We could use this strategy, for example, if we were interested in retrieving from a database all references containing the keywords "hearing loss" OR "oti-

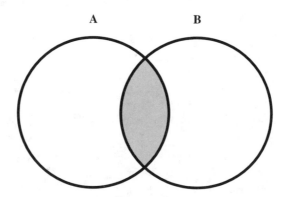

FIGURE 4-3   A single AND search strategy.

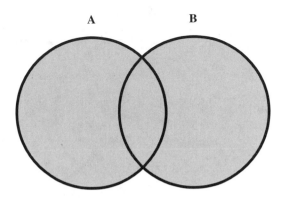

FIGURE 4-4   An inclusive OR search strategy.

tis media" OR both of these. All such computer databases support an OR search strategy that functions in this manner.

Some of them also support an *exclusive* OR search strategy (see Figure 4-5), which will not retrieve references containing both keywords. Because you usually would not want to exclude such references, the *inclusive* OR strategy is used far more often than this one. An example of where you might want to use the *exclusive* OR strategy is for retrieving references dealing with "dysarthria without aphasia" and "aphasia without dysarthria." The two keywords here would be dysarthria and aphasia.

The AND NOT search strategy is illustrated in Figure 4-6. (In some systems it may be referred to as the NOT or BUT NOT one.) It will retrieve references that mention one keyword that do not mention a second keyword. It can be used, for example, to retrieve all references on hearing loss that do not mention otitis media. This strategy should be used with caution because it will eliminate all references that mention the excluded keyword, including those that only do so in passing.

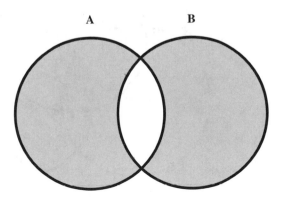

FIGURE 4-5   An exclusive OR search strategy.

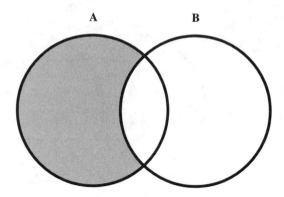

FIGURE 4-6 An AND NOT search strategy.

A search strategy can involve more than two keywords. A multiple AND search strategy that involves three keywords is illustrated in Figure 4-7. It can be used for retrieving references in which three keywords are mentioned. It could be used, for example, for finding papers dealing (at least in part) with "hearing loss" in "children" resulting from "otitis media." This search strategy—which can use more than three keywords—is one of the most useful ones.

Another type of search strategy that involves more than two keywords combines the AND and AND NOT logical connectors (see Figure 4-8). It can be used for retrieving references that mention two keywords that do not mention a third. It could be used, for example, for finding papers dealing with "hearing loss" in "children" that do not mention "otitis

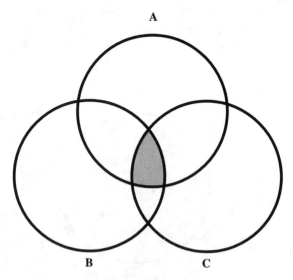

FIGURE 4-7 A multiple AND search strategy.

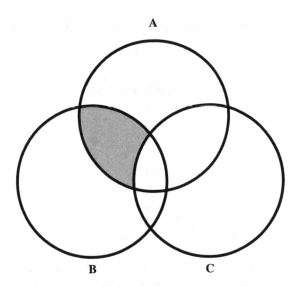

FIGURE 4-8   A compound AND and AND NOT search strategy.

media." The problem mentioned in the discussion of the AND NOT search strategy affects this one also.

A third type of search strategy that involves more than two keywords combines the AND and OR logical connectors (see Figure 4-9). When using it, two keywords are connected to each other by OR and these in turn are connected to another keyword by AND.

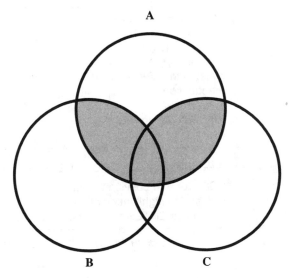

FIGURE 4-9   A compound search strategy in which two keywords are connected to each other by OR and these in turn are connected to another keyword by AND.

This strategy could be used, for example, to locate papers dealing with "children" in which either "otitis media" or "hearing loss" is mentioned.

Conducting an Online Search

If a database you decide to search is one that can be searched at your institution by an enduser, you can begin the search after you have formulated a strategy for doing so. The first step in the process is "logging on," or "signing on," to the computer on which the database is stored. If the database is stored on CDs on a microcomputer that cannot be accessed remotely, the enduser would log onto that computer. On the other hand, if the database is stored on a mini- or mainframe computer, the enduser would log on to it using a terminal or a microcomputer that was programmed to simulate one. Most logon procedures involve keyboarding your name and a password when requested to do so. The password, which is issued by the institution where the computer being accessed is located, may not be displayed on the screen while it is being keyboarded for security reasons.

When the logon procedure is completed, you are given access to the database's main menu (see Figure 4-10). This menu may also give you access to a tutorial that provides basic information about the commands and procedures used for searching that database (see Figure 4-10). It is a good idea to go through the tutorial at least once, particularly if you do not have access to a manual that provides this information.

The second step in the process is actually executing the search. This is done by selecting the appropriate item from the main menu (it would be "search for information" in Figure 4-10) and by sending commands to the computer. Commands may be sent by activating

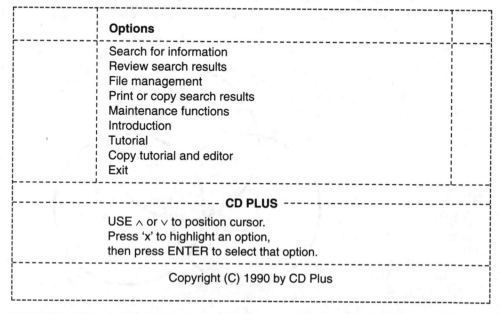

Options

Search for information
Review search results
File management
Print or copy search results
Maintenance functions
Introduction
Tutorial
Copy tutorial and editor
Exit

------------------------------ **CD PLUS** ------------------------------

USE ∧ or ∨ to position cursor.
Press 'x' to highlight an option,
then press ENTER to select that option.

Copyright (C) 1990 by CD Plus

FIGURE 4-10   A representative main menu screen for a computer database intended for enduser searching.

Number	Search Sets	Results

-------------------- **Medline <1987 forward>** --------------------

Enter subject, then press ENTER

__ :   hearing loss

^A Help	^F Limit Set	^J Browse Set
^B Search Text Words	^G Combine Sets	^K Print/Download Set
^E End Session	^I Save/Change Files	^L Additional Options

FIGURE 4-11   A representative screen for entering the subject of a search.

single keys or combinations of ESCAPE or CONTROL keys and other keys. For example, X may be used for highlighting an option on a menu (see Figure 4-10), CONTROL J (abbreviated as ^*J*) for instructing the computer to browse through a set (see Figure 4-11), and ESCAPE E for instructing it to move to the last line of a citation. Unfortunately, the commands used for accessing databases have not been standardized. The same command may be used in two databases but have a different meaning in each.

The search is initiated by entering the "string" containing the keywords that is to be used for it (see Figure 4-11). The string entered for the example diagrammed in Figure 4-2 would be the following:

hearing loss

The computer after searching will indicate whether there are any items in the database that can be indexed by the string and, if so, how many. If there are many, it may indicate ways that you can eliminate some (i.e., narrow the search) by focusing more directly on the specific information you want. It may do this by adding a Boolean AND and keyword to the search. For example, it may permit you to limit the items selected to those dealing with partial hearing loss or hearing loss occurring during middle age (see Figure 4-12). After you have made a decision about whether you are interested in all the items or a more limited set, you will be informed how many items there are and possibly given the opportunity to limit the search further by restricting it to articles in which the keyword (index term) is a main focus (see Figure 4-13). After making this decision you may be presented with another menu of subhead-

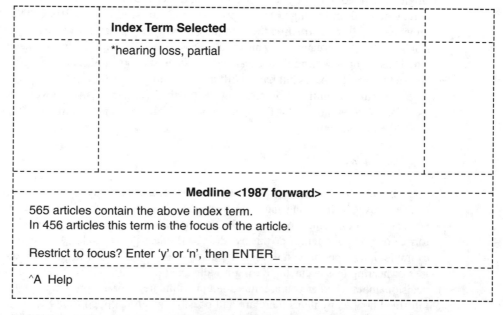

```
┌─────────────────────────────────────────────────────────────────────────┐
│          Medical Subject Headings          Line 1 of 10                   │
├─────────────────────────────────────────────────────────────────────────┤
│          hearing loss, sensorineural                                      │
│          hearing loss, noise-induced                                      │
│          hearing loss, partial                                            │
│          hearing disorders                                                │
│          cochlea                                                          │
│          neomycin                                                         │
│          evoked potentials, auditory                                      │
│          audiometry, evoked response                                      │
│          occupational disease                                             │
│          middle age                                                       │
├──────────────────── Medline <1987 forward> ───────────────────────────────┤
│   Press 'x' to mark the single most relevant subject heading, then        │
│   press ENTER. Or press ENTER to pick no heading, or ^A for help.         │
├───────────────────────────────────────────────────────────────────────────┤
│   ^A  Help                                                                │
│   ^B  Scope Note                                                          │
└───────────────────────────────────────────────────────────────────────────┘
```

FIGURE 4-12   A representative screen menu of subject headings for limiting a search by adding a Boolean AND and a keyword.

```
┌───────────────────────────────────────────────────────────────────────────┐
│          Index Term Selected                                              │
├───────────────────────────────────────────────────────────────────────────┤
│          *hearing loss, partial                                           │
│                                                                           │
│                                                                           │
│                                                                           │
│                                                                           │
│                                                                           │
├──────────────────── Medline <1987 forward> ───────────────────────────────┤
│   565 articles contain the above index term.                              │
│   In 456 articles this term is the focus of the article.                  │
│                                                                           │
│   Restrict to focus? Enter 'y' or 'n', then ENTER_                        │
├───────────────────────────────────────────────────────────────────────────┤
│   ^A  Help                                                                │
└───────────────────────────────────────────────────────────────────────────┘
```

FIGURE 4-13   A representative screen for limiting a search by restricting it to articles in which the keyword (index term) is a main focus.

Subheadings	Line 1 of 20	Results
chemically induced		33
complications		15
congenital		7
diagnosis		69
drug therapy		9
epidemiology		11
etiology		113
genetics		16
history		1
immunology		1

v More v

Medline <1987 forward>

The subheadings shown above may be applied to refine your search.
Press 'x' to mark as many as are relevant, then press ENTER.
To restrict to no particular subheading, simply press ENTER.

^A	Help
^B	Explain subheading

FIGURE 4-14 **A representative screen menu of subheadings for limiting a search by adding a Boolean AND and a keyword.**

ings that will allow you to further limit (focus) the search if you want to do so (see Figure 4-14). After you respond to this menu, the number of items in the search set is indicated and you are given the opportunity to "browse" through them (see Figure 4-15)—that is, to view them one at a time on the screen (see Figure 4-16). If you want an item included in the printout, you can issue a command (e.g., ^{E}) after viewing it (see Figure 4-16).

If the computer indicates that there are no items containing the keywords you selected, the reason may be that you have chosen the wrong ones. Each database has a printed thesaurus, as a reference tool, that lists the keywords to which it will respond—that is, ones that are in its index.

The final steps in the search process are printing relevant items and logging off. You may be given choices about the format in which you want the bibliography printed, including whether you want abstracts included, if available. If you are using a microcomputer as a terminal, you probably will be given the option of downloading the bibliography to it for saving as a file that can be edited and printed with a word-processing program. After the bibliography is printed or transferred to the microcomputer and saved as a file, you are expected to log off unless you plan to do another search immediately. Doing so usually involves sending a command indicating that you want to quit and possibly keyboarding a sequence of characters such as LO (for "logging off").

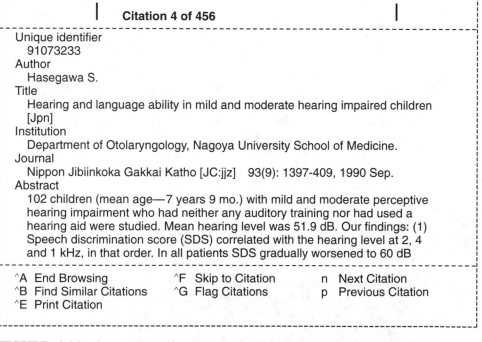

Number	Search Sets	Line 1 of 1	Results
01	*hearing loss, partial		456

-------------------------------- **Medline <1987 forward>** --------------------------------

Mark set to browse, then press ENTER.
Press ENTER to browse last set.

^A Browse Selected Fields

FIGURE 4-15   A representative screen for selecting a search set to browse.

	Citation 4 of 456	

Unique identifier
  91073233
Author
  Hasegawa S.
Title
  Hearing and language ability in mild and moderate hearing impaired children
  [Jpn]
Institution
  Department of Otolaryngology, Nagoya University School of Medicine.
Journal
  Nippon Jibiinkoka Gakkai Katho [JC:jjz]   93(9): 1397-409, 1990 Sep.
Abstract
  102 children (mean age—7 years 9 mo.) with mild and moderate perceptive
  hearing impairment who had neither any auditory training nor had used a
  hearing aid were studied. Mean hearing level was 51.9 dB. Our findings: (1)
  Speech discrimination score (SDS) correlated with the hearing level at 2, 4
  and 1 kHz, in that order. In all patients SDS gradually worsened to 60 dB

^A End Browsing	^F Skip to Citation	n Next Citation
^B Find Similar Citations	^G Flag Citations	p Previous Citation
^E Print Citation		

FIGURE 4-16   A representative screen when citations are being browsed. You could have the remainder of the abstract displayed by typing a command.

Some computerized databases support searches other than keyword topic ones. For example, they may allow you to identify items by a particular author or those published by authors at a particular institution.

Literature Searching Using Abstracts Journal

The abstracts journals that cover the field of communicative disorders include *dsh Abstracts* (1960–1984), *Dissertation Abstracts* (1952–), *Index Medicus* (1960–), *Linguistics and Language Behavior Abstracts* (1967–), and *Psychological Abstracts* (1927–). There was no abstract journal when this chapter was revised (1996) that comprehensively covered the field. The journal *dsh [deafness, speech, and hearing] Abstracts* did so between 1960 and 1984, and hence, is a valuable resource for doing literature searches that include these years. The journal *Linguistics and Language Behavior Abstracts* was titled *Language and Language Behavior Abstracts* between 1967 and 1984.

Representative abstracts and index pages from abstracts journals are reproduced in Figures 4-17 and 4-18 respectively.

Begin a literature search with the last issue of the most recent complete volume of the journal. An index in the back of this issue covers the entire volume (i.e., all four issues for a quarterly journal). You look up your keywords in this index. If you do not find them, you look up synonyms. Then you scan the abstracts of papers that may contain relevant information. Finally, you write down references to those that appear to contain such information.

This process is repeated with the next most recent volume of the abstracts journal and continues until you have covered the number of years you want to include in your search. If the most recent volume of the abstracts journal is *incomplete*, you can check the table of contents of each issue for sections in which there may be papers that contain relevant information.

Exercises and Discussion Topics

1. Use both a single keyword and a single AND strategy (p. 40) to search a computerized database.

2. Search the literature on a topic using both an abstracts journal and a computerized database. How similar are the bibliographies yielded by each?

1678. SEMPLE, J. E. Hearing-impaired preschool child. Springfield, Ill.: Charles C Thomas, 1970. Pp 86.

Designed for parents, the book first describes the problems parents face in coping with their hearing-impaired child and suggests some solutions to these problems. The next two chapters deal with hearing aids and with language and speech development. The last and major chapter presents a series of daily home lesson plans to be used by the parent to assist the child in developing speech and language. The appendixes include reading materials, children's books, an outline for an auditory training program, and suggestions for auditory training.—*I. M. Ventry*

1679. SHARRATT, J. Teaching deaf children to read. *Teacher Deaf*, 68, 1970, 42–44.

Some of the experiences of a teacher of young deaf children during her first three years' teaching.—*K. W. Kritz*

1680. THAN, A. M. (Roy. Nat. Inst. Deaf, 105 Gower St., London W.C. 1, England) Education of the deaf in Burma. *Hearing*, 25, 1970, 108–111.

After a very brief geo-political description of the Union of Burma, the history of services to handicapped children in that country are described. Considers present audiological and educational facilities, and indicates "that by late 1970, two E.E.N.T. specialist doctors and the author will open the first audiology clinic in the country . . ." Goes on to provide some statistics on incidence and services.—*S. E. Gerber*

1681. TRUFFAUT, B. La préparation des jeunes sourds au C.A.P. de dessinateur en construction mecanique. (Training of young deaf as draftsmen.) *Rev. gen. Enseigne. deficients auditifs*, 61(4), 1969, 28–31.

For 10 years the Institute of Saint-Jean-de-la-Ruelle has trained draftsmen, both hearing and deaf. The average age of admission is 16 years. Selection is empirical. The course is of three years' duration. Despite certain difficulties, most deaf graduates obtain satisfactory employment.—*P. J. Wevrick*

1682. VAN UDEN, A. (U. St. Michielsgestal, The Netherlands) Johann Vatter, a German teacher of the deaf. *Teacher Deaf*, 68, 1970, 21–34.

The work and philosophy of this teacher of the deaf is discussed. Pure oral instruction in a residential setting is advocated. Language learning is based on conversation.—*K. W. Kritz*

1683. WRIGHT, D. Deafness. New York, N.Y.: Stein and Day, 1969. Pp 213.

David Wright, the author of this book, is a poet who became profoundly deaf at age seven. In the first section of the book (eight chapters) he provides a biographical account of the impact of deafness on his life, with special emphasis on conveying the feelings of a deaf person as he participates in a variety of activities. The second section (five chapters) is a history of education of the deaf. A short appendix by K. Murphy summarizes basic hearing physiology, hearing pathology, and related research trends. The author indicates that when he wrote this book he had in mind the predicament of parents who have a deaf child.—*J. B. Chaiklin*

ETIOLOGY AND PATHOLOGY

1684. ANDERSON, H. (Karolinska Hosp., Stockholm, Sweden), FILIPSSON, R., FLUUR, E., KOCH, B., LINDSTEN, J. and WEDENBERG, E. Hearing impairment in Turner's syndrome. *Acta otolaryngol.*, Suppl. 247, 1969. Pp 26.

The hearing was studied in 79 clinically and cytogenetically analyzed patients with Turner's syndrome. Middle ear infections had occurred in 68% of the patients. Conductive or mixed losses were found in 22%. Cephalometric analysis showed the external auditory meati to be caudally displaced which resulted in abnormal orientation of the Eustachian tube, a condition that may explain the predisposition to middle-ear infections. Sensorineural hearing impairment with recruitment was found in 64% of the patients. Vestibular findings were normal for the nine patients who were given vestibular tests. The etiological significance of the abnormal sex chromosome constitution for the hearing impairment is discussed.—*Authors, edited*

FIGURE 4-17   A representative page of abstracts from an abstracts journal.

FIGURE 4-18   A representative index page from an abstracts journal.

Part **II**

Asking and Answering Questions

Choosing a Research Project: Asking Questions That Are Both Relevant and Answerable

The first four chapters were intended to set the stage for our discussion of research design. My primary objective in this chapter and the seven that follow is to provide basic information about the process of asking and answering questions that a speech-language pathologist or audiologist needs to function as a clinician-investigator. This chapter will deal with selecting and formulating questions for research. It also will be concerned with selecting a topic, or area, to research. The topic selected, of course, determines the questions asked.

A speech-language pathologist or audiologist who chooses to function as a clinician-investigator must first decide what to investigate—what question or questions to try to answer. This decision is important because it will influence both the impact of his or her research and the likelihood that the research will be completed. By *impact* here is meant the effect that answering a particular question or group of questions is likely to have on clinical process in speech-language pathology and audiology. Unfortunately, the amount of impact that answering a particular question is likely to have on clinical process is quite difficult to predict. As Murray Sidman has pointed out,

> It is necessary . . . to be wary about using the presumed importance of data as a criterion for evaluating them. Science, like fashion, has its fads and cycles. A discovery that lies outside the current stream of interest may be unrecognized and eventually forgotten, perhaps to be rediscovered at some later date. On the other side of the coin, we often find experiments acclaimed as significant because they resolve a problem of great contemporary concern, but of little lasting interest. It

is a characteristic of science that we are seldom able to predict its future course of development. Many of the exciting issues of today will be forgotten tomorrow as the stream of scientific progress shifts into new channels. (Sidman, 1960, p. 2)

Sidman's comments obviously have relevance for assessing the probable impact of answers to questions (i.e., experimental results) on clinical process in speech-language pathology and audiology. While the criterion of "importance" will always be of concern to investigators, it will not be particularly useful either for selecting questions to answer or for evaluating answers to questions.

An investigator's choice of questions to answer influences the likelihood that he or she will complete the research, for several reasons. The first is the *time required to make the necessary observations.* The longer you take to make these observations, the less likely you are to complete your research. As long as the time necessary does not exceed a year, this probably would not be an important consideration. While I do not wish to imply here that investigators should avoid questions that take longer than a year to answer—since there are probably many such questions that would be worthwhile answering—you should realize that when you attempt to answer such questions you are less likely to complete your research. This may be one of the reasons, incidentally, why so little longitudinal research has been reported.

A second factor likely to influence the probability that research will be completed is the *complexity of the procedures required to make the necessary observations.* The more complex such procedures, the less likely an investigator is to complete the research. If you need electronic instrumentation (particularly, complex electronic instrumentation) to make your observations, you may have difficulty getting the instrumentation to function well enough to make them. The author experienced such difficulty in his own research with a miniature voice-actuated white-noise generator that was designed to be used with stutterers. About 50 percent of the time the device would not function properly, and several electronics technicians who tried to repair it were unsuccessful. While I am not attempting to discourage investigators from answering questions that require instrumentation to answer, you should realize that problems can arise when you attempt to answer such questions.

A third factor is the *availability of subjects.* If subjects are not available in sufficient numbers *within a reasonable time period,* the probability that the research will be completed can be reduced. It should be noted, however, that speech-language pathologists and audiologists have successfully completed research that has taken a number of years to observe a sufficient number of subjects. Berry and colleagues (Berry, Darley, Aronson, & Goldstein, 1974), for example, required fifteen years to observe a sufficient number of persons with Wilson's disease to be able to describe the speech deviations associated with it.

A fourth factor is the *time available for the purpose.* Some questions require more time to answer than others. Before beginning a piece of research, therefore, you should at least roughly estimate both the time required to complete it and the time you are likely to have available for the purpose.

A fifth factor is the *availability of supporting personnel (including consultants) and services.* To make the observations necessary to answer a question may require the cooperation or assistance of persons with expertise in various areas, and such persons may not be available. For example, a study of the effect of a therapy program on persons who have vocal nodules may require the services of an otolaryngologist to do indirect laryngoscopy on the subjects before and after participating in the program. The investigator may be unable to locate an otolaryngologist who would be willing to provide this service. This possibility should be considered before beginning a piece of research.

A sixth factor that should be considered is *available funding*. To answer some questions, a research grant is needed, and to answer others, only minimal funding (less than $100) is required. Many questions of interest to speech-language pathologists and audiologists, incidentally, require only minimal funding to answer: Funding may only be needed for supplies, such as postage stamps or test forms. Before you commit yourself to answering a particular question, or questions, you should be reasonably certain that available funding will be adequate.

Generating Relevant Questions for Research

Now that we have considered some factors to think about when choosing questions to answer, we will consider some strategies that can be used to generate relevant questions for research. By a "relevant question" we mean one for which a response to the "so what" or "who cares" question can be provided—in other words, a question for which *a need* for answering can be established. This is referred to as establishing *scientific justification* (see the next section and Chapter 13).

Need for Selecting Questions That Are Likely to Be Regarded as Being Relevant

Though the scientific method does not require it, you will find it advantageous to select questions to answer that you feel are relevant and that others will think are relevant for several reasons. First, your research is more likely to be publishable if you select such questions. In the introductory section of a research report for a professional journal, such as the *American Journal of Audiology*, the *American Journal of Speech-Language Pathology*, the *Journal of Speech and Hearing Research*, and *Language, Speech, and Hearing Services in Schools*, the author is expected to establish scientific justification for the research reported. That is, the author is expected to demonstrate the importance of answering the question or questions proposed. If you understand why it is important and can communicate this to readers of your report, you will increase the probability that your report will be accepted for publication.

A second reason to select questions that both your peers and the administrators to whom you are responsible will regard as relevant is to increase the possibility that you will receive the support you need for your research. You are more likely to have peer support and secure funding for research you can justify as relevant than for research for which you can provide no such justification. Also, you are more likely to receive approval from administrators for "released time" for research if they view your research as satisfying an important need, particularly for their institution. The need it satisfies could be enhancing the prestige of the institution for marketing purposes. Gaining such approval would be particularly important for speech-language pathologists and audiologists who are employed in clinical settings and whose primary responsibilities are clinical.

Identifying a Problem Area

What should you take into consideration when attempting to identify a problem area from which to generate relevant questions for research? Several factors need to be considered. These factors include: (1) personal interests, (2) competencies, (3) the potential value of the research, (4) the available equipment and facilities for making observations and analyzing data, (5) the "populations" available for study, (6) the financial resources available, (7) the amount of time available, and (8) the possibilities for consultation. Several of them were discussed in a different context earlier in this chapter.

The first factor you should consider when attempting to identify a problem area for research is *personal interests*—you should attempt to identify problem areas within the field of communicative disorders that are of particular interest to you. An area could be defined partially by a symptom complex such as aphasia, stuttering, defective articulation, or conductive hearing loss. An area could also be defined partially by a management strategy such as impedance audiometry, augmentative communication, or language testing. You should attempt to identify as many such areas as you can and roughly order them on the basis of your interest in them. It is desirable to identify more than one area initially, since factors may be present that would make it quite difficult to pursue certain areas. Several such factors will be discussed in this section.

As already indicated, you should select an area to research in which you have some interest. Your interest in the research will influence both how positively reinforcing you will find the experience and the probability that you will complete it. We all tend to pursue activities we find positively reinforcing and avoid those we find "punishing."

A second factor that you should consider when selecting a problem area for research is deficiencies in your training or experience. The probability that you will be successful in your research endeavors may be greater if you avoid certain problem areas. If you had no training or experience in aphasia testing, for example, you might be wise to avoid questions that required the administration of aphasia tests to answer. While you could probably learn to administer such tests, it might require a considerable investment of time before you would be sufficiently competent to administer them with adequate reliability for your purposes. Of course, you might be able to find someone with whom to collaborate on the research who is competent in aphasia testing. This illustrates one way an investigator can reduce the consequences of a deficiency in training or experience. It is not unusual, incidentally, for two or more persons to collaborate on a piece of research. In fact, more than 80 percent of the papers in five randomly selected issues of the *Journal of Speech and Hearing Research* were authored by two or more persons. It is desirable, therefore, when attempting to evaluate a potential problem area for research, to specify as completely as you can the competencies necessary to pursue the research and to judge whether you possess each one. If you do not possess some necessary competencies and cannot find a collaborator (or collaborators) who does, you might be wise not to pursue research in the area, particularly if overcoming such deficiencies would require large investments of money and/or time.

A third consideration when attempting to identify a problem area for research is the *potential value* of the research. As already indicated, it is difficult to predict the impact a piece of research will have on a discipline. Nevertheless, this is almost always a consideration when an investigator chooses an area of research. You will usually choose a problem you regard as worthwhile to investigate. For this reason, you may choose a problem with immediate relevance—for example, you may attempt to evaluate a therapy program that you are presently using or are contemplating using. Such research could have considerable impact on your own caseload and, if it is communicated to other clinicians, on their caseloads as well.

A fourth factor is the *availability of equipment and facilities for making observations and analyzing data.* An investigator may not be able to pursue a research area of interest because the necessary facilities, equipment, or both, are lacking. From one frame of reference this factor could restrict an investigator in exploring certain problem areas. From a second frame of reference additional possible problem areas for research might be suggested. Investigators with equipment and facilities that are not generally available may wish to exploit them—that is, to define a problem area based on questions they would permit to be answered. An audiologist, for example, who possessed some pieces of testing equipment not generally available might choose to ask questions that could be answered through the use of this equipment. Or a speech-language pathologist who is employed in a clinic that has sophisticated instrumentation for augmentative communication might choose to exploit it in a similar manner. As an investigator, therefore, you might find it worthwhile to prepare an inventory of the equipment and facilities available to you as a preliminary step in defining a problem area for research. Such an inventory could assist you in assessing problem areas you are considering and in identifying additional possible problem areas.

A fifth factor is the *"populations" available for study.* Before you begin to try to identify a research area, you might find it worthwhile to inventory relevant attributes of persons who might be available and willing to serve as research subjects. Relevant attributes might include: (1) sex, (2) whether they have particular communicative disorders, (3) chronological age, (4) physical status, (5) intellectual and emotional status, (6) socioeconomic status, and (7) therapy history—whether they have previously had therapy and if they have, what kind or kinds. Such an inventory could provide two types of input into the selection process. First, it could alert you, the investigator, to research areas you would be wise to avoid because subjects who have the necessary attributes would probably not be available to you in sufficient numbers. A speech clinician employed in a school setting, for example, might have a difficult time obtaining adequate numbers of laryngectomized geriatric subjects for a research project. Second, the inventory could suggest problem areas you might want to consider. If you had subjects available in fairly large numbers who were relatively homogeneous in some attribute (e.g., deaf children or mentally retarded children) or if you had small numbers of subjects available who were unusual in some way (e.g., persons with rare diseases or conditions that influence communicative behavior), you might be able to define a problem area in which you could use observations made on such subjects to answer questions. A single subject, incidentally, who is unusual in some regard might be used in this manner for an individual case study.

A sixth factor is the *financial resources available.* As already indicated, while some research requires only minimal funding, other research can be quite costly. To do research that required more than minimal funding, an investigator would probably have to secure a research grant from a government (state or national) agency, private organization, or private foundation. Many such agencies, organizations, and foundations have funded research on communicative disorders. Nevertheless, a person who is considering applying for such a grant should be aware that they are usually quite competitive. More applications are ordinarily submitted than can be funded. Investigators who have demonstrated research competence by publishing are usually favored for the larger grants; they also are favored for many relatively small grants. A beginning investigator, therefore, would probably be wise to select a project that only requires minimal funding. However, after demonstrating research competency by publishing the results of several such projects, you can consider projects that require external funding if you so desire. The topic of research funding is discussed further in Chapter 16.

A seventh factor is the *amount of time available*. Before you decide to do a particular research project, it is a good idea to estimate roughly both the amount of time it would take to complete and the amount of time that is likely to be available. If the amount of time necessary grossly exceeds the time available for the purpose, you have several options as an investigator: (1) You can try to locate one or more professional colleagues who would be interested in collaborating with you on the project and sharing the work; (2) you can enlist the aid of persons who are not speech-language pathologists or audiologists, such as spouses or secretaries, for parts of the project that do not require competence in these areas; (3) you can secure a grant and hire full- or part-time research assistants to gather data and assist with data analysis; (4) you can attempt to arrange your schedule to have adequate time available for the project; (5) you can reduce the magnitude of the project—ask fewer questions and/or use fewer subjects; or (6) you can decide not to pursue the project. Many projects, incidentally, require a time investment that would not exceed that available to most clinicians. Among these are projects for which data could be gathered in conjunction with ongoing clinical activities, for example, therapy evaluation studies.

An eighth factor is the *possibilities for consultation*. If, to do a research project, you must consult with persons who have expertise in certain areas such as electronics, computer programming, or mental measurement, you should be reasonably certain before beginning that such persons will be available for consultation. As I have already indicated, faculty members at local colleges and universities who have the required expertise may be willing to serve as consultants—possibly even unpaid ones.

Generating Relevant Research Questions

After a problem area has been selected, the next task is to generate one or more questions to answer that are relevant to the area. These questions, implicitly or explicitly, define the research topic. They indicate what the investigator is trying to find out. They also indicate the kinds of information that are apt to result from the research. Since most research questions only can be answered in a finite number of ways, we usually can infer from a question what the possible answers could be. If, for example, the question we sought to answer was, "Do most elementary-school stutterers avoid talking?" our research could lead to three possible answers: (1) It could indicate unequivocally that the majority of elementary-school stutterers avoid talking; (2) it could indicate unequivocally that the majority of elementary-school stutterers do not avoid talking; or (3) it could lead to an equivocal result. Finally, the questions asked specify, at least partially, what has to be done to answer them. Suppose, for example, we asked the question, "How likely are persons who are employed as firemen for more than ten years to develop noise-induced hearing losses?" To answer this question, we would have to measure the hearing acuity of persons who have been employed as firemen for more than ten years using methods that were sufficiently reliable and valid to detect noise-induced hearing losses if they were present.

What approaches can be used for selecting a research topic within an area—that is, generating questions to answer? Several approaches can be used for this purpose. One is to do a careful review of the literature in the area to identify: (1) questions that have been formulated but only partially answered, (2) questions that have been formulated but not answered, and (3) questions that have not been formulated but should be.

Many questions about communicative disorders have been formulated but only partially answered. A question is rarely answered unequivocally on the basis of a single set of observations for several reasons. First, in many cases (perhaps most) the observations that were used to answer a question were *not* made on a random sample of subjects from the population referred to by the question. To illustrate this point, let's again use the question, "How likely are persons who are employed as firemen for more than ten years to develop noise-induced hearing losses?" The population referred to by this question consists of all firemen who have more than ten years' experience. For a sample from this population to be random, all such firemen would have to have an equal chance of being selected. However, it would be unusual for an investigator who sought to answer this kind of question to use a random sample. He or she would most likely use a "nonrandom" one, such as a local group of firemen with more than ten years' service who volunteered to have their hearing tested. The likelihood of the subjects in such a sample having noise-induced hearing losses may differ systematically from that for firemen in general. In other words, the answer to the question could be different for this sample than it would have been for a random sample. Consequently, the generality of an answer based on a nonrandom sample would be uncertain (see Chapter 12). In cases where a question has been answered through the use of a nonrandom sample, therefore, the answer should be regarded as equivocal until the observations have been replicated on other samples of subjects from the population. This would be true even if the results were statistically significant. One assumption that underlies almost all tests of statistical significance is that the subjects observed were a random sample from the population of interest. (This concept is further discussed in Chapter 12.)

A second reason why a question may not have been answered unequivocally on the basis of a single set of observations is that they were *not* adequately *reliable, valid*, or both (see Chapter 12). If the observations were not sufficiently reliable, the investigator may not have been able to observe the phenomenon with sufficient clarity to answer the question accurately. Returning to the fireman example again, if the audiometer used had not been properly calibrated, if the person who administered the test or tests had not been sufficiently proficient, or if the room in which the testing was done had not been adequately sound treated, the thresholds recorded could have been sufficiently in error that the effect of noise on firemen's hearing might not be detected—particularly if the resulting hearing loss was a mild one. On the other hand, if the observations used to answer a question were not sufficiently valid, the answer *might* be incorrect. We use the word *might* here because an investigator could arrive at the right answer for the wrong reason (e.g., Gall's conclusion that the anterior portion of the brain is dominant for speech, discussed in Chapter 3). In our fireman example, an investigator could conclude through the use of an invalid testing procedure (e.g., one that was thought to be able to detect noise-induced hearing losses but was not sensitive to such losses) that the firemen did not have noise-induced hearing losses when they did, or that they had noise-induced hearing losses when they did not.

A third reason why a question may not have been answered unequivocally on the basis of a single set of observations is *random*, or chance, *sampling error*. This can influence research results derived from random samples of subjects by methods that were adequately reliable and valid. What happens here is that by chance the behavior of the subjects in the sample is not representative of that in the population from which they were selected, even though appropriate sampling procedures were used. While random sampling is more likely to result in a sample that is representative of the population than are other sampling methods, it does not always produce such a sample. A random sample will not be representative of the population from which it was selected a certain percentage of the time. (The reason for this phenomenon is discussed in Chapter 12.) The observations that were made on such a sample of subjects could be sufficiently biased to cause an investigator to answer a question incorrectly. Because of this possibility, research findings should be regarded as suspect until they have been replicated. A question should not be regarded as having been answered unequivocally until the same answer has been obtained with several samples of subjects.

A fourth, and final, reason why a question may not have been answered unequivocally on the basis of a single set of observations is *experimenter bias*. An investigator's expectations and theoretical biases can influence his or her observations without the investigator being conscious of it (Barber, 1976; Rosenthal, 1976). If you expect a question to be answered in a particular way or if your theoretical biases suggest that a question should have a particular answer, you may unconsciously "filter" your observations to obtain the answer you expect. This is particularly apt to be a problem when an investigator has considerable ego-involvement in a theoretical position relevant to the questions he or she is attempting to answer. This problem is extremely difficult to deal with. With regard to our concern here—selecting questions to answer—the relevance of experimenter bias is that if a question has only been answered by a single investigator (particularly one with an ego investment in the answer), the answer should probably not be regarded as unequivocal unless it has been replicated by other investigators unlikely to have the same theoretical biases.

In addition to helping identify questions that have been formulated but only partially answered, a search of the literature in an area of interest may reveal questions that have been *formulated but not answered*. There are several places in which such questions might be found. One is the "discussion" section of research reports in the area. Frequently in this section the author or authors will indicate some implications they feel their findings have for future research. They may even specify a question or two that they feel need to be answered and provide "scientific justification" for answering them.

Another source of questions that have been formulated but not answered is review papers in the area of interest. A review paper is one that summarizes and integrates the research in a particular area. Such papers usually suggest some information that is needed to improve our understanding of the area—that is, questions that need to be answered. Review papers have been published for many areas of interest to speech-language pathologists and audiologists. They have appeared in journals and monographs as well as in books. One way to locate a review paper on a topic of interest that was published in a journal or monograph (if one has been written) is to use an abstracts journal or computer database (see Chapter 4).

Abstracts of papers relevant to the topic can be scanned to determine if they are review papers. If you are using an abstracts journal rather than a computer database (e.g., Medline), it would be wise to begin a literature search with the most recent volume and work backward. This procedure would maximize the odds of finding the most recent review paper on a topic, if there has been more than one.

Thus far, we have considered how a review of the literature in the area of interest can help to identify questions that have been formulated but only partially answered and questions that have been formulated but not answered. We now will consider how such a review can suggest *questions that have not been formulated but should be*. The strategy here would be to: (1) do a careful search of the literature in the area to determine what is known (what questions have been answered), and (2) formulate questions that, if answered, would be likely to increase our understanding of the area.

The first task, the literature search, can be expedited by the use of abstracts journals and computer databases (see Chapter 4). The reference lists of all papers found should be checked for relevant research reports that were not identified. Such reports would include those published prior to the year in which the literature search began; those that appeared in limited circulation journals such as state speech and hearing journals; those that were presented orally at state, national, and international professional and scientific meetings; those that were reported in unpublished master's theses and doctoral dissertations; and those that were reported in unpublished papers, including technical reports.

The research reported should be organized in a manner to make it apparent what is known about the area. One approach that can sometimes be used for this purpose is to define a *dependent variable* and indicate what *independent variables* have been shown to influence it. One example of a dependent variable is speechreading ability; examples of independent variables that have been shown to influence it include visual acuity and training in speechreading. Another example of a dependent variable is extent of recovery from aphasia. Independent variables that would be expected to influence it include chronological age, extent and location (e.g., right or left hemisphere) of lesion, and amount of language stimulation received.

After the available data has been organized to make it apparent what is known about the area, the next task is to formulate questions that, if answered, would be likely to increase our understanding of it. What is required here is first to formulate as many questions as possible and then to select from these one or more to answer. Organized in this way, the information available on a topic would facilitate the question formulation process. This would be particularly true if a dependent variable had been defined and independent variables that have been shown to influence it cataloged. One would then attempt to identify independent variables not yet studied that might be relevant. A question, or questions, could be formulated about each such variable. If the dependent variable, for example, were speechreading ability and an independent variable that had not been investigated were telepathic ability, one question that might be asked would be, "Do persons who earn relatively high scores on a Duke University card-guessing telepathy task exhibit greater speechreading ability than those who earn relatively low scores on this task?"

How can we identify uninvestigated independent variables that may influence a particular dependent variable? This question is difficult to answer since the process of discovery is not fully understood. Perhaps our ability to identify such independent variables involves what Michael Polanyi (1967) has referred to as "tacit knowing." According to Polanyi,

> *. . . we can know more than we can tell. This fact seems obvious enough; but it is not easy to say exactly what it means. Take an example. We know a person's face, and can recognize it among a thousand, indeed among a million. Yet we usually cannot tell how we recognize a face we know. (Polanyi, 1967, p. 4)*

Polanyi states that tacit knowing guides the scientist to problems worth investigating—that is, to questions worth answering. Hunches and intuitions resulting from tacit knowing may be the mechanism by which we identify relevant independent variables.

While the process used to identify relevant independent variables is not fully understood, there is a strategy that may facilitate it. This strategy is to identify independent variables that have been shown to influence other dependent behavioral variables that have not been investigated with regard to the dependent variable of interest. Chronological age is an example of an independent variable that has been shown to influence many dependent behavioral variables of interest to speech-language pathologists and audiologists. If such an independent variable had not been investigated with regard to the dependent behavioral variable in which you are interested, it might be worthwhile for you to do so. The author worked for several years as a research associate on a project that investigated the variability of stuttering frequency (dependent variable) in school-age children under the same conditions it had previously been investigated in adults. The question we sought to answer was, "Do conditions that have been shown to influence (reduce or increase) stuttering frequency in adults also do so in school-age children?"

A second general approach for identifying relevant research questions is to examine your clinical experience in the area of interest for questions that seem worth answering and then to search the relevant literature to determine whether they have been answered. You should ask yourself the following question: "To what clinically relevant questions have I sought answers for which I know of no data to answer?" You also should ask yourself, "To what clinically relevant questions do I feel I have answers where the validity and reliability of the data on which the answers are based is uncertain?" That is, "What questions am I assuming have been adequately answered empirically that may not have been?" Things are frequently done clinically not because they have been shown to be effective empirically, but because they have either been recommended by an authority, "make sense" theoretically, or are *traditional*. What I mean by being traditional can be illustrated by the frequency and duration of therapy sessions assigned to clients. It may be traditional in a particular clinical setting for clients with a particular communicative disorder to be scheduled for therapy a particular number of sessions per week, each of which is a particular number of minutes in duration. One might ask whether this number of sessions per week of this length is optimal for reducing the severity of these clients' communicative disorders. Perhaps the sessions either are: (1) longer and more frequent than necessary, or (2) longer but not more frequent than necessary, or (3) less frequent but longer than necessary, or (4) shorter and less frequent than necessary. One way to answer this question—to determine whether the frequency and duration of therapy sessions are optimal—would be to vary systematically the frequency and duration of sessions for clients who have a given communicative disorder and observe whether better results are obtained when a different frequency or duration is used. Questions such as these were particularly relevant when this chapter was revised because of the widespread acceptance of the "managed care" philosophy.

One approach that can be used for identifying questions that have answers based on "authority" or "tradition" rather than on empirical data is to subject information on which you operate clinically to the "how do I know?" question. How do I know, for example, that a therapy procedure does what it is supposed to do? If there were no unequivocal empirical evidence that a therapy procedure did what it was supposed to do, this circumstance would suggest questions for research. The available data on clinical procedures of interest can be located through the use of computer databases and abstracts journals (see Chapter 4).

A third approach for generating questions that might be worth answering is brainstorming with colleagues about their clinical experience in the area and then searching relevant literature to determine whether the questions suggested have been answered unequivocally. The procedure here is much the same as that described for the second approach. The only difference is that questions are abstracted from informal discussions with colleagues about their clinical experience rather than from the clinician's own experience.

What specifically might colleagues say that would suggest potential research questions? They might indicate concern over the effectiveness of a particular diagnostic or therapeutic procedure. They might state that they failed to obtain the results reported for this procedure in the literature. Assuming that they appeared to have applied it as described in the literature, one might ask whether the results reported in the literature can be replicated. Such could be the genesis of a piece of clinical research.

A colleague may also raise questions about the organization of a clinical program for which no data-based guidelines exist in the literature. Such questions may relate to any of a number of areas, including intake procedures, dismissal procedures, follow-up procedures, and the utilization of paraprofessionals.

Furthermore, a colleague may raise questions about the accuracy of certain "answers" (findings) reported in the literature. He or she may state, for example, that the incidence of a particular communicative disorder appears to be considerably higher or lower than reported in the literature. Or he or she may indicate that most of those clients who have a particular communicative disorder fail to exhibit some aspect or aspects of the symptomatology reported in the literature as characteristic of this disorder.

Structuring Research Questions to Make Them Answerable

The question considered thus far in this chapter has been, "How can we generate relevant questions for research?" In this section we will consider the question, "How can we structure research questions to make them as answerable as possible?" By an answerable question we mean one that can be answered by observations and that implicitly or explicitly (preferably the latter) specifies the observation or observations needed to answer it.

Not all questions of interest to speech-language pathologists and audiologists are equally answerable empirically. One reason is that a question may be formulated in a way that makes it uncertain what observations have to be made to answer it. Consider, for example, the following questions:

1. Is hypnosis effective in treating stuttering?
2. Is the post-hypnotic suggestion, "You will not stutter anymore," effective in reducing stuttering frequency?

These questions are not equally answerable. The second specifies the observations that would have to be made to answer it more explicitly than the first and consequently, is more answerable empirically.

A question may not be answerable empirically because it is not possible to make the observations needed to answer it. In some cases the reason is that appropriate observational methods have not as yet been developed. When they are, the question will no longer be unanswerable. In other cases, a question may be unanswerable because the instruments required to make the observations are not available to the investigator. While such a question would be unanswerable for him or her, it might not be for someone else (someone who has the necessary instruments).

How does one structure a question to make it answerable? According to Wendell Johnson,

> *One cannot get a clear answer to a vague question. The language of science is particularly distinguished by the fact it centers around well-stated questions. If there is one part of a scientific experiment that is more important than any other part, it is the framing of the question that the experiment is to answer. If it is stated vaguely, no experiment can answer it precisely. If the question is stated precisely, the means of answering it are clearly indicated. The specific observations needed, and the conditions under which they are to be made, are implied in the question itself. (Johnson, 1946, pp. 52–53)*

For a question to be answerable, therefore, it cannot be vague or ambiguous. The meanings of all words must be made explicit and, if possible, defined operationally. If a question we wished to answer were "Do persons with cleft palates have normal intelligence?" we would have to specify as precisely as possible what segment of the cleft palate population we were referring to (i.e., those with a cleft of the soft palate only, those with clefts of both hard and soft palates, or both groups) and what we meant by intelligence (i.e., performance on what task or test). The question would be more answerable, for example, if it were structured as follows: "Are 5-year-old children who have clefts of the palate only more likely to have below normal intelligence as measured by the Stanford-Binet than 5-year-old children who do not have this condition?"

To further illustrate what an answerable question consists of, pairs of questions are presented in Table 5-1 in which the members of each pair differ in the degree to which they are answerable. The member in column one is less answerable than that in column two.

TABLE 5-1   Pairs of Questions That Differ in the Degree to Which They Are Answerable

Less Answerable Version	More Answerable Version
How much can aphasics be expected to improve between one month and one year following trauma?	How many points can receptive aphasics be expected to gain, on the average, on the Western Aphasia Test between one month and one year following trauma?
Does drinking alcoholic beverages reduce stuttering?	Does drinking a six-pack of beer in a period of an hour reduce stuttering frequency?
Are home assignments helpful for correcting phonological errors?	Is a particular home assignment at a particular stage of therapy for a particular phonological error helpful for correcting that error?
Is a particular ear-protector effective for preventing noise-induced hearing loss?	Is a particular ear protector effective for preventing a temporary threshold shift if used in the presence of noise of a particular intensity with a particular spectrum for a particular period of time?

Exercises and Discussion Topics

1. Determine whether each of the following questions is answerable by attempting to specify the observations necessary for answering it. If you feel that a question is not as answerable as it could be, rewrite it to make it more answerable and specify the observations you would make to answer the question as you have rewritten it.
   a. Do aphasics benefit from therapy?
   b. Can lateral emission during /s/ production be eliminated by training in auditory discrimination?
   c. How accurately can classroom teachers identify children in their classrooms who have hearing losses?

2. Formulate an answerable question about clinical process (i.e., evaluation or therapy) you could answer using observations you made while working with a specific client during your practicum experience. Describe these observations.

Chapter 6

Single Subject and Group Designs

After an investigator has formulated research questions, the next task is to select an appropriate design for making the observations needed to answer them. There is no one design appropriate for gathering the data needed to answer all questions. This chapter will describe the two main types of designs that are used for this purpose: those in which the data are descriptions of the attributes of *single* subjects or those in which they are descriptions of the attributes of the *typical* member of a group. Before doing so, we will consider some of the terminology used for describing them.

Terminology Used for Describing Group and Single Subject Research Designs

Group and single subject research designs have been categorized in a number of ways and a terminology has developed for describing them. Some terms that have been used for doing so are defined below. Others are defined elsewhere in the chapter.

- **Counterbalanced design.** A group experiment design in which all the conditions are administered to all subjects, but not in the same order. Subjects are divided into approximately equal size groups, the number being equal to the number of conditions. For example, suppose we wanted to determine in which of two conditions (A or B) stutterers tended to stutter most severely. We would obtain a speech sample from each stutterer under each condition. Half would speak under *Condition A* first and half under *Condition B*. This design allows us to control for *order effects*, which are described elsewhere in this chapter.
- **Ex post facto design.** A group or single subject research design in which causation is studied by an analysis of past events. This has also been referred to as both a *causal-comparative* and a *correlational* design. The latter term is used when the analysis involves the computation of correlation coefficients (see Chapter 9). This is the type of design that

was used for generating the data indicating that smokers are more at risk than nonsmokers for developing a number of health problems. The data used were from medical case *histories* of smokers and nonsmokers. It is also the type of design that is used for studying causation (e.g., inferring the impacts of a therapy program) in individual case studies in which the data utilized are abstracted from material in the client's clinic file.

- **Experiment.** A group or single subject research design in which an investigator *manipulates* one variable and watches the effect on another. An example would be watching the effect of manipulating stress level on stuttering frequency.

- **Factorial design.** A group research design in which it is possible to determine the impacts of more than one independent variable (factors) on a dependent variable. Real-world outcomes usually are the result of a number of factors. In research on the effect of an aphasia therapy, for example, we might want to assess the impacts of two independent variables: age and number of months post-trauma. This would allow us to determine whether the age of the client and/or the length of time he or she has been aphasic influences therapy outcome.

- **Longitudinal design.** A group or single subject research design in which observations are made of the same persons for a relatively long period of time, usually years. An example would be observing for a number of years young children judged to be "at risk" for developing a particular communicative disorder to determine how many develop it.

- **Natural experiment.** A group or single subject research design in which it is possible to observe the effect that one variable (usually some type of abnormality) has on others without having to produce it. It is also referred to as an *investigation*. An example would be determining the function of a portion of the right cerebral cortex by observing the behavior of one or more persons who have a lesion in it.

- **Pretest–posttest design.** A group or single subject research design in which the impact of an intervention strategy is judged from the difference between pretreatment and posttreatment measures.

- **Randomized controlled trials (RCTs).** A group design used for treatment outcome research in which clients are randomly assigned to two groups—those in one receive the treatment being assessed and those in the other do not. The person doing the assigning is not told to which group a particular client is assigned until after the assignment is made in order to prevent any of his or her conscious or unconscious biases from influencing assignment decisions (e.g., wanting the therapy to be effective and, therefore, assigning clients with the best prognosis to the treatment group). This methodology has been used for evaluating aphasia therapies (Howard, 1986).

- **Replication.** A research design that is the same as that of an earlier study. It is used for evaluating the reliability and/or generality of the findings of that study. A *systematic replication* is the same as a replication except that one aspect of the design is changed—for example, males are used instead of females. If the findings from the modified design are the same as those from the earlier study, their generality is increased. If the findings are not the same, it could be either because those of the earlier study are not reliable or that the change in design made a real difference. Hence, systematic replications are risky!

- **Retrospective design.** A group or single subject research design for collecting reports of observations made at an earlier point in time. An example would be the parental interview data reported by Johnson and Associates (1959) on the speech of children at the "moment" they were initially regarded as beginning to stutter by their parents. It differs from the *ex post facto design* in that the data generated may be used to describe events rather than explain them.

　　• **Static-group comparison design.** This design compares the status of a group that has received an experimental treatment to one that has not. The first is referred to as the *experimental* group and the second the *control* group. This is one of the most frequently used designs in speech, language, and hearing research.

　　• **Time-series design.** A group or single subject research design in which observations (e.g., measurements) are made at periodic intervals and there is an experimental treatment between two of them. The treatment is judged to have had an effect if there is a change from the observation immediately before to the one immediately after its introduction. These designs are used frequently in therapy outcome research.

Differences between Single Subject and Group Research Designs

A single subject design permits the performance of single subjects under the experimental condition or conditions to be *reliably* determined. Reliable conclusions can be reached concerning the effects of an experimental condition on the behavior of a single subject. The question, "Has a client improved following a period of therapy?" would require a single subject design to answer. The simplest such design would be one that permitted relevant "before and after" measures (e.g., pretherapy and posttherapy measures) to be made.

　　Single subject designs are *not limited to studies in which there is only one subject.* They can be used in studies in which there is almost any number of subjects. However, when they are used, the data from each subject is reported separately (usually in a graph or table). That is, data from individual subjects are not combined and averaged.

　　A group design *reliably* permits the average (mean, median, or mode) performance of the subjects in a group under the experimental condition or conditions to be determined. Reliable conclusions can be reached concerning the effects of an experimental condition on the behavior of the average, or "typical," member of a group. The question, "Are elementary-school stutterers able to predict their moments of stuttering as accurately as adult stutterers?" would require a group design. To answer it, the average (i.e., mean or median) performance of a group of elementary-school stutterers on a stuttering prediction task could be compared to that of a group of adult stutterers on the same task.

　　Thus far, these two types of designs have been discussed as if they were mutually exclusive. This is not the case. Some studies use designs that generate both types of data. They permit the average performance of a group as well as the performance of the individual subjects in that group under the experimental condition or conditions to be *reliably* determined. Such designs are useful when it appears likely that subjects will respond differently to an experimental condition. In fact, they permit the investigator to determine whether subjects do, in fact, respond differently to such a condition. It might be suspected, for example, that a particular approach to teaching speechreading would be more effective with some hard-of-hearing persons than with others. It probably would be worthwhile, therefore, to gather sufficient data on each person with whom the approach is used so that the amount each learned could be *reliably* estimated. From these data could be determined:

(1) the amount the "average" person in the group learned, and (2) the degree of variability in the amount learned. Also, if considerable variability occurred, an attempt could be made to identify the factor or factors responsible through the use of correlational procedures. (These are described in Chapter 9.)

Considerable emphasis has been placed here on the word *reliability*, particularly with regard to the single subject design. The types of data usually gathered when group designs are used—that is, each subject run only once under each experimental condition—usually are not sufficiently reliable for determining the responses of single subjects to experimental conditions. A subject may not always respond to an experimental condition in the same manner, because of the effects of extraneous variables that have not been controlled and in many cases would be quite difficult to control even if we wished to. A subject's emotional state and degree of motivation would be examples of such variables.

Another reason for the lack of reliability of such data is that descriptions of behavior (both numerical and verbal) are subject to error of various kinds. The human observer is not an error-free describer of events. The more observations on which a description is based, the more reliable it is apt to be. Suppose that we wished to determine the effect of speaking in the presence of masking noise on stuttering. Our description would probably be more reliable if each stutterer spoke five times without masking noise and five times with masking noise and stuttering frequencies during the five speeches under each condition were averaged than it would be if each spoke only once under each condition.

To clarify the distinction between single subject and group designs, we have indicated in Table 6-1 eight of the more important differences between them. The order in which they appear in the table is not necessarily related to their importance.

One of the more important differences between these two designs is the nature of the data provided. Single subject designs provide data on the *typical* responses of *individual subjects* to an experimental condition. The typical response referred to here would be the mean, median, or most frequently occurring (modal) response. Group designs, on the other hand, provide data on the mean, median, or most frequently occurring (modal) response(s) of the *members of a group*—that is, the response(s) of a typical group member.

With both designs, it is possible for the typical response to an experimental condition not to be typical. This is particularly likely to occur when the mean is used. With a single subject design, a subject's mean response to an experimental condition may represent behavior that did not occur even once. This has been demonstrated, for example, with the mean response of individual aphasics to aphasia test items (Silverman, 1974).

The typical response to an experimental condition also may not be typical when a group design is used. The mean response of the typical group member may not correspond to that of any group member. The mean number of stutterings produced by twenty-five stutterers during their reading of a 100-word passage, for example, might be 10.5. Since no stutterer could stutter a fraction of a stuttering, this stuttering frequency would not correspond to that produced by any of the twenty-five stutterers. The lack of "representativeness" of mean data would be of considerable importance for answering some questions since it would lead to incorrect answers.

A second difference between single subject and group designs is the necessity of assuming that subjects respond similarly to an experimental condition—that is, the necessity of assuming that observed differences in the responses of subjects to an experimental

TABLE 6-1   Differences between Single Subject and Group Designs

Single Subject Designs	Group Designs
Provide data concerning the "typical" behavior of individual subjects under an experimental condition	Provide data concerning the behavior of the "typical" member of a group under an experimental condition
Not necessary to assume that subjects respond similarly to an experimental condition	Necessary to assume that the subjects in a group respond similarly to an experimental condition
Necessary for subjects to be run more than once under each experimental condition	Not necessary for subjects to be run more than once under each experimental condition
Generalize to "typical" behavior of individual studied under experimental condition	Generalize to "typical" behavior of mean or median group member under experimental condition
May not be relatively easy to control for order and sequence effects	Usually relatively easy to control for order and sequence effects
Statistical procedures for assessing the reliability of research findings are not as well developed as for "typical" subject designs	Statistical procedures for assessing the reliability of research findings are well developed
Minimum number of subjects necessary is 1	Minimum number of subjects necessary is usually more than 10
Generalize to population from which subjects are selected on logical basis	Generalize to population from which subjects are selected on statistical basis

condition result from the effects of extraneous variables or from "chance" (random) fluctuation rather than from real differences in their responses to that condition. While single subject designs do not require such an assumption, group designs implicitly or explicitly do. Without such an assumption, it would not be particularly meaningful to talk about the typical response of a group to an experimental condition. This would be particularly true when an experimental condition had opposite effects on different persons. An example of such a condition would be consecutive readings of a passage. This condition has been shown to result in some stutterers becoming progressively more disfluent (adaptation effect) and others becoming progressively more fluent (Bloom & Silverman, 1973). The only circumstance under which it would probably be meaningful to talk about a typical response to an experimental condition when people differ in their responses to that condition is when the differences are of degree rather than kind—that is, when an experimental condition changes the behavior of all subjects in the same direction but to different degrees. A particular obturator may reduce the hypernasality of all persons with cleft palates who are fitted with it, but not to the same degree. It would be meaningful, therefore, to talk about the effect of this obturator on the speech of the typical person who was fitted with it.

A third difference between single subject and group designs is the minimum number of times it is necessary to run a subject under each experimental condition. With a group design, reliable results are frequently obtainable when a subject is run only once under each such condition. With a single subject design, on the other hand, reliable results would rarely be obtainable if a subject were run only once under each condition. The reason for this difference is that with a group design, factors that reduce reliability (e.g., measurement error, effects of extraneous variables, and random fluctuation) can usually be kept from biasing the results by using as a measure of performance (criterion measure) the average of the measures from a number of subjects under each condition. Such factors are unlikely to bias the performance of the majority of subjects in a group under an experimental condition in the same manner.

With a single subject design, the previously mentioned factors that can reduce reliability can be prevented from biasing the results by using as a measure of individual performance (i.e., as a *criterion measure*) under each condition the average of the measures made under each condition. These factors usually will not repeatedly affect measures of a subject's performance under a given experimental condition in exactly the same manner. Consequently, answers to questions will tend to be more reliable with a single subject design if they are based on a subject's average performance under a condition rather than on any single performance under it.

A fourth difference between single subject and group designs is what the answers to questions can be used to predict. For research findings to be useful, they usually must be applicable outside of the experimental situation in which they were generated. With a single subject design, the behavior of a subject under an experimental condition can be used to predict his most probable behavior under that condition.

With a group design, the behavior of the mean or median group member under an experimental condition can be used to predict the most probable behavior of the mean or median member of such a group under such a condition. It can also be used to predict the response to an experimental condition of the mean or median member of a population from which a group (sample) of subjects was selected, if it was randomly selected from that population. A *population* consists of all individuals who are classified in a particular manner. Thus, the population referred to by the question, "Are adults who have anomia helped by a particular therapy?" consists of all adults who have anomia. If a group of subjects were not randomly selected from a population, this type of generalization would be questionable. (The rationale and methodology for random sampling are described in Chapter 10.)

A fifth difference between single subject and group designs is related to the control of order and sequence events. An *order effect* is one that systematically improves or impairs a subject's performance on a series of tasks. An example of an order effect that could impair performance would be fatigue. If an aphasic were to perform a series of ten tasks one after the other, his or her performance might systematically worsen as a function of fatigue. This could occur regardless of the ordering of the tasks. An example of an order effect that could enhance a subject's performance on a series of tasks would be learning. Clients may score higher on a test following a period of therapy than they did on it prior to therapy not because they improved, but because of what they learned during their first exposure to the test.

A *sequence effect* occurs when a subject's performance on a task is enhanced or impaired by his or her doing another task before it. An investigator who sought to determine the effect of a drug on stuttering would have to obtain samples of stutterers' speech both while they were and while they were not under the influence of the drug. If both speech samples were elicited during the same day, it might make a difference whether the "drug" or "no-drug" speech sample was elicited first. If the "drug" speech sample was made first and if the effects of the drug had not worn off completely before the "no-drug" sample was made, this could result in a different stuttering frequency during the "no-drug" condition than probably would have occurred if it had come first. For a sequence effect, then, the ordering of tasks, or experimental conditions, is critical. One ordering may result in sequence effect contamination, while a second ordering may not.

Both order and sequence effects are easier to eliminate in a group design than in a single subject design. In a group design, they can be controlled by administering only one experimental condition to each subject. An investigator who wished to determine the effect of a drug on stuttering could take a group of stutterers and randomly assign them to one or two conditions—that is, speaking without being under the influence of the drug and speaking while under the influence of the drug. Since each subject would only speak under one condition, there would be no possibility of order or sequence effect contamination.

Order and sequence effect contamination is always a possibility with a single subject design, since subjects are run under more than one condition and often more than once under each condition. These effects can sometimes be prevented by having fairly long intervals between treatments. An investigator who wished to determine the effect of a drug on stuttering with a single subject design could separate drug and no-drug speech samples by 24 hours. This would prevent a sequence effect if the effects of the drug wore off in less than 24 hours. Some order effects, such as fatigue, could probably be eliminated with this same strategy.

A sixth way that single subject and group designs differ is related to statistical procedures for assessing the reliability of research findings. These are less well developed for single subject than for group designs.

A seventh way that single subject and group designs differ is in the minimum number of subjects necessary. With a single subject design, research can be done with a single subject (N of 1). Therapy outcome research, for example, can be done with an N of 1 (though a larger N usually would be desirable). "Pure" research also is sometimes possible with an N as small as 1. In some of the research on teaching "language" to chimpanzees, only a single chimpanzee was used. Though research with this type of design can be done with only one subject, many studies that utilize it have more than one (McReynolds & Kearns, 1983; Tawney & Gast, 1984).

The minimum number of subjects necessary when a group design is used almost always exceeds that necessary for a single subject design. Studies that use a group design usually require an N of greater than 10. The minimum N necessary for a particular study is a function of several factors, including how reliable answers to questions have to be. The more reliable they have to be, the larger the N required. An investigator who wished to determine whether a particular therapy resulted in a particular behavioral change would need a larger N if he or she wished to be 99 percent certain of the accuracy of the conclusion than if it were adequate to be 95 percent certain. (Factors that should be considered when estimating the N necessary for a particular study are discussed in Chapter 10.)

The eighth, and final, difference between single subject and group designs to be considered here is the basis on which generalizations are made to the population from which subjects are selected. A group design usually does so on a statistical basis, and a single subject design usually does so on a "logical" basis. In a group design, if the sample of subjects selected approximates a random sample from the population to which one wishes to generalize, then one could generalize to the population through the use of *inferential statistical procedures*. (These are discussed in Chapter 10.) These procedures permit us to infer characteristics of a population from characteristics of a sample (or samples) from that population. If the population of interest were speech-language pathologists who hold the Certificate of Clinical Competence in Speech-Language Pathology from the American Speech-Language-Hearing Association, and the sample consisted of a group of speech-language pathologists randomly selected from the population (from the American Speech-Language-Hearing Association Membership Directory), the attitudes of speech-language pathologists in the population could probably be inferred reliably from those in the sample through the use of inferential statistics, provided that the sample was large enough (Hsu, 1989).

In a single subject design, generalizations to the population from which subjects are selected usually are made on a "logical" rather than statistical basis. While a single subject from a population cannot be assumed to respond to an experimental condition similarly to the majority of persons in the population, it is unlikely that the person is the only one in the population who would respond to the condition in this way he or she did. Consequently, the behavior of this subject is representative of that of a segment of the population. The size of this segment, however, cannot be specified from the performance of only one subject. After data on the performance of other persons in the population under the experimental condition are gathered, some inferences can be made about the size of this segment. If the majority of subjects perform in essentially the same way under the experimental condition, it is likely that this segment is relatively large. That is, it is unlikely if this segment were relatively small that a high percentage of the subjects tested would perform in the way that they did.

Advantages and Disadvantages of Each Design

Advantages and disadvantages of single subject and group designs are summarized in this section. Much of this discussion is based upon material in Table 6-1.

Single Subject Design

Advantages

The single subject design has several advantages. First, this design makes it possible to detect individual differences. It does not require an investigator implicitly or explicitly to assume that all persons in a population respond similarly to particular experimental conditions. In fact, it offers a means of testing this assumption. If subjects respond differently to an experimental condition and their responses are adequately reliable, this is evidence that the assumption that all persons in a population respond similarly to an experimental condition is not viable. This characteristic of single subject designs is of particular importance in therapy outcome research since most clinicians are usually not willing to assume a priori that particular therapies affect all clients with similar communicative disorders in the same manner.

A second advantage of the single subject design is that it permits generalization to real persons in a population rather than an abstraction—that is, the "typical" member of a population—who might not exist. A speech-language pathologist may never encounter an aphasic who responds to a particular stimulus as does the "typical" aphasic. This is because of the problem with mean data discussed previously.

A third advantage of the single subject design is that it does not require a large *N*. The *N* needed, in fact, may be as few as 1.

Disadvantages

Several characteristics of the single subject design may be disadvantageous under certain circumstances. The first, and perhaps most important, is that the design may be difficult to control for order and sequence effects. The possibility of such effects should be considered when you are planning a study that could be done with either a single subject or group design. If they seem possible and it seems unlikely they can be controlled with a single subject design (e.g., by spacing experimental conditions), you should probably use a group one.

A second possible disadvantage is that statistical procedures may not be available for assessing the reliability of answers. These are available for a wider variety of group designs than single subject ones. Before deciding to use a single subject design, you would probably be wise to determine whether an appropriate statistical procedure is available for assessing the reliability of answers, *assuming that you feel it necessary to do so statistically*. In some types of research (e.g., operant conditioning research), this is rarely done (McReynolds & Kearns, 1983; Tawney & Gast, 1984).

A third possible disadvantage is that generalizing to a population may not be "neat" if appropriate statistical procedures are unavailable.

Group Design

Advantages

The two main advantages of group designs are that statistical procedures usually are available for assessing the reliability of answers and for generalizing to the population from which subjects are selected. Also, such designs usually make it possible to control for order and sequence effects and, through randomization, for the effects of extraneous variables. Furthermore, it is often possible to infer from these data characteristics of the "typical" member of a population or characteristics of the majority of members of a population (statistical procedures for doing both are described in Chapter 10).

Disadvantages

A group design *may* be disadvantageous for several reasons. First, it *usually* requires an investigator implicitly or explicitly to assume that all members of a population respond similarly to an experimental condition. Observed differences in response are regarded as a function of extraneous variables, random fluctuation, measurement error, and so on, rather than differences in response to the condition. Without this assumption, it would not make sense to average together the responses of individual subjects. The qualifier *usually* was used here because a few group designs—such as multivariate analysis of variance—do not require this assumption for certain variables (see Chapter 10).

A second possible disadvantage of a group design is that it may require more subjects from a particular population to answer a particular question than are available. A speech-language pathologist who wished to determine the impact of a particular therapy on elementary-school stutterers and had only six such children in his or her caseload would probably have too small an N to use a group design. This *N* would probably be adequate, however, for a single subject design.

A third possible disadvantage of group designs is that the characteristics of a "typical" subject may not be typical. Mean measures of the characteristics of the subjects in a sample may not be similar to those of most, if not all, subjects in that sample. Suppose we wished to evaluate the effects of an articulation therapy on the speech of ten children who had multiple articulation errors. As a criterion measure, we might use the number of errors each child made on an articulation test before and after receiving therapy. Suppose the numbers of articulation errors produced by these children before and after therapy were as shown in Table 6-2. It would be reasonable to conclude from these means that the typical child in this group had fewer articulation errors following therapy than before therapy. Actually, the therapy only appeared to influence the articulation of two of the ten children and the magnitude of the effect for these children was considerably more than one error. Thus, the mean performance of the children in this group is not representative of the "typical" performance of these children.

A fourth possible disadvantage of the group design pertains to generalizing to the population from which subjects are selected on statistical grounds. If a sample of subjects who were observed did not at least closely approximate a random sample from the population of interest, the accuracy of generalizations to this population through the use of statistical inference would be uncertain and possibly misleading. If, for example, the children in a kindergarten classroom did not approximate a random sample of kindergarten children in general, attempts to generalize the results of a speech improvement program conducted in this classroom to the population of kindergarten children through the use of statistical inference could lead to erroneous conclusions. The children in a particular classroom may not approximate a random sample because the suburbs or the inner city are underrepresented. A speech improvement program that is effective in the suburbs may not be in the inner city, and vice versa.

TABLE 6-2   Numbers of Articulation Errors Produced by Ten Children before and after Therapy

Subject Number	Number of Errors before Therapy	Number of Errors after Therapy
1	3	3
2	11	4
3	4	4
4	1	1
5	3	3
6	9	6
7	2	2
8	2	2
9	4	4
10	1	1
Mean	4	3

Categories of Single Subject Designs

Thus far two basic types of designs have been described, differences between them pointed out, and advantages and disadvantages of each summarized. Some of the variations possible within the single subject design are described in this section and some of those possible within the group design in the next.

The ABC notation is used here for describing single subject designs. This notation has been utilized for a number of years by behaviorally oriented psychologists, speech-language pathologists, and others for describing them (McReynolds & Kearns, 1983; Tawney & Gast, 1984). The symbols from it that are used in this section are defined below:

A   A baseline condition in which the independent variable is not present—that is, one in which there is no treatment or intervention.

B   The first treatment or intervention condition.

C   The second treatment or intervention condition that is different from the first.

A-B A dash is used for separating adjacent conditions.

A_1 The subscript indicates whether this was the first, second, third, and so on time that the baseline was measured.

B_1 The subscript indicates whether this was the first, second, third, and so on time that the treatment was introduced.

Other notations that have been used for this purpose include those of Campbell and Stanley (1966) and of Glass, Wilson, and Gottman (1975).

The A-Only Design

The A-only design is one in which attributes of behaviors of individual subjects are observed and described as they occur naturally. No attempt is made to manipulate them. Consequently, the resulting study is an investigation rather than an experiment. Observations used may have been made by the investigator or communicated to him or her by an informant (or informants). What was observed may be described using words (qualitatively), numbers (quantitatively), or a combination of the two. Those studies in which observations are described mostly using words sometimes are referred to as case studies (Bromley, 1986). The investigator in studies utilizing the A-only design is sometimes referred to as a participant-observer (McCall & Simmons, 1969)—he or she attempts to observe and describe behavior without influencing it (Tawney & Gast, 1984). This type of design has been used for what are referred to as longitudinal diary studies of language acquisition (McReynolds & Kearns, 1983). These are studies in which attributes of a child's language behavior in his or her natural environment are described at periodic intervals. It also has been used for studies of preschoolers' normal speech disfluency (e.g., Silverman, 1972).

The A-only design also has been used for *post hoc* analyses. It was used, for example, to determine whether there is any reason to believe that the incidence and prevalence of stuttering changed during this century (Van Riper, 1982). This was done by comparing incidence and prevalence figures reported in the literature for various years during this century.

The A-only design is not strictly speaking an experimental one, because the identification of functional relationships between dependent and independent variables is not possible. Nothing is manipulated or varied. Ongoing behavior is merely described. Consequently, it is not possible with this design to reach conclusions about how particular dependent variables are influenced by particular independent ones. For example, it would not be possible using it to identify factors (independent variables) that cause preschoolers to repeat syllables (dependent variable) more frequently in one situation than in another.

The B-Only Design

With the B-only design, as with the A-only one, attributes of behaviors of individual subjects are observed and described under a single condition. While with the A-only design this condition is one in which they occur naturally, with the B-only design it occurs during or soon after an intervention (treatment, introduction of an independent variable)—not before (which would be an A-only design). Observations of a target behavior with this design, as with the A-only one, can be made more than once. An audiologist probably would depend on this type of design to gather data needed for preparing periodic progress reports about how a client is adapting to the use of a hearing aid. And a speech-language pathologist probably would do so for assessing how a severely communicatively impaired client is adapting to the use of an augmentative communication device. With this type of design, a client's status prior to intervention *would not* be compared systematically to that during or immediately following it. However, it would be with the design that is considered next—the A-B one.

The B-only design can be used for assessing therapy outcome, but it has several limitations when utilized for this purpose. While it can be used to describe attributes of a client's communication behavior at certain points during or at termination of therapy, it cannot be used to determine how he or she has changed as a result of therapy. To do so it would be necessary to compare these to what they were before therapy began. A second limitation is that the effects of therapy cannot be differentiated from those due to other factors that occurred while it was taking place, such as maturation. The need for a design that allows the effects of a therapy to be differentiated from those of maturation is particularly important when assessing the impacts of language intervention strategies on young children (McReynolds & Kearns, 1983).

The A-B Design

The A-B design, sometimes referred to as the "simple time series design" (Birnbrauer, Peterson, & Solnick, 1974), combines elements of the A-only and B-only designs. With it, attributes of behaviors are observed and described both when they occur naturally and during (or immediately following) some intervention. Behavior observed under the intervention (B) condition is compared to that observed under the baseline (A) one to determine if it had an effect. The design requires that the dependent variable (the target behavior) be measured and/or described using words repeatedly under both conditions. After doing so several times under the baseline (A) condition, the intervention (B) one is introduced. It is necessary to observe the target behavior more than once under the baseline condition to ensure that measurements and/or word descriptions of it will be reliable. The target behavior is repeatedly observed during the intervention condition to monitor changes in it that occur *over time* (which is why the design is referred to as a "time series" one). Hence, behavior occurring at a point during the intervention condition can be compared to that occurring at one prior to or following it as well as to that occurring during the baseline condition. In most studies using this design, changes in the target behavior (dependent variable) are described quantitatively.

This design can be used instead of the B-only one for assessing therapy (intervention) outcome. In fact, it is the one (which has been referred to as the "before and after" design) that speech-language pathologists and audiologists appear to use most often for this purpose clinically (McReynolds & Kearns, 1983). The target behavior would be observed and described prior to therapy as well as during it and when it is terminated. To determine whether the client has improved and, if so, how much, the status of the target behavior would be compared to what it was before therapy. While this design is superior to the B-only one for assessing therapy outcome because it provides baseline (pretherapy) data, it has a limitation when used for this purpose. If the target behavior changes during intervention, it is not possible to tell whether the change was due to intervention or to something else that occurred during this period. This limitation is of particular concern when it appears likely that a target behavior will be affected by something other than intervention such as *maturation* when assessing the effects of a language intervention program on young children or *spontaneous recovery* when assessing the effects of one on adult aphasics.

The A-B design sometimes is referred to as a "quasi-experimental" one (Campbell & Stanley, 1966; Kratochwill, 1978). Because there is no return to the baseline condition (as there would be in a "true" experimental design) following intervention, it cannot be determined empirically whether the change observed in the target behavior in the B-condition resulted from intervention (i.e., the independent variable that was used) or something else. The A-B design can be transformed into a true experimental one by adding a baseline condition, thereby creating the design discussed next—the A-B-A one.

The A-B-A Design

The A-B-A design is the simplest single subject one for demonstrating cause-effect relationships empirically. It is similar to the A-B design in that the target behavior is observed and described periodically under both baseline (A_1) and intervention (B) conditions. However, it differs in that following intervention the baseline condition is reintroduced (A_2) and the target behavior is again periodically observed and described. Descriptions of the target behavior when this design is used are almost always quantitative, that is, involving measurement.

This design has been classified as a *withdrawal* one (Sidman, 1960). The reason is that it allows you to determine empirically if a target behavior is different in the intervention than it was in the baseline condition and whether the difference was due to the intervention. This is done by withdrawing the intervention—thereby creating the baseline condition a second time—and again observing and describing (measuring) the target behavior. If it returns to approximately what it was during the initial baseline condition, this would be evidence that the change in the target behavior resulted from the intervention. This design is most appropriate for assessing the impacts of interventions that would be expected to affect the target behavior only while they are present. Hence, it would not be appropriate for assessing therapies having impacts that would be expected to persist for a long period of time (hopefully, permanently) following intervention. One type that it usually would be appropriate for assessing is drug therapy (e.g., on stuttering). If A_2 is delayed until the effect of the drug has worn off, it can be inferred whether changes observed in the target behavior (e.g., reduced stuttering) resulted from it.

While this design provides stronger evidence than the A-B one that changes in a target behavior resulted from intervention, the design we will consider next—the A-B-A-B one—can provide even stronger evidence that this is the case.

The A-B-A-B Design

The A-B-A-B design has been one of the most frequently used single-subject ones in behavior modification research (Kratochwill, 1978). There is repeated introduction and withdrawal of an intervention strategy. This design provides stronger evidence that changes in a target behavior result from intervention than does the A-B-A one because it provides for a direct replication (Sidman, 1960) of the effects of the intervention on the target behavior—that is, the last two conditions (A_2-B_2) replicate the first two (A_1-B_1). Based on these characteristics it has been referred to as the "reversal design" (Baer, Wolf, & Risley, 1968), "withdrawal design" (Leitenberg, 1973), and "equivalent time series design" (Campbell & Stanley, 1966).

While this design is an excellent one for "laboratory demonstrations" of the effects of independent variables (interventions) on dependent ones (target behaviors), there can be ethical concerns about its use clinically for assessing therapy outcome (Tawney & Gast, 1984). The reason is that it requires therapy to be terminated for a period of time after the client has improved so that the target behavior will return to what it was during baseline (A_1)—that is, so that the client will relapse. In fact, the design requires the client to relapse almost completely—that is, to have the status of the target behavior in A_2 be approximately what it was in A_1.

The A-B-A-B design, of course, is appropriate only if it is reasonable to assume that the effects of the intervention on the target behavior can be reversed. If intervention resulted in the target behavior being learned *very well*, this probably would not be a reasonable assumption. For example, if as a result of intervention a client learned to produce /r/ correctly in words and had been doing so for a while, it is unlikely that he or she would relapse to baseline (A_1) if therapy was terminated.

The B-A-B Design

The B-A-B design is a variation of the A-B-A-B one that can be used when it is not possible to measure the target behavior (i.e., collect baseline data) prior to intervention. It could be used by a speech-language pathologist or audiologist for determining the amount a client is benefiting from an intervention strategy, particularly one that he or she was using when first seen. An audiologist, for example, could use it for determining the amount a client is being helped by the hearing aid he or she is currently using; the client's hearing would first be tested with the aid, then without it, and then with it again. While this design does not provide as strong a demonstration of intervention effectiveness as does the A-B-A-B one, it tends to provide a stronger one than the A-B-A design because it provides two opportunities to demonstrate it.

Multitreatment Designs

The designs discussed thus far are used for assessing the impact of a single intervention strategy (independent variable) on the target behavior (dependent variable). Multitreatment ones are used when it is desired to assess the impact of two or more intervention strategies on it, singly or in combination. They can be particularly useful for determining which of two intervention strategies has the greater impact on it or whether the combination has a greater one than either by itself. An example of a multitreatment design that can be used for determining which of two treatments has the greater impact on a target behavior is the A-B-A-B-C-B-C one. This is an A-B-A-B design to which a second intervention (C) has been added. And an example of a multitreatment design that can be used for determining whether the combination of two treatments has a greater impact than either by itself is the A-B-A-B-BC-B-BC one. This, like the A-B-A-B-C-B-C design, can be viewed as an extension of the A-B-A-B one.

If there are no order or sequence effects, each of the designs mentioned in the preceding paragraph can be used for answering two questions. Those that the A-B-A-B-C-B-C design can be used for answering are the following:

- Does intervention strategy *B* affect the target behavior?
- Do intervention strategies *B and C* differ with regard to the amount they affect the target behavior?

And these are the ones that can be answered using the A-B-A-B-BC-B-BC design:

- Does intervention strategy *B* affect the target behavior?
- Does the combination of intervention strategies *B and C* affect the target behavior more than *B* by itself?

Abbreviated versions of the multitreatment design have been used in behavioral research. The A-B-A-B-BC-B-BC design, for example, has been abbreviated to A-B-BC-B-BC (Tawney & Gast, 1984).

Multiple Baseline Designs

The designs discussed thus far are single baseline ones because the status of only one target behavior is observed and described. With multiple baseline designs (Baer, Wolf, & Risley, 1968) this is done for two or more target behaviors. One of the most significant advantages of multiple baseline designs is that they can demonstrate the impacts of intervention strategies on target behaviors without it being necessary to withdraw intervention as it is with the A-B-A-B design (Kratochwill, 1978). That is, with these designs it is not necessary to cause a person to "relapse." It should not be surprising, therefore, that these designs have been used clinically for assessing the impacts of intervention strategies.

There are several types of multiple baseline designs. One that can be useful for evaluating intervention strategies has been referred to as the multiple baseline design across behaviors (Tawney & Gast, 1984). With this type of design two or more target behaviors that appear to be functionally independent and should respond to the same intervention strategy are observed and described (measured). The intervention strategy is applied to one but not to the other. If the only target behavior that changes is the one to which it is applied, this is evidence that the strategy is effective. The evidence, of course, would be stronger if this result was replicated on a number of subjects.

An example of the use of this type of multiple baseline design to demonstrate the effectiveness of an intervention strategy is in the study reported by Elbert, Shelton, and Arndt (1967). Two target behaviors were observed and measured periodically: correct production of /r/ and correct production of /s/. The target behavior that the intervention strategy was expected to modify was the articulation error being treated. Thus, when it was produced correctly a higher percentage of the time following intervention and the other was not, this was interpreted as evidence for the effectiveness of the strategy.

The variations of the single subject design discussed in this section should be regarded as representative rather than exhaustive. There are a number of books and papers that describe other variations and further discuss the ones presented here in the reference list (Barlow & Hayes, 1979; Barlow & Hersen, 1973, 1984; Birnbrauer, Peterson, & Solnick, 1974; Campbell, 1963; Campbell & Stanley, 1966; Connell & Thompson, 1986; Cook & Campbell, 1979; Cuvo, 1979; Davidson & Costello, 1969; Dukes, 1965; Edgar & Billingsley, 1974; Gottman, 1973; Holtzman, 1963; Horner & Baer, 1978; Jerger, 1964b; Kazdin, 1981, 1982a, 1982b; Kearns, 1986; Kendall, 1981; Kratochwill, 1978; Kratochwill & Brody, 1978; Kratochwill & Levin, 1980; McCullough, 1984; McReynolds & Kearns, 1983; McReynolds & Thompson, 1986; Merriam, 1988; Pring, 1986; Rickels, Schweizer, & Case, 1988; Rusch & Kazdin, 1981; Sidman, 1960; Stanley, 1985; Strain & Shores, 1979; Tawney & Gast, 1984; Watson & Workman, 1981; Wolery & Harris, 1982; and Yin, 1984).

Categories of Group Designs

Hundreds of designs have been devised that can be classified as group designs. Many of the ones that are usable for research on communicative disorders are described in books by Ferguson (1989), Hays (1973), Lindquist (1953), Siegel (1988), and Winer (1991).

Two general categories of group designs can be identified: (1) those intended to determine whether a *difference* exists, and (2) those intended to determine whether a *relationship* exists. The designs in these categories permit different kinds of questions to be answered. Those in the first category permit the answering of such questions as:

1. Is vocal rest effective in reducing the size of vocal nodules?
2. Does hearing aid *A* tend to result in better speech discrimination ability for persons with conductive hearing losses than hearing aid *B?*

Designs in the second category, on the other hand, permit the answering of such questions as:

3. Is auditory discrimination ability positively related to articulation proficiency?
4. Are scores of audiometric test *A* negatively related to scores on audiometric test *B?*

The first of these questions can be answered by determining whether there is a *differ-ence* in the average (mean or median) size of the vocal nodules of a group of persons fol-lowing vocal rest. The second can be answered by determining whether there is a *difference* in the average (mean or median) speech discrimination scores of a group of persons who have conductive hearing losses when hearing aid *A* and hearing aid *B* are used. The third can be answered by determining whether there is a *positive relationship* between scores on auditory discrimination tests and scores on tests of articulation proficiency—that is, it would be necessary to determine whether persons who earn high scores on one tend to earn high scores on the other. Finally, the fourth question can be answered by determining whether persons who earn *high* scores on audiometric test *A* tend to earn *low* scores on audiometric test *B*, and vice versa.

Designs for Detecting Differences

To answer some questions, it is necessary to determine whether one or more differences exist. These differences can be of several kinds. They can, for example, be differences between percentages (or proportions), as in these questions:

1. Are stutterers more likely to have articulation errors than nonstutterers?
2. Do more children who have hearing losses fail audiometric screening test *A* than audio-metric screening test *B*?

The first question can be answered by determining whether a higher percentage (or proportion) of stutterers than nonstutterers have articulation errors; the second, by deter-mining whether the same percentage (or proportion) of children who have hearing losses fail audiometric test *A* as audiometric test *B*.

Other kinds of differences that can be detected by a group design are those between means, or medians, as in these questions.

1. Do kindergarten children tend to have fewer articulation errors after participating in a particular speech improvement program than before?
2. Does the level of academic achievement of elementary-school stutterers tend to differ from that of their nonstuttering peers?

The first question can be answered by comparing the mean (or median) number of articulation errors of a group of kindergarten children after participating in the program to that before participating in the program; the second, by comparing the mean (or median) academic achievement scores of a group of elementary-school stutterers with that of a matched group of nonstutterers. Note that the first requires a comparison between two mea-sures made on the *same* subjects and the second requires a comparison between single mea-sures made on *different* subjects.

The questions that illustrated group designs for detecting differences involved com-parisons between two measures. Such designs also can be used to compare more than two measures. Suppose we wanted to determine whether there were any differences in the percentages of children in kindergarten through sixth grade who had chronic hoarseness. A group design could be used for comparing these seven percentages. Similarly, such a design could be used to compare mean auditory discrimination scores earned by a group of persons who have conductive hearing losses while using five different hearing aid models.

Group designs for detecting differences differ in several dimensions, including: (1) the type of measure for which they are appropriate, (2) the number of measures that can be compared, and (3) their appropriateness for related measures, independent measures, or a combination of the two. The type of measure for which a design is appropriate refers to the nature of the criterion measure—whether it is a percentage, a proportion, a frequency count, a mean, a median, a mode, or some other derived measure. A design that is appropriate for detecting differences between percentages may not be appropriate for detecting differences between means.

A third dimension in which these designs differ is their appropriateness for related measures, independent measures, and combinations of the two. Related measures are measures made on the same subjects or on extremely well matched groups of subjects (e.g., two groups in which there is one member of a number of pairs of identical twins in each). Independent measures are measures made on unmatched groups of subjects. "Before and after" therapy measures would be examples of related measures, since they are made on the same persons. Measures made on unmatched groups such as stutterers and nonstutterers would be examples of independent measures.

Some designs only are appropriate for related measures or independent measures, and others are appropriate for combinations of the two. A design appropriate for related measures would be necessary to answer this question: "Do dysarthrics who have been fitted with a palatal lift prosthesis tend to be more intelligible with the device than without?" Such a design would be needed because two measures on the same subjects would have to be compared—one with the prosthesis and one without it.

Answering other questions requires a design appropriate for independent measures. Consider the question, "Do dysarthrics who have been fitted with palatal lift prostheses tend to be more intelligible than those who have had pharyngeal flap surgery?" A design appropriate for comparing independent measures would be needed here because two groups are being compared, one consisting of dysarthrics who have been treated surgically and the other consisting of dysarthrics who have been fitted with a prosthesis.

To answer some questions, a design appropriate for both related and independent measures is necessary. For example, consider the question, "Do palatal lift prostheses tend to increase the intelligibility of the speech of dysarthrics who have inadequate velopharyngeal closure more than do pharyngeal flaps?" One design appropriate for answering this question, known as the Type I analysis of variance design (Lindquist, 1953), can be diagrammed as shown in Figure 6-1. If this design were used, measures of the intelligibility of the speech of two groups of dysarthrics would be made before and after physical management. Between-group comparisons would involve independent measures, and "before and after" treatment comparisons would involve related measures. Note that this design has an advantage over the one described in the preceding paragraph because it is possible to determine whether the groups differed in degree of intelligibility prior to intervention.

Dependent Measures

	Before Management	After Management
Palatal Lift Group		
Pharyngeal Flap Group		

(Independent Measures)

FIGURE 6-1   **Analysis of variance design for assessing the effects of palatal lift prostheses.**

Designs for Detecting Relationships

Answering some questions requires a design for detecting relationships rather than differences. There are several kinds of questions about relationships that such designs can help to answer if relationships are found to exist, including those related to: (1) the *direction* of the relationships (positive or negative), (2) the *strength* of the relationships, and (3) the *nature* of the relationships (linear or nonlinear). Suppose you wished to describe the relationship between children's speech disfluency levels in two situations—that is, you wished to determine whether those who tended to be the most disfluent in one situation also tended to be the most disfluent in the other, and vice versa. You might sample the speech of ten children in the two situations and determine the frequency of speech disfluency per 100 words spoken by each child in each situation. Suppose the disfluency frequencies you obtained were as shown in Table 6-3. To permit the relationship between the disfluency frequencies in the two situations to be visualized, they were plotted on a two-dimensional graphical display known

TABLE 6-3   Frequencies of Speech Disfluency Exhibited by Ten Children in Two Situations

Child	Situation I	Situation II
1	6.3	10.1
2	5.6	9.4
3	4.5	10.1
4	9.0	22.5
5	4.5	8.7
6	3.9	6.1
7	6.8	17.5
8	5.5	10.4
9	12.5	35.4
10	3.4	5.6

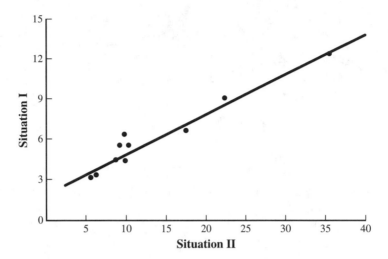

FIGURE 6-2   Scattergram depicting a relatively strong positive relationship between two variables.

as a *scattergram* (see Figure 6-2). The configuration of this scattergram provides data for answering the following four questions (assuming the answer to the first is yes):

1. Does a relationship exist between these children's disfluency frequencies in the two situations?
2. What is the *direction* of the relationship between the disfluency frequencies in the two situations?
3. Does the relationship appear to be *linear* or *nonlinear?* If nonlinear, what does the *nature* of the relationship appear to be?
4. How *strong* does the relationship between the disfluency frequencies in the two situations appear to be?

What would be the answer to each question based on the configuration of the scattergram in Figure 6-2? The answer to the first question would be yes, since the points are not randomly distributed on the scattergram but are confined to a relatively small segment of it. The configuration of Figure 6-3, incidentally, illustrates what a scattergram might look like if little or no relationship existed between the variables. The points are not confined to a segment of the graph, they are scattered throughout the graph. A child who had a relatively high disfluency frequency in one situation would be about as likely to have a relatively high as a relatively low frequency in the other.

From the configuration of the points in Figure 6-2, it would appear that the *direction* of the relationship between the children's disfluency frequencies in the two situations is "positive." The ordering of the children with regard to disfluency frequencies is quite similar in the two situations. Children who had relatively high disfluency frequencies in one tended to have relatively high disfluency frequencies in the other, and vice versa. If the direction of the relationship had been "negative," the configuration of the points might have been similar to that in Figure 6-4.

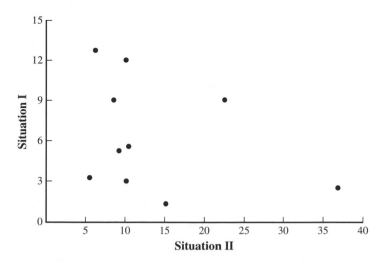

FIGURE 6-3 **Scattergram depicting little or no relationship between two variables.**

To answer the third question, it would seem reasonable to assume from the configuration of the points in Figure 6-2 that the relationship between the disfluency frequencies in the two situations for these children is *linear*. The line that could be drawn on the scattergram from which the points would deviate least and which could be the least complex would be a straight line. When two variables are linearly related, an increase (or decrease) in the magnitude of one is associated with a *proportional* increase (or decrease) in the magnitude of the other. This proportional increase (or decrease) will occur throughout the range of possible values. If two variables are *not linearly related*, on the other hand, an increase

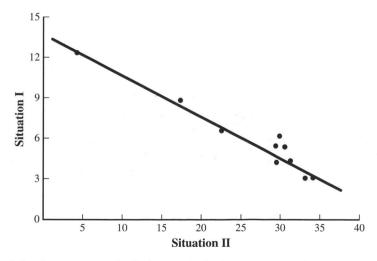

FIGURE 6-4 **Scattergram depicting a relatively strong negative relationship between two variables.**

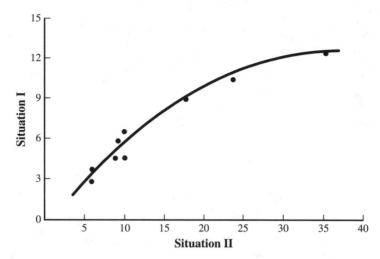

FIGURE 6-5   Scattergram depicting a relatively strong curvilinear relationship between two variables.

(or decrease) in the magnitude of one will not be associated with a proportional increase (or decrease) in the magnitude of the other throughout the range of possible values. Two common nonlinear relationships between variables are depicted in Figures 6-5 and 6-6. The relationship depicted in Figure 6-5, which is *curvilinear*, is the least complex of the possible nonlinear relationships between variables. That depicted in Figure 6-6, which is *cubic*, is one step up in complexity from curvilinear.

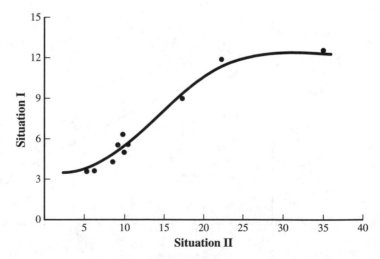

FIGURE 6-6   Scattergram depicting a relatively strong cubic relationship between two variables.

To answer the fourth question, it would appear from the configuration of points in Figure 6-2 that the relationship between the relative disfluency frequencies in the two situations for these children is *fairly strong*. The points are not scattered very much; they deviate little from the straight line that best describes the relationship between them. The greater the deviation of the points in a scattergram from the line that best describes the nature of the relationship between two variables, the weaker the relationship between them. The scattergrams in Figure 6-7 illustrate two degrees of linear relationship. The relationship depicted in the scattergram on the top is stronger than that depicted in the scattergram on the bottom.

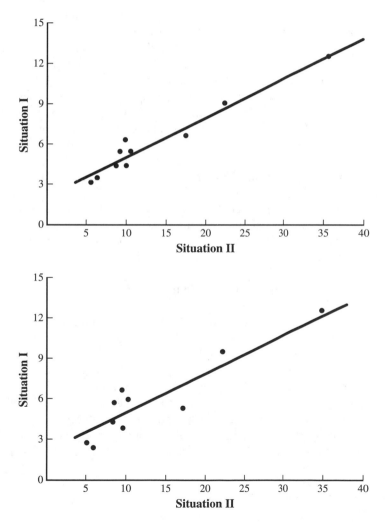

FIGURE 6-7 **Scattergrams depicting two degrees of linear relationship. The relationship depicted in the scattergram on the top is stronger than that depicted in the one on the bottom.**

The discussion thus far has been limited to detecting and describing relationships between two variables. There are group designs for detecting and describing more complex relationships—that is, those involving more than two variables. Such designs could be used for answering such questions as:

1. How well do clinicians agree on how severe stutterers are?
2. What factors influence how severe a stutterer is perceived as being?
3. What factors best differentiate the speech of a child beginning to stutter from that of his peers?

The first question could be answered by determining the extent to which a sample of clinicians would order a group of stutterers in the same manner in the severity of their stuttering. The second could be answered by identifying factors that are related to judgments of stuttering severity. And the third could be answered by identifying factors that are more likely to be related to the speaking behavior of peers who have no history of a stuttering problem. Statistical procedures that could be used to answer these questions (the Kendall coefficient of concordance, multiple regression and correlation, and the discriminant function analysis for questions one through three respectively) are discussed in Chapter 10.

Which Type of Design Should You Use?

It should be fairly apparent from the discussion in this chapter that usually a number of factors must be considered when you decide whether to use a single subject or group design to answer a question. For some questions, however, only one of these two types would be appropriate because of a single consideration. Such questions include those:

- That state unequivocally whether they refer to individuals or to typical members of groups
- For which all treatments could not be administered to individual subjects
- For which an insufficient N would be available for a group design

For questions where the choice is not clear cut, you must weigh the advantages and disadvantages of each design and select the one that seems most likely to yield data of adequate validity, reliability, and generality to answer the question (see Chapter 12). If neither design seems likely to yield data of adequate validity, reliability, and generality to answer a question (or questions), it might be wise to search for some other question (or questions) for which the prospects of collecting such data seem better.

Exercises and Discussion Topics

1. Indicate whether you would use a single subject or a group design to answer each of the following questions and state the reasons for your decisions.

Also describe the subjects you would observe to answer each question (indicating attributes they would and would not possess) and specify the observations you would make on these subjects and the conditions under which you would make them.

a. What impact does learning to use a communication board have on aphasics?

b. Which of two methods of teaching speech-reading tends to produce the best results with hard-of-hearing adults?

c. Do persons who have sensorineural hearing losses tend to respond differently to a particular hearing test than those who have conductive hearing losses?

2. Using the ABC notation, diagram a design you have used during your clinical practicum experience for assessing (auditing) therapy outcome. What limitations does this design have and how could it be improved?

3. Order and sequence effects are discussed in this chapter from the perspective of their possible detrimental impacts on clinical research. How could they also adversely affect the outcome of a diagnosis and/or a therapy session?

Chapter 7

Types of Data

This chapter deals with the observations, or data, that are the "raw material" from which answers to questions are arrived at. They are regarded as raw material because they usually have to be organized in some manner before they can be used for this purpose. The process by which they are organized (and consequently converted from raw material to a form that can be used to answer questions) is described in Chapters 9, 10, and 11.

What Are Data?

Data can be viewed as an abstraction from the observational process. When you observe an event to answer a question, you do not attend to, or abstract, all attributes of it. You simply attend to a small number (in some cases, only one) that are relevant for answering that question. If, for example, you wished to determine whether a child had articulation errors, you could administer an articulation test. Most such tests require the child to say a number of words in which the phonemes of the language occur in various positions. The child's production of each word constitutes an event. This event would have a number of attributes, including accuracy of production of each phoneme, voice quality, pitch level, intensity. During a child's production of each word, you would probably attend only to the phoneme (or possibly two phonemes) the word was included in the test to sample. This illustrates what is meant by abstracting only those attributes of an event that are relevant for answering a question, which in this case would be: "Is the phoneme (or are the phonemes) that the word was intended to sample produced correctly in the position in which it occurs in the word?" The information abstracted about the accuracy of production of the phoneme could serve as *data* for answering this question.

There may be more than one attribute of an event that, if abstracted, could serve as data for answering a particular question. The accuracy of production of a phoneme in a word, for example, could be described in several ways. First, it could be described on the basis of how it sounds to an observer (or observers). Second, it could be described on the basis of how accurate the postures of the articulators look during production of the phoneme through the use of cinefluorography (i.e., X-ray motion pictures). Third, it could be described on the basis of action potentials recorded from the speech musculature during production of the phoneme by means of electromyography. Finally, it might be described on the basis of oral and nasal pressure and flow measurements made during production of the phoneme through the use of appropriate transducers and electronic amplifiers and recording devices. (The use of instrumentation for observing attributes of events is discussed in Chapter 8.)

Strictly speaking, data are symbolic representations of attributes of events. They are not what is abstracted from events but abstractions of what is abstracted from events. As the general semanticists have pointed out (e.g., Johnson, 1946), you cannot express in words or numbers everything you observe. If, for example, the event you were observing was a child telling a story about a picture and the attribute you were attending to was phonological development, the data resulting would be your description of what you observed—in words, or numbers, or both. It would not be what you observed per se.

What relationship should exist, then, between the symbolic representation of what is observed (data) and what is observed? The answer is that the two should be similar in structure. By this we mean that the relationship between data and what is observed should be analogous to that between a *map* and the *territory* it represents. If a map that included Illinois and Wisconsin were similar in structure to the territory represented, Chicago, Illinois, would be north of Champaign, Illinois, and Milwaukee, Wisconsin, would be north of both Champaign and Chicago. If the map indicated that Milwaukee was south of Chicago, the structure of the map would not be similar to the territory. (For further discussion of the man-territory analogy, see Johnson, 1946, pp. 131–133.)

The relationship between map and territory, or between what is observed and its symbolic representation, can be further illustrated by means of the relationship between a pure-tone audiogram and what it depicts. A pure-tone audiogram can be regarded as a *partial* symbolic representation of one attribute of hearing, that is, threshold for pure tones. It is a partial representation because thresholds are not plotted for all frequencies in the audio range (e.g., they are not plotted for 562 Hz or 1079 Hz). If the configuration of the audiogram is similar in structure to the territory it is supposed to depict—that is, a person's thresholds for pure tones at selected frequencies—it will accurately indicate the person's thresholds at the frequencies tested. The ordering of these frequencies for threshold would correspond to the person's relative ability to detect the presence of pure tones at the frequencies tested. Not only would the ordering of frequencies for threshold correspond to that in the territory, but the relative degrees of hearing loss at the frequencies tested would also. If a pure tone of one frequency had to be made 10 dB louder than a pure tone of a second frequency to be detected, this would be indicated by the configuration of the audiogram.

A second illustration of the map-territory relationship that is relevant to communicative disorders is the relationship between articulation test results and articulation errors. For articulation test results to be similar in structure to the territory they are supposed to depict—that is, the articulation errors of the person tested—they have to indicate the speech sounds that are produced incorrectly and how they are produced incorrectly (i.e., omitted, distorted, or substituted for).

The extent to which a data map is similar in structure to the territory it represents determines its validity. The greater the structural similarity, the more valid the data. A description of something is valid if it accurately describes that which it is intended to describe.

Aphasia test results are valid to the extent that they accurately describe attributes of an aphasic's language deficits. Assessing the validity of data, therefore, involves estimating the degree of structural correspondence between map and territory—between the description of an attribute and the attribute itself.

Speech-language pathologists and audiologists use many types of data for answering questions. The following data, for example, were reported in a single issue of a journal published by the American Speech-Language-Hearing Association:

- Transcriptions of samples of stuttered speech
- Linguistic analyses of normal speech disfluencies
- Children's scores on the Environmental Language Inventory
- Anecdotal reports of parents functioning as language trainers
- Numbers of syllables spoken per minute
- Judgments of "normalcy" of speech
- Stutterers' self-ratings of reactions to speech situations
- Personality test scores
- Frequency of use of specific syntactic structures
- Scores on the Elicited Language Inventory
- Verbal descriptions of expressive language
- Chronological ages
- Scores on Porch Index of Communicative Ability
- Pure-tone audiometric test results
- Verbal descriptions of apraxics' use of American Indian Sign
- Mean values of temporal integration in dB
- Verbal descriptions of "cocktail party speech" accompanying myelomeningocele and shunted hydrocephalus
- Auditory localization test scores
- Verbal description of a person with contact granuloma of the vocal cords
- Measures of respiratory function (e.g., tidal volume)
- Measures of speaking pitch level
- Verbal descriptions of X-rays
- Verbal descriptions of the communicative behavior of a young deaf child
- Nasality scores
- Articulation error frequencies

Actually, thousands of different kinds of verbal and numerical descriptions have been used by speech-language pathologists and audiologists to map territories—that is, attributes of events.

Qualitative and Quantitative Data

There are two basic types, or classes, of data—qualitative and quantitative. *Qualitative* data are *verbal* descriptions of attributes of events, and *quantitative* data are *numerical* descriptions of attributes of events. Both are used by speech-language pathologists and audiologists to answer questions.

Qualitative Data

Some attributes of events can be more adequately described ("mapped") by words than by numbers. Verbal descriptions of such attributes could be less abstract—that is, could convey more information—than numerical ones. Suppose, for example, you wanted to describe the response of an aphasic to an aphasia test item. A highly abstract description of such a response would be to assign it a *1* if it were appropriate and a *0* if it were inappropriate. A less abstract description would be to assign it a number that would indicate how close it was to being appropriate, for example, a number from 0 to 16 as is done with the PICA scoring system (Porch, 1971). The level of abstraction could be reduced even more by describing the aphasic's behavior when the item was presented in as much detail as possible. (Excellent examples of such descriptions of aphasics' response to aphasia test items can be found in Head's classic work, *Aphasia and Kindred Disorders of Speech*, published in 1926.)

Verbal descriptions of attributes of events vary in the degree to which they are similar in structure to the territory they are intended to map. As I indicated earlier in this chapter, this topic has been dealt with in depth by the general semanticists (e.g., Johnson, 1946). They have indicated how the use of language can cause some verbal maps to be more similar in structure to the territory being mapped than others. The following sets of statements illustrate several of the ways in which verbal descriptions of attributes of events can vary in the extent to which they are similar in structure to the territory they are intended to depict. The second statement in each set would probably be judged to be more similar in structure than the first.

1a. John said his first word when he was 10 months old.
1b. John's parents first remembered hearing him produce sounds that they interpreted as a meaningful word when he was 10 months old.
2a. John is a moderately severe stutterer.
2b. John's stuttering was judged moderately severe in the situation in which he was observed.
3a. John's study was rejected by the *Journal of Speech and Hearing Research* because it was poorly designed.
3b. An associate editor for the *Journal of Speech and Hearing Research* felt that John's study was poorly designed and rejected it.
4a. John is a good clinician.
4b. John behaves in a manner that is consistent with my internal standard regarding what constitutes a good clinician.
5a. Stutterers do not stutter when they are alone.
5b. Some stutterers report they do not stutter when they are alone.
6a. The articulation test results indicated that John had a relatively severe articulation problem.
6b. Based on the articulation test results, I felt that John had a relatively severe articulation problem.

Qualitative data (i.e., verbal descriptions of attributes of events) vary with regard to level of validity, reliability, and generality. The greater the structural similarity between the description of an attribute of an event and what occurred, the more valid the description. The "b" descriptions in the preceding paragraph, therefore, would probably be regarded as more valid than the "a" descriptions.

The level of reliability of qualitative data is a function of the interaction between the observer and the observed. Some persons tend to be more reliable observers than others. They are more able to attend to (abstract) the relevant attributes of an event. And they have fewer biases that would tend to distort their observations.

The level of generality of qualitative data is a function of the representativeness of the sample of events observed. Samples selected by a random procedure (i.e., table of random numbers) that are relatively large usually are the most representative. They permit relatively accurate inferences to be made regarding the class of events of which they are representative. If you wished to determine the distribution of attitudes of ASHA certified speech-language pathologists and audiologists toward a piece of legislation before the Congress, you could select a random sample of such individuals from the most recent American Speech-Language-Hearing Association Directory and ask each to complete a questionnaire. Assuming your sample was adequately large, the distribution of attitudes in the sample would probably correspond closely to that in the population (i.e., the total group of ASHA certified speech-language pathologists and audiologists). The distribution of attitudes in the sample would serve, therefore, as a fairly accurate "map" of the distribution of attitudes in the population. The data in the sample thus would have some generality.

Is qualitative data less objective—less scientific—than quantitative data? While there is no reason for regarding one form of data as intrinsically more objective and scientific than the other, the answer to this question would depend on the territory being described. Verbal descriptions would yield maps more similar in structure to some territories than would numerical descriptions. For such territories, verbal descriptions would be superior to numerical ones. On the other hand, some territories can probably be described more precisely through numbers than through words. For such territories, qualitative data would be inferior to quantitative data. Consequently, an investigator's choice should be determined by which he or she feels provides the most accurate map for a territory. This choice, however, should not always be an either-or one. For describing some territories, a more accurate map would be yielded by a combination of the two than by either one alone. Both are often used, for example, for describing attributes of clients' language disorders in evaluation reports.

Quantitative Data

Some attributes of events can be described more accurately by numbers than by words. This is particularly true for attributes that involve quantities, or magnitudes. Consider the following statements that concern the frequency of occurrence of an articulation error:

1. During the session John produced /s/ correctly most of the time.
2. During the session John produced /s/ correctly 80 percent of the time.

You would probably regard the second as more adequately describing John's production of /s/ during the session than the first, since the meaning of "80 percent" is less ambiguous than that of "most." Consequently, the second would be a more adequate map of the territory than the first.

The defining characteristic of quantitative data is that they consist of number symbols, or numerals. Numerals function semantically in the same manner as words—that is, they have *assigned* meanings. Meanings are assigned to both classes of symbols; they do not exist in nature. To identify the meanings that have been assigned to a given word, you can look it up in a dictionary. If it has more than one meaning, its meaning in a particular situation has to be inferred from context. Numerals function similarly in that each can be assigned several meanings; to determine their meaning in a given situation you have to know the context in which they are being used. The numerals 10, 20, and 30, for example, would have different meanings in the following five contexts:

1. They could be used to designate types of communicative disorders.
2. They could be used to designate positions in a rank ordering for hypernasality.
3. They could be used to designate points on an equal-appearing interval scale of articulation defectiveness.
4. They could be used to designate frequencies of occurrence of stuttering.
5. They could be used to designate degrees of hearing loss in dB.

The first context illustrates the *nominal* meaning of numerals, or number symbols. In this context they are used merely to designate, or label, categories. Letters of the alphabet, words, or other symbols could be substituted for them. The numeral 10, for example, could be used to designate spastic dysphonia, 20 to designate Broca's aphasia, and 30 to designate conductive hearing loss. The numerals on the backs of football players' jerseys also have this meaning.

The second context illustrates the *ordinal* meaning of numerals. In this context they are used to designate locations in a rank ordering. They indicate the relative amount of an attribute each individual possesses relative to that possessed by the other individuals ranked. The numeral 10, for example, could be used to designate the individual in a group of three who was most hypernasal and 30 the one in the group who was least hypernasal.

The third context illustrates the *interval* meaning of numerals. In this context they designate points on a continuum that have equal amounts of the attribute being measured between them. If the numerals 10, 20, and 30 had interval meaning, the amount of increase in articulation defectiveness between a speech sample assigned the numeral 10 and one assigned the numeral 20, for example, would be equal in magnitude to the amount of increase in articulation defectiveness between a sample assigned the numeral 20 and one assigned the numeral 30. If these numerals had ordinal rather than interval meaning, the amount of increase in articulation defectiveness between them would not be assumed equal.

The fourth context illustrates the *ratio* meaning of numerals. In this context they designate points on a continuum that both have equal amounts of an attribute between them and are related to an absolute zero. Because of the presence of an *absolute* zero, the magnitudes between points, as well as those represented by the points themselves, have meaning. A speech sample assigned the numeral 20, for example, would contain articulation that is twice as defective as one assigned the numeral 10. And one assigned the numeral 10 only would be one-third as defective in articulation as one assigned the numeral 30. These relationships would not hold for numerals with ordinal or interval meanings, since such numerals are not related to an absolute zero.

The fifth context illustrates the *logarithmic* meaning of numerals. In this context numerals designate points on a continuum that have *unequal*, but known, mathematically defined amounts of an attribute between them. These amounts become progressively smaller as the numbers become larger. Since the numerals on the decibel scale have logarithmic meanings, a person who had a 30 dB hearing loss would hear less well than a person who had either a 20 dB or 10 dB one, and the magnitudes of the differences between these amounts of hearing loss could be estimated.

These five meanings for numerals (nominal, ordinal, interval, ratio, and logarithmic) will be discussed further in the final section of this chapter, which is concerned with measurement.

Quantitative data, like qualitative data, vary in validity, reliability, and generality. The factors that influence these are the same for quantitative data as for qualitative data.

The validity of quantitative data is a function of the degree of structural similarity, or isomorphism, between the meanings of the numerals used to describe, or quantify, attributes of events and the attributes being described. The more valid the data, the greater the degree of similarity, or isomorphism. If ordinal numerals are used to describe the ordering of a group of individuals on the basis of a particular attribute and the individuals are orderable on the basis of that attribute in the manner designated by the numerals, then the numerals are isomorphic to the attribute being described and hence validly describe that attribute. Suppose you had five stutterers who varied considerably in severity in relation to the others, with 1 designating mildest stuttering and 5 most severe stuttering. The numerals would be isomorphic to the territory and hence valid if, for example: (1) The stutterer assigned the numeral 2 was more severe than the stutterer assigned the numeral 1 and less severe than the stutterers assigned the numerals 3, 4, and 5; (2) the stutterer assigned the numeral 5 was more severe than any of the others; and (3) the stutterer assigned the numeral 1 was less severe than any of the others. For the numerals to be a valid map of the territory, therefore, they would have to rank order the stutterers in a manner that would be consistent with the relative severities of their stuttering.

The reliability level of quantitative data, like that of qualitative data, is a function of the interaction between the observer and the observed. The factors mentioned as influencing this interaction in the discussion of qualitative data also apply here. The main difference between the two is that the level of reliability of quantitative data can usually be estimated more precisely than that of qualitative data.

The factors mentioned as influencing the generality of qualitative data also influence the generality of quantitative data. Random sampling and a sufficiently large N maximize the probability of adequate generality for both types of data. The main difference between the two for generality is similar to that for reliability—that is, the generality of quantitative data usually can be estimated more precisely than that of qualitative data. Statistical inference, which is the approach used to estimate the generality of quantitative data, is discussed in Chapters 10 and 11.

Measurement-Related Properties of Quantitative Data

The measurement-related properties of the five most frequently encountered types of quantitative data in speech-language pathology and audiology research—nominal, ordinal, interval, ratio, and logarithmic—were summarized briefly in the preceding section. These properties will be dealt with here in greater depth. It is essential for speech-language pathologists and audiologists to develop as good an intuitive understanding of them as they can. Without such an understanding, quantitative data cannot be interpreted accurately or utilized appropriately for answering questions.

The Nature of Measurement

Measurement can be defined as *the assignment of numerals to attributes of (objects and) events according to rules*. This definition is a slightly modified version of one formulated by the late S. S. Stevens (1951, p. 1), who was a pioneer in psychological and psychophysical measurement. There are several terms in this definition to which particular attention should be paid. The first is the term *numeral*. Numerals, as was indicated earlier in this chapter, are number symbols. Their meanings are determined by the rules used to assign them. Numerals on nominal, ordinal, interval, ratio, and logarithmic scales have different meanings because they are assigned by different rules. Therefore, it is necessary to know the rules by which a particular set of numerals was assigned to grasp their meaning.

The second important aspect of this definition is that numerals are assigned to *attributes* of objects and events rather than to objects and events themselves. As I have previously indicated, when you describe an object or event, you only describe certain attributes of it, not all possible ones. Objects and events possess infinite numbers of attributes (Johnson, 1946).

The third, important point of this definition is that the term *objects* is in parentheses, to indicate that it could be deleted from the definition. Objects can be classified as events. What you abstract as an object on the macroscopic (observable) level would be classified as an event on the submicroscopic (molecular) level since its configuration would be constantly changing (Johnson, 1946). The eventness, or process nature, of objects is apparent even if they are observed on the macroscopic level over a relatively long period of time (Johnson, 1946). The author's 1982 Toyota did not have the same attributes in 1995 when he sold it that it had when it was new (e.g., one of the doors would no longer open). The attributes (or characteristics) of a hearing aid after two years of use are unlikely to be identical to what they were when it left the factory. Since the attributes of phenomena classified as objects vary as a function of time on both macroscopic and submicroscopic levels, they are not sharply differentiable from phenomena classified as events. It would appear justifiable, therefore, to classify them as events rather than to place them in a separate category.

The rules used for assigning numerals to attributes of events on nominal, ordinal, interval, ratio, and logarithmic scales are presented and discussed in the following sections.

Nominal Scales

Numerals on a nominal scale are assigned to categories, or subclasses, of attributes of events by means of the rule that states "do not assign the same numeral to different classes or different numerals to the same class" (Stevens, 1951, p. 26). They merely label, or identify, such categories or subclasses. The particular numeral assigned to a particular category or subclass is *arbitrary*. It is desirable, however, that the categories or subclasses be *mutually exclusive* and *exhaustive* with regard to the attribute being scaled. That is, all events that possess the attribute being scaled should be (1) assignable to only one category or subclass, and (2) assignable to a category or subclass. Suppose the attribute you wished to scale was articulation errors. The following three categories, or subclasses, could be used for this purpose, and a numeral could be assigned arbitrarily to identify each:

1. Sound substitutions
2. Sound omissions, additions, and inversions
3. Sound distortions

These categories would probably be regarded as both mutually exclusive and exhaustive, since individual articulation errors would be assignable to only one category and all such errors could be assigned to a category. The specific ordering of the numerals that is used to label the three categories is completely arbitrary. Any of the six—that is, $(N)(N-1)$—possible permutations of these three numerals (see Figure 7-1) would serve equally well.

The events assigned to any one category must be equivalent with regard to the attribute being scaled, or fall within the defined domain of that category. They do not have to be equivalent, however, with regard to any other attributes. The relation between such events for the attribute scaled is referred to as *equivalence* and is symbolized by the familiar sign =. The equivalence relation is defined logically as being *reflexive* ($x = x$ for all values of x), *symmetrical* (if $x = y$, then $y = x$), and *transitive* (if $x = y$ and $y = z$, then $x = z$). These qualities are further defined in the section on ordinal scales.

Nominal scales have been constructed for a variety of attributes of interest to speech-language pathologists and audiologists. Some such scales are an end in themselves and others are a means to an end. Several examples of the first type would be Angle's (1907) three classes of malocclusion—that is, Class I (Neutrocclusion), Class II (Distocclusion), and Class III (Mesiocclusion); Jerger's four types of Békésy audiogram tracings (Jerger, 1960); and Schuell's five major diagnostic categories of aphasia (Schuell, Jenkins, & Jimenez-Pabon, 1964). The second type would include instances where qualitatively defined categories, or subclasses, are arbitrarily assigned numerals to facilitate computer analysis. The category "male," for example, might be assigned the numeral 1, and "female" the numeral 2. Or the numeral 1 might be assigned to conductive hearing loss, 2 to sensorineural hear-

123
321
132
231
213
312

FIGURE 7-1   Permutations of numerals on a nominal scale.

ing loss, and 3 to mixed hearing loss. Various statistical analyses can be performed on observations that have been categorized in this way, including determining the number and percentage of total observations that fall into each category.

Ordinal Scales

Numerals on an ordinal scale are assigned to N categories, or subclasses, of events to designate a *rank order*. The categories, or subclasses, ordered may contain only a single event (e.g., a person). While the ordering of the N numerals designates the ordering of the N categories with regard to the amount of the target attribute they possess, it is arbitrary whether 1 or N is used to designate the greatest amount of the attribute. Thus, if 10 events (e.g., speech samples) were rank ordered, the one with the greatest amount of the target attribute (e.g., hypernasality) could be assigned either the numeral 1 or the numeral 10.

With an ordinal scale, the differences in the amount of the target attribute between the categories ranked are not necessarily the same. There are not necessarily equal intervals between scale points. This is illustrated in Figure 7-2. The difference in the amount of the target attribute between the category assigned the numeral 1 and the category assigned the numeral 2 in this figure is greater than the difference between the category assigned the numeral 2 and that assigned the numeral 3. If the 10 numerals on this scale had been assigned to 10 samples of speech to designate an ordering on the basis of articulation defectiveness, the difference in degree of articulation defectiveness between the sample assigned the numeral 1 and that assigned the numeral 2 would be greater than the difference in degree of articulation defectiveness between the sample assigned the numeral 2 and that assigned the numeral 3.

Categories on an ordinal scale can be labeled by words and certain other symbols rather than (or in addition to) numerals. The labels "mild," "moderate," and "severe" can be attached to categories on an ordinal scale, as can the labels "poor," "fair," "good," "very good," and "excellent"; "strongly disagree," "moderately disagree," "undecided," "moderately agree," and "strongly agree"; and A, B, C, D, E. The labels "correct" and "incorrect"; "+" and "−"; and "+", "±", and "−" also can be attached to categories to define ordinal scales.

For a scale to have ordinal properties, the numerals have to be assigned by rules that result in a specific relationship between the categories ranked. This relationship, according to Hempel (1952, pp. 58–62), is based on the relations of *coincidence* (sharing the same place or being equal to another) and *precedence* (being less than or greater than another). For the relationship between categories on a scale to be ordinal, Hempel states that the two relations have to meet the following conditions.

1. Coincidence must be *transitive;* that is, whenever x stands in coincidence to (or in the same category as) y and y stands in coincidence to (or in the same category as) z, then

FIGURE 7-2   An ordinal scale.

x stands in coincidence to (or is included in the same category as) *z*. In other words, if John lives in the same state as Jim and Jim lives in the same state as Joe, then John lives in the same state as Joe.

2. Coincidence must be *symmetric;* that is, whenever *x* stands in coincidence to (or is included in the same category as) *y*, then *y* stands in coincidence to (or is included in the same category as) *x*. In other words, if John lives in the same state as Jim, then Jim lives in the same state as John.

3. Coincidence must be *reflexive;* that is, any event *x* stands in coincidence to (is includable in the same category as) itself with regard to the attribute being measured. Another way of stating the same thing is that *x = x* for all values of *x*. In other words, all events included in a category are equivalent with regard to the attribute on the basis of which they were assigned to the category. Thus, all individuals classified as having a conductive hearing loss would have pathology in the outer and/or middle ear.

4. Precedence must be *transitive;* that is, if *x* stands in coincidence to *y* and *y* stands in precedence to *z*, then *x* stands in precedence to *z*. In other words, if Bloodstein's (1987) Phase II stuttering is more severe than his Phase I stuttering, and his Phase III stuttering is more severe than his Phase II stuttering, then his Phase III stuttering should be more severe than his Phase I stuttering.

5. Precedence must be *coincidence-irreflexive;* that is, if *x* stands in coincidence to (or is equal to) *y*, then *x* does not stand in precedence to *y*. In other words, if John has the same threshold for a 1000 Hz tone as Jim, then John does not have a higher threshold or lower threshold for this tone than Jim.

6. Precedence must be *coincidence-connected;* that is, if *x* does not stand in coincidence to (or is not equal to) *y*, then *x* stands in precedence to *y* or *y* stands in precedence to *x*. In other words, if John does not have the same threshold for a 1000 Hz tone as Jim, then John either has a higher threshold or a lower threshold for this tone than Jim.

There are six conditions, then, that Hempel indicates need to be satisfied for numerals to have ordinal properties. The first three, incidentally, also must be satisfied for numerals to have nominal properties (see section on nominal scales).

Ordinal scales are the type that has probably been used most frequently to measure, or quantify, attributes of events of interest to speech-language pathologists. There are at least three reasons for the frequent use of this type of scale. First, ordinal scales are simpler to construct than other types that indicate magnitudes, or quantities (i.e., interval, ratio, and logarithmic scales). The reason for this is that the other types require the six conditions for ordinal measurement to be satisfied in addition to some others. (These additional conditions are indicated in the sections in which the three types are discussed.)

A second reason for the frequent use of ordinal scales is that ordinal level measurement is all that is required for answering many questions. Such questions often are similar in form to one of the following:

- Does Person A (or Group A) *have more of (or less of) an attribute* than Person B (or Group B)? Other phrases that could occur instead of the italicized one include: (a) have a higher (or lower) score on a task, (b) have a longer (or shorter) response time, and (c) exhibit a higher frequency (or lower frequency) of a behavior.

- Do persons who exhibit a relatively high level (or relatively low level) of an attribute under one condition (or on one task) also tend to exhibit a similar level under one or more other conditions (or on one or more other tasks)? Another way of phrasing this question would be: Does Condition A (or Task A) tend to rank order persons in the same manner as Condition B, etc. (or Task B, etc.)?

A third probable reason for the frequent use of ordinal scales is that some attributes, or dimensions, do not lend themselves to higher than ordinal level measurement—that is, they do not lend themselves to interval or ratio level measurement. An example would be a scale in which the categories, or points, include several dimensions, such as Bloodstein's (1987) four-phase scale for describing the development of stuttering. It would be extremely difficult, if not impossible, to construct such a scale so there would be equal intervals between points for all dimensions included.

Interval Scales

Numerals on interval scales are assigned by the same rules as those on ordinal scales, *plus* one additional rule: They must be assigned in such a manner that the interval widths between successive numerals are equal in magnitude with respect to the attribute being scaled. This requirement is graphically portrayed in Figure 7-3 for the attribute "distance." The distance between the numerals 1 and 2 in this figure is equal to that between the numerals 2 and 3, 3 and 4, 4 and 5, 5 and 6, 6 and 7, 7 and 8, 8 and 9, and 9 and 10. The equality of these interval widths can be checked with a ruler.

Interval scales can be constructed for psychological attributes as well as physical ones. In addition to equal physical distances between points, there can be *equal-appearing* perceptual distances between points—distances that appear approximately equal based on observer judgments. The Lewis-Sherman Scale of Stuttering Severity (Lewis & Sherman, 1951) represents an attempt to develop a scale on which the perceptual distances between points are equal appearing. This scale consists of nine sets of speech segments, each of which has been assigned a numeral between 1 and 9. The segments assigned the numeral 1 contain the mildest stuttering and those assigned the numeral 9 the most severe. The segments were selected from a larger group that were rated by the method of equal-appearing intervals for "degree of stuttering severity." This method, which is described in Chapter 8, is thought to result in measurement that approximates interval level. Theoretically, differences in stuttering severity between speech segments assigned the numeral 1 and those assigned the numeral 2 would be approximately equal to those between speech segments assigned the numerals 2 and 3, 3 and 4, 4 and 5, 5 and 6, 6 and 7, 7 and 8, and 8 and 9. The interval widths on this scale, incidentally, were estimated by means of a rating procedure and with a few exceptions were found to be fairly equal (Berry & Silverman, 1972).

$$
\begin{array}{cccccccccc}
1 & 2 & 3 & 4 & 5 & 6 & 7 & 8 & 9 & 10
\end{array}
$$

FIGURE 7-3   An interval scale.

Because of the equality of interval widths, the *differences* between numerals on interval scales can be manipulated arithmetically. That is, they can be added, subtracted, multiplied, and divided. The difference in the amount of an attribute between events designated by the numerals 1 and 3 would be twice that between events designated by the numerals 1 and 2 and half that between events designated by the numerals 1 and 5. If these numerals were points on an interval scale of stuttering severity, the difference in severity of stuttering between a speech segment designated by the numeral 1 and one designated by the numeral 3 would be twice that between speech segments designated by the numerals 1 and 2 and half that between speech segments designated by the numerals 1 and 5.

While the differences between numerals on an interval scale can be manipulated arithmetically, this cannot be done with the numerals themselves. The reason for this restriction is that the numerals on such a scale are not related to an absolute, or "true," zero. Consequently, a speech segment that was assigned the numeral 2 would not necessarily contain stuttering that was twice as severe as that in a segment assigned the numeral 1 nor half as severe as that in a segment assigned the numeral 4.

Scales that have been regarded either implicitly or explicitly as having interval properties have been developed for a number of attributes of interest to speech-language pathologists and audiologists. Such scales would include those which were constructed by the method of equal-appearing intervals, for example, the Lewis-Sherman Scale of Stuttering Severity (Lewis & Sherman, 1951). They also might include scales based on age ratios such as IQ (i.e., MA/CA × 100). Numerals on IQ scales could be regarded as having either ordinal or interval properties. The interpretation would depend on whether you were willing to assume, for example, that the increase in "intelligence" from an IQ of 60 to an IQ of 70 is equivalent to the increase from a IQ of 95 to one of 105. If you were willing to assume that the intervals between points on the IQ scale are approximately equal throughout the *entire* range of possible IQs, then you would be justified in regarding numerals on this scale as having interval properties. On the other hand, if you would not be willing to make this assumption, it would be safest to regard such numerals as having ordinal properties.

Scales that are claimed to have interval properties should probably be regarded as having ordinal properties unless it has been demonstrated unequivocally that the equal interval assumption is viable. Regarding them as such in most instances would probably not cause any problems.

Ratio Scales

Numerals are assigned by the same rules on ratio scales as on interval scales with the exception that they are required to be related to an absolute, or true, zero. This requirement is portrayed graphically for the attribute "distance" in Figure 7-4. Because ratio scales have as their origin a true zero point, the numerals on such scales, as well as the intervals between them, are isomorphic to the structure of arithmetic and can be manipulated arith-

FIGURE 7-4   A ratio scale.

metically. A speech segment assigned the numeral 4 on a ratio scale of stuttering severity would contain stuttering that is twice as severe as that in a speech segment assigned the numeral 2 on this scale. A ratio scale theoretically could be constructed for the attribute stuttering because it would be possible to have a speech segment that contained zero stuttering. It might not be possible, on the other hand, to construct a ratio scale for the attribute "intelligence" because it would be difficult to define zero intelligence.

The decision on whether a scale has ratio properties may not be unequivocal. Frequency of articulation errors would probably be regarded as a scale with ratio properties if it were viewed as a *frequency* scale, since the numeral 4, for example, would indicate twice as many articulation errors as the numeral 2. On the other hand, it would probably not be regarded as a ratio scale of *articulation defectiveness*, since four errors would not necessarily be judged to represent twice the degree of articulation defectiveness as two errors. It would probably not be regarded even as an interval scale of articulation defectiveness since interval widths between successive numerals are unlikely to be judged equal. The change from one to two articulation errors, for example, would probably be judged to represent a greater increase in articulation defectiveness than would the change from fifteen to sixteen such errors. Hence, a scale of articulation defectiveness based on frequency of articulation errors would probably be regarded as having ordinal properties.

While one measure of a particular attribute might not result in a scale that has ratio properties, another such measure might result in a scale with these properties. It might be possible, for example, to construct a ratio scale of articulation defectiveness by using a psychological scaling procedure such as *direct magnitude-estimation* (see Chapter 8) rather than frequency counts of articulation errors. With this approach, each of a group of speech segments that contained a wide variety of frequencies and types of articulation errors would be assigned a number by a panel of listeners that would be instructed to indicate how defective the articulation was in it as compared to the articulation in a "standard" speech segment. The standard speech segment would be arbitrarily assigned a point value, for example, 100. Each listener would be instructed to assign a point value to each speech segment that would indicate how defective he or she considers the articulation in it to be as compared to that in the standard speech segment. A listener who felt, for example, that the articulation in a particular speech segment was twice as defective as that in the standard segment would assign that segment 200 points. On the other hand, a listener who felt the articulation in a particular speech segment was half as defective as that in the standard segment would assign it 50 points. The listener could assign any number of points desired to a speech segment as long as it reflected a judgment on how defective the articulation was in it as compared to that in the standard segment. The mean of the point values assigned to each segment could be computed and used as its *scale value*—that is, the point, or value, on the scale to which it is assigned. Assuming the listeners *rated the speech segments as instructed*, the resulting scale should at least come close to having ratio properties. A segment with a mean point value of 100, for example, would be approximately twice as defective in articulation as one with a mean point value of 50, and approximately half as defective in articulation as one with a mean point value of 200.

The unit of measurement of a ratio scale is arbitrary. For the attribute "length," for example, you can convert from inches to feet (or from feet to inches) by multiplying (or dividing) all numerals by the *positive constant* 12. The conversion, or transformation, from one unit of measurement to another by *multiplying* or *dividing* all numerals by a positive constant does not influence the ratio properties of a scale.

Ratio scales for attributes of interest to speech-language pathologists and audiologists have been developed from several types of measures including the following:

- Frequency counts. One attribute that has been scaled by this measure is frequency of phonological errors.
- Temporal (time) measures. One attribute that has been scaled by this type of measure is duration of moments of stuttering.
- Length (distance) measures. The amount of opening between the posterior surface of the velum and the anterior surface of the posterior pharyngeal wall during the production of /a/ has been measured in millimeters from lateral headplates (X-rays) to assess velopharyngeal closure.
- Voltage measurements. Output voltages from some types of electroacoustical instrumentation used in audiology (e.g., Békésy audiometers) are recorded and measured.
- Observer judgments. Scales for attributes of communicative behavior which at least approximate ratio measurement have been constructed through the use of psychological scaling methods such as direct magnitude-estimation. (Several such scales are described in Chapter 8.)

Logarithmic Scales

Logarithmic scales, like ratio scales, are constructed from numerals that meet the conditions for ratio level measurement. To construct a logarithmic scale from such numerals you multiply each by a particular *base* number. (Only numerals with ratio properties can be used to construct logarithmic scales because numerals with nominal, ordinal, and interval properties cannot be manipulated arithmetically.) The base numbers used most often for scaling attributes of communicative behavior are 2 and 10. Relationships between ratio scale values and logarithmic scale values for the base numbers 2 and 10 are illustrated in Table 7-1.

TABLE 7-1   Relationships between Ratio Scale Values and Logarithmic for the Base Numbers 2 and 10

Ratio Scale Value	Logarithmic Scale Value (Base 2)	Logarithmic Scale Value (Base 10)
0	(2^0) 1	(10^0) 1
1	(2^1) 2	(10^1) 10
2	(2^2) 4	(10^2) 100
3	(2^3) 8	(10^3) 1000
4	(2^4) 16	(10^4) 10000
5	(2^5) 32	(10^5) 100000
6	(2^6) 64	(10^6) 1000000
7	(2^7) 128	(10^7) 10000000
8	(2^8) 256	(10^8) 100000000
9	(2^9) 512	(10^9) 1000000000

FIGURE 7-5   A logarithmic scale.

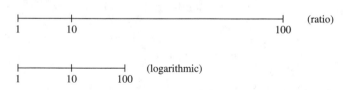

FIGURE 7-6   Comparison between ratio and logarithmic scales.

These relationships demonstrate one of the main advantages of logarithmic over ratio scales. A logarithmic scale can present data more compactly than a ratio scale. Scale values up to 10,000 are included in the logarithmic scale depicted in Figure 7-5 in the same space as for scale values up to 10 in the ratio scale depicted in Figure 7-4. The compactness of logarithmic scales in comparison to ratio scales is illustrated further in Figure 7-6.

Because logarithmic scales are derived from numerals with ratio scale properties, the numerals on such scales can be manipulated arithmetically. Logarithmic scales can be transformed into ratio scales for the same reason.

Logarithmic scales have been used to quantify a number of attributes of interest to speech-language pathologists and audiologists, including the intensities and fundamental frequencies of voices and pure-tone audiometric thresholds in decibels. They also have been used to record the effects of speech therapies on articulation errors over time (e.g., Mower, 1969).

Exercises and Discussion Topics

1. How does a clinical evaluation report serve as a "map" of a "territory"?
2. Specify two types of qualitative and two types of quantitative data that an audiologist might gather during a hearing aid evaluation.
3. Indicate what *attribute* of what *event* you would attempt to describe verbally or numerically to answer the following questions. For each, specify two ways you could describe this attribute of this event that probably would be sufficiently reliable and valid for answering the question.
   a. How much does production of /s/ tend to improve after ten weeks of daily therapy using a particular program?
   b. How much better does a particular hard-of-hearing child tend to understand speech while he or she is using a hearing aid than while he or she is not using it?
   c. How intelligible is the esophageal speech of a person who has had a total laryngectomy?
4. You are to evaluate the numerical properties of the scores yielded by three diagnostic tests. Indicate what measurement scale you feel the scores from each are on and give your reasons.

Chapter 8

Strategies for Generating Data

The strategies that have been used most often for observing attributes of communicative behavior are described in this chapter. It is important that you develop an intuitive understanding of these strategies and the types of questions they can answer, as well as the factors you should consider when designing and evaluating the findings of studies that utilize them. Without such an understanding, you will have little or no idea of the amount of confidence you can have in the accuracy of answers to questions in which the data utilized were generated by them.

Role of the Observer in the Data Generating Process

Before beginning our discussion of strategies for describing attributes of events of interest to speech-language pathologists and audiologists, we will consider the data-generating process itself, particularly the role of the observer in this process. The observer is a component of all schemes for generating data, since all of them rely on observer judgment to some extent. With psychological scaling (rating) procedures, which are discussed elsewhere in this chapter, the importance of the observer in the process is obvious because the data are observer judgments. It may not be as obvious, however, for physical measurement, that is, measurement of physical attributes of events that utilizes electronic or other types of instrumentation. Examples of such instruments would be rulers and voltmeters that have dials with pointers rather than digital readouts. Both may appear to result in "objective" measurement, that is, measurement not influenced by observer judgment; distances may appear to be indicated by the marks on rulers and voltages by the position of the pointer on voltmeter dials. Rulers and voltmeters do not read themselves, however. Someone has to decide which mark on a ruler corresponds to the distance being measured and which number of the voltmeter dial the indicator is pointing at. Also, the accuracy of the calibration of such devices obviously influences the accuracy of the measurement it is possible to obtain from them. And the accuracy of their calibration is partially a function of observer judgment, since they are calibrated by some human agent. For these reasons, observer judgment is an unavoidable component of any data-generating process or scheme.

The presence of an observer (or observers) in the measurement process introduces error into it. A group of observers who measure the same thing, for example, may not record the same measurement. This can be demonstrated by means of a relatively simple task such as measuring the length of a line with a ruler. How long is this line?

_____

To answer this question, ten students at Marquette University were handed a card on which a line of this length had been drawn and a foot ruler graduated in sixteenths of an inch. All measured the line with the same ruler. They were told to measure the line and record their measurement on a blank card that they had been given. Their length estimates ranged from 1.88 inches to 2.25 inches, with a mean of 2.07 inches. While the differences between estimates are relatively small, they could be large enough in some instances to make a difference that would result in a difference in an answer to a question.

The presence of an observer in the process can introduce two types of error: random and systematic. Both were mentioned in Chapter 7. *Random error*, as indicated previously, is present to some degree in all data-generating processes. It can arise from several sources, including insufficient accuracy in making and in recording (writing down) observations. If, for example, you were measuring distances with a ruler, random error could result occasionally from not placing the ruler at the exact point from which you wished to begin to measure, or from reading distances from the ruler incorrectly, or from writing down distances inaccurately after you had read them. The nature of random error is such that if you were to describe again an aspect of an event (or object) after you had made an error (or errors), you would be unlikely to make the same error (or errors). Because random error does not replicate itself—that is, does not occur whenever a data-generating process is repeated—it does not bias the resulting data. It does not, for example, cause numbers from a measurement process to be consistently larger or smaller than they should be. While random error can be reduced by such means as making all measurements twice, it is doubtful whether it ever can be completely eliminated.

The second type of error, *systematic error*, is usually of more concern to investigators than the first because it *biases* the resulting data. For example, it causes the numerals generated by a measurement process to be consistently larger or smaller than they should be. In the case of measuring distances with a ruler, systematic error could result from consistently placing the end of the ruler at a point that was not the one from which you wished to begin to measure, or consistently misreading the ruler in the same manner (e.g., interpreting the gradations as occurring every $\frac{1}{16}$ inch rather than every $\frac{1}{8}$ inch), or consistently recording distances incorrectly after reading them (e.g., indicating inches rather than millimeters after numerals).

Observer-related systematic error can be introduced from several sources, including:

• *A measuring "instrument" or process being improperly administered or conducted.* An investigator, for example, may not administer an educational or psychological test in the manner in which it was supposed to be administered. An investigator who deviated from the instructions in the test manual for administering the test might obtain scores that are biased—that is, consistently higher or lower than they should be.

• *Subjects not performing a task as instructed.* They may, for example, not make the judgment they were instructed to make. Suppose a group of subjects were told to rate a series of speech segments from cleft palate speakers for degree of nasality, thus requiring them to ignore articulation errors and other deviations of speech, voice, and language usage. They may not be able to keep the other deviations present in the speech segments from influencing their nasality ratings, which would cause these ratings to be biased.

• *Experimenter bias.* An experimenter's outcome expectations or hypotheses can bias the measurements he or she makes (Rosenthal, 1976). For example, a speech-language pathologist who expected a particular treatment to be effective in reducing word-finding difficulties might rate aphasics as less severe after the administration of the treatment than before more often than the effects of the treatment would justify. Such errors would not represent deliberate, or conscious, attempts to deceive but "wishful thinking." (This topic is further discussed in Chapter 11.)

• *Subject bias.* This phenomenon is closely related to, and is sometimes the result of, experimenter bias. Subjects may respond to experimental conditions in the manner that they feel the experimenter either would like them to respond or expects them to respond. That is, they have thoughts about an experiment that can influence their performance on an experimental task. As Orne has pointed out:

> *Insofar as the subject cares about the outcome, his perception of his role and of the hypothesis being tested will become a significant determinant of his behavior. The cues that govern his perceptions—that communicate what is expected of him and what the experimenter hopes to find—can therefore be crucial variables. . . . They include the scuttlebutt about the experiment, its setting, implicit and explicit instructions, the person of the experimenter, subtle cues provided by him, and of particular importance, the experimental procedure itself. All of these cues are interpreted in the light of the subject's past learning and experience. (Orne, 1969, p. 146)*

If clients were asked, for example, to describe the effects a particular therapy had on them as part of a study of the effectiveness of that therapy, and if they surmised that the person who was conducting the study either expected (or hoped) to find it effective in certain ways, they might be more likely to indicate that it had at least "a little" effect in these ways than they would if they had had no information concerning the expected (or hoped for) outcome. Hence, at least some of their statements could be biased.

Data-generating schemes used by speech-language pathologists and audiologists can be divided into two groups. The first includes those that use an "instrument" to supplement observer judgment. The instrument helps the observer to "abstract" the attribute he or she wishes to describe. A speech-language pathologist who wished to describe the extent of increase in sympathetic nervous system activity in response to a feared stimulus as part of a desensitization procedure could use a psychogalvanometer to assist in observing and measuring this activity. Or an audiologist who wished to describe thresholds for pure tones could use a pure-tone audiometer to help abstract this phenomenon.

An instrument used to supplement observer judgment need not be electronic. Most, if not all, educational and psychological tests could probably be used for this purpose. So also could tests of communicative ability such as articulation tests, aphasia tests, language development scales, auditory discrimination tests, and tests of speechreading ability. Other "instruments" that could be used for this purpose include questionnaires and structured interviews.

The second group of data-generating schemes includes those that rely primarily upon observer judgment. The observer is the most important component of such schemes. Psychological scaling techniques, which have been used a great deal by speech-language pathologists and audiologists for quantifying attributes of communicative behavior, are representative of the schemes in this group. These techniques require the observer to make various kinds of judgments, including the following:

- Deciding to which of a group of categories an event should be assigned
- Deciding which member of each of a series of pairs of events possesses the greater amount of an attribute
- Rank ordering a group, or series, of events on the basis of the amount of an attribute they possess
- Assigning numerals between 1 and a specified upper limit (usually 7 or 9) to events on the basis of the amount of some attribute they possess, so that the intervals between successive numerals will be equal-appearing with respect to an attribute
- Assigning numerals between 1 and a specified upper limit (usually 7 or 9) to events on the basis of the amount of some attribute they possess, so that each event is assigned the numeral of the category on the scale that comes closest to indicating the amount of the attribute it possesses (the amount of the attribute possessed by each category on the scale would be specified either verbally or nonverbally)
- Assigning points to each of two events that sum, or add up, to a particular constant (e.g., 100) so that the points assigned to each of the two correspond to the relative amount of the attribute being measured that it possesses in relation to that possessed by the other (e.g., if one member of a pair were judged to possess twice the amount of an attribute as the other, it would be assigned 66.67 points and the other would be assigned 33.33 points)
- Assigning points to events on the basis of the amount of an attribute they possess as compared to that possessed by a "standard" event, or stimulus (this is the type of direct magnitude-estimation judgment described in Chapter 7)

Each of these tasks is associated with a psychological scaling technique that is described elsewhere in the chapter.

Several data-generating strategies of each type are described in this chapter. While these are not the only ones that have been used in speech and hearing research, they include those that have been used most often.

Strategies That Utilize an Instrument to Supplement Observer Judgment

Strategies that utilize an instrument to supplement observer judgment can be divided into two groups. The first consists of those that utilize electronic or other instruments for physical measurement; and the second, those that do not utilize such instruments—for example, those that utilize tests, structured tasks, and questionnaires.

Strategies That Utilize Electronic Instrumentation

Various types of electronic instrumentation schemes are used by speech-language pathologists and audiologists to measure physical attributes of communicative behavior. Information about them and their components can be found in books by Code and Ball (1984), Cudahy (1988), Curtis and Schultz (1986), Decker (1989), and McPherson and Thatcher (1977).

These schemes measure attributes of events that are electrical signals or can be transduced (i.e., converted) into electrical signals. Their components are diagrammed in Figure 8-1. The task performed by each of them is described in this section.

Detection

The first step in the measurement process is *detection*. Its purpose is to detect the presence (and absence) and possibly the magnitude of the signal of interest. If the phenomenon being observed is not an electrical signal, it is transduced into one.

The detection component of the instrumentation used for measuring speech and other acoustical signals consists of a microphone and possibly a preamplifier. The microphone transduces (translates) acoustical signals into weak electrical signals. The function of the

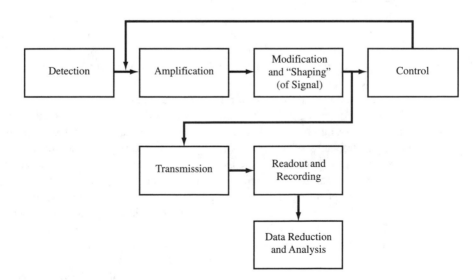

FIGURE 8-1   Instrumentation scheme for measurement.

preamplifier is to amplify the weak electrical signals (i.e., voltages) generated by the microphone, with minimal distortion, to the point where their magnitude is within the sensitivity range of the amplifier component.

The detection component of the instrumentation for measuring biological electrical signals such as those resulting from muscle action potentials, brain waves, and changes in skin resistance consists of electrodes that either would be attached to the surface of the skin (i.e., surface electrodes) or inserted into muscle fibers or other tissue (i.e., needle electrodes) and an appropriate preamplifier. The function of the preamplifier here would be to increase the magnitudes of the weak electrical signals detected by the electrodes, with minimal distortion, to the point where their magnitude is within the sensitivity range of the "amplifier" component.

While these two types of detection stages are probably the ones that have been used most frequently in speech and hearing research, several other types have also been used. These would include: (1) strain gages that transduce mechanical pressures, or stresses, into electrical signals, (2) pneumotactographs that transduce rates of air flow into electrical signals, and (3) photoelectric cells that transduce light intensities into electrical signals. An appropriate preamplifier would be fitted to each such transducer.

Amplification

The second step in the measurement process is *amplification*. Its function is to increase the magnitude of the electrical signal from the preamplifier to the point where it is within the sensitivity range of the readout and recording device being used. The electrical signal from the detection stage may have to be passed through a series of amplifiers, rather than a single amplifier, to increase its magnitude to the point where it is within the sensitivity range of this device.

Modification and Shaping

A third step that may be present in the measurement process is the *modification and shaping* of the electrical signals generated by the amplifier(s). Its purpose is to remove "noise" (extraneous information to what is being measured) from these signals—that is, to make the figure, or what the investigator wishes to observe, stand out better from the background (other information in the signal).

The instrumentation used for removing extraneous information from an electrical signal usually contains a filter network. There are three basic types of filter networks—high pass, low pass, and band pass. Their function is to emphasize or deemphasize specific frequency components of a signal. A *low pass* filter network is used to reduce or eliminate from a signal frequency components *above* a specified frequency. A low pass filter network thus would emphasize the low frequency components of a signal. A *high pass* filter network is used to eliminate from a signal frequency components *below* a specified frequency. A high pass filter network thus would emphasize the high frequency components of a signal. A *band pass* filter network is used to reduce or eliminate from a signal *both* frequency components above a specified frequency and below a specified frequency; it consists of a high pass and a low pass filter network. A band pass filter network thus would emphasize a particular "band" of the frequency components of a signal—those between specified upper and lower frequency limits.

Control

The next step in the measurement process is *control*. Its function is to keep the amplitude or some other attribute of the electrical signal outputed by the amplification stage (or the modification and shaping stage, if one is used) *within certain limits*. This is a feedback component that functions in much the same manner as a thermostat on a furnace and an automatic record level on a tape recorder. It measures the average amplitude (or other attribute) of the output signal from the amplification or shaping instrumentation. If the amplitude (or value of some other attribute of the signal) is too great, it adjusts the amplification stage to attenuate, or weaken, it. If, on the other hand, the magnitude is insufficient, it adjusts the amplification stage to increase it. This process keeps the amplitude (or other attribute) of the signal within the sensitivity range of the device used to record the signal.

A microcomputer is frequently used now to perform this task and the remaining ones in the measurement process. Software is available for microcomputers that utilize the Macintosh and Windows operating systems that enables them to simulate the instrumentation required to do these tasks (see Chapter 12 in Silverman, 1997). However, because the only type of information that computers can process is digital information, the electrical ("analog") signals from the amplifier or shaping instrumentation must be converted to digital form. The digital conversion process is accomplished by passing the electrical signals through a device known as an *analog-to-digital converter* (see Chapter 12 in Silverman, 1997). Many microcomputer systems contain such devices.

Transmission

The signals from amplification or shaping instrumentation or an analog-to-digital converter have to be transmitted to a readout and recording device to be measured. The simplest device for transmitting such signals is an electrical cable (i.e., jumpcord) that connects the amplifier(s), the modification and shaping device, or an analog-to-digital converter to the readout and recording device being used. Radio telemetry instrumentation also could be used for this purpose. The output signals from the amplifier(s), the modification and shaping device, or an analog-to-digital converter would be fed into a radio transmitter and beamed to a radio receiver that could be anywhere from a few feet to hundreds of thousands of miles (e.g., astronauts in space) away. The radio receiver would be connected to the readout and recording device.

Recording and Reading Out

The next, and possibly last, step in the measurement process consists of *recording and reading out*, or displaying, the output signals from the transmission stage. There are two basic types of devices can be used for this purpose. The first are real instruments and the second are computer simulations of them. Both yield the same information.

Let's begin with the simplest type—the *meter*. Meters indicate the value of the attribute of the signal being measured by means of a pointer (Figure 8-2) or a digital display (Figure 8-3). A computer can simulate either type of meter on a monitor screen.

Another class of readout and recording devices that can be used in such schemes consists of *oscillographic recorders* (see Figure 8-4) and *strip chart recorders* (Figure 8-5). Both will indicate changes in the configuration of a signal during a specified period of time by means of a continuous line drawn on a strip of paper. The primary difference between

FIGURE 8-2   A meter that indicates values of the attribute being measured by a pointer.

them is that an oscillographic recorder can handle a wider range of rates of change in the configuration of a signal than a strip chart recorder can. Strip chart recorders are most useful when the rate of change in the configuration of a signal is relatively slow. The line may be drawn in ink by a pen, by a light on photosensitive paper, or by a heated stylus on heat-sensitive paper. The strip of paper may be in a roll or in a Z-fold pack (i.e., folded in a fan-like manner similar to computer readout paper). Some such recorders have more than one channel—that is, they can indicate changes in the configurations of several signals simultaneously on the same strip of paper.

A computer can be programmed to simulate a multichannel *oscillographic recorder* or *strip chart recorder*. Fluctuations in the configuration of a signal during a specified time period can be stored in a computer and reproduced with a dot-matrix printer or plotter.

FIGURE 8-3   A meter that indicates values of the attribute being measured by a digital display.

FIGURE 8-4   A multichannel oscillographic recorder.

FIGURE 8-5   A single-channel strip chart recorder.

Almost any such fluctuations can be displayed in this manner: Extremely rapid ones can be stored in the computer and sent to the printer or plotter at a rate it can handle.

A third class of devices for displaying changes in the configurations of electrical signals are *oscilloscopes* (Figure 8-6). The oscilloscope display is similar to an oscillographic recorder display. The only real difference is that the signal is "painted" with light on a screen, not inscribed on a strip of paper. A signal displayed on an oscilloscope screen can be photographed if a permanent record of it is desired.

A microcomputer can be programmed to simulate an oscilloscope. Changes in the configurations of electrical signals would be displayed on its monitor screen.

A fourth class of devices used for this purpose are ones that *record changes in the configurations of electrical signals on a magnetic medium.* There are two types of magnetic media that are used for this purpose. The first is magnetic tape. The type of device that is used most often for recording on such tape is referred to as an *instrumentation tape recorder* (Figure 8-7). These can be used to record both biological electrical signals and electrical signals from transducers (e.g., strain gages). They usually have more than one channel and consequently, can record signals from several sources simultaneously.

A second type of magnetic medium that is used for the purpose is a computer disk (Silverman, 1997). A microcomputer (e.g., an IBM compatible or a Macintosh) would be used for recording the electrical signal data on the disk. Signals recorded in this manner can be displayed graphically (in whole or part) on a monitor screen and/or printed. They also can be subjected to various statistical analyses, with the results displayed on a monitor screen and/or printed.

The final class of devices that will be mentioned here for displaying changes in the configurations of electrical signals are *X-Y recorders* (Figure 8-8). These recorders automatically plot the value of an independent variable versus a dependent variable directly on

FIGURE 8-6   An oscilloscope.

FIGURE 8-7   An instrumentation magnetic tape recorder.

FIGURE 8-8   An X-Y recorder.

sheets of graph paper. Electrical signals from two transmission stages are inputed into the recorder. Plots produced by X-Y recorders can provide information concerning the *nature* of the relationship (e.g., linear or nonlinear), the *direction* of the relationship (i.e., positive or negative), and the *strength* of the relationship (i.e., degree of correlation) between the two signals, or variables, being measured. A plot from such a recorder could, for example, provide information about how a client's thresholds for pure tones (X) vary as a function of their frequency (Y).

A microcomputer, with appropriate hardware and software, can produce X-Y plots. While a plotter would be the most desirable device to use for printing them, a dot-matrix or other type of computer printer may be usable for the purpose (see Silverman, 1997 for descriptions of these devices).

The readout and recording devices mentioned here are not the only such devices that have been used in instrumentation schemes for measuring attributes of events relevant to speech-language pathology and audiology. However, they are the ones that have been used most often for this purpose.

Computer Data Reduction and Analysis

Readout and recording is the final step in some instrumentation schemes for measuring electrical signals. In others, there is an additional step—*data reduction and analysis*. The output of the "readout and recording" device is digitized and analyzed with a computer. Computer data reduction and analysis is particularly likely to be incorporated into an instrumentation measurement scheme that produces too many signals to be measured by an observer "by hand" in a relatively short period of time, or when the statistical analyses to be made of the data are relatively complex. Signals that are to be analyzed in this manner may be recorded on a magnetic medium—tape or disk—prior to doing so.

A Clinical Example

Now that the functions of individual components of instrumentation schemes for measuring electrical signals have been described, we can indicate how such a scheme might be used to measure an attribute of communicative behavior. Suppose we wished to measure a stutterer's anxiety level in certain situations outside the clinic. One measure of this that could be used would be the galvanic skin response (GSR). To *detect* changes in skin resistance (associated with changes in anxiety level) electrodes could be attached to the stutterer's skin in an inconspicuous place. The electrical signals from the electrodes could be fed into a miniature *preamplifier, amplifier*, and from there into a miniature *radio transmitter*. The preamplifier, amplifier, and radio transmitter circuitry could be fitted into a very small case and attached to the stutterer's body or clothing so that it would not be visible. The signals from the transmitter could be picked up by a *radio receiver* located at the clinic (providing the clinic was not too far away). They could be fed into an *amplifier* (or series of amplifiers) to increase their magnitude to the point where they would be within the sensitivity range of a strip chart recorder. A *control* device could be used to keep the level of the signals within the sensitivity range of the device. If the baseline magnitude of the signals transmitted became weaker because the stutterer moved farther away from the location of the radio receiver, the degree of amplification would be increased. On the other hand, if the baseline magnitude of these signals became stronger because the stutterer moved closer to the location of the radio receiver, the degree of amplification would be reduced. The signals from the amplifier might be fed through a *filter* before being transmitted by means of an electrical cable to the *strip chart recorder* (or a computer simulation thereof). The function of the filter would be to remove extraneous signals, or "noise," from the output of the amplifier stage. This would be likely to "simplify" the strip recorder plot, thereby making it easier to interpret.

This instrumentation scheme, of course, is not the only one that could be used for measuring changes in skin resistance that occur outside a clinic setting. It is merely intended to illustrate how such a scheme might function.

Measuring Readouts from Instrumentation Schemes

This section will describe how quantitative data are abstracted from meter dials, oscilloscope screens, and the displays from such devices as strip chart recorders, oscillographic recorders, and X-Y recorders, as well as computer simulations thereof.

The quantification of electrical signals involves the assignment of numerals to one or more of their attributes (i.e., their amplitudes, frequencies, phase relationships, etc.). The numerals assigned usually have *ratio* properties and for this reason can be manipulated arithmetically. The process by which numerals are assigned may be relatively simple. This is usually the case when the readout device is some sort of meter, for example, a VU meter. VU meters are used by both speech-language pathologists and audiologists to measure the loudness levels of auditory signals, including speech ones. Some have a dial with numerals around its perimeter ranging from –20 to +3 and a pointer. The position of the pointer indicates the numeral that corresponds to the loudness level of the signal. This numeral is used to designate its loudness level at that moment in time. Since the loudness level of a signal may vary considerably during a relatively short period of time, the pointer may be moving almost continuously. The fact that the loudness level of a signal may not remain constant can create problems when it is necessary to assign a single number to designate it for a particular period of time. One approach that could be used to generate such a value would be to average the numerals indicated by the pointer at specified intervals during this period of time. If this time interval were 60 seconds, for example, the dial might be read every 5 seconds and the mean of these values computed.

The measurement of electrical signals displayed by strip chart recorders, oscillographic recorders, X-Y recorders, oscilloscopes, or computers that have been programmed to simulate one of these devices usually involves a *distance measuring*, or *frequency counting*, or *both* a distance measuring and frequency counting operation.

A *distance measuring operation* involves determining how far (in inches or millimeters) a particular point in a display deviates from a baseline. The numeral assigned to that point is this value. The *baseline* could be the magnitude, or level, of the phenomenon being measured prior to the administration of an experimental treatment. The baseline for measuring the degree of reaction to a feared stimulus through changes in skin resistance, for example, could be the level of skin resistance immediately prior to the presentation of this stimulus. The deviation from a baseline can be estimated in several ways. It can be measured with a ruler, or by counting the number of squares in the grid printed on the readout paper between the baseline and the point on the display you wish to measure. The amount of deviation from a baseline following administration of a treatment is apt to vary to some extent. If it is necessary to assign a single number to designate the amount of deviation from a baseline during a specific period of time, the mean of a series of deviation measures made during this period of time could be used. The amount of change in skin resistance during a 1-minute period following the presentation of a feared stimulus could be designated by the mean amount of deviation from the baseline measured at 5-second intervals. It would be necessary to attach + and − signs to the deviation measures if they occurred in both directions from the baseline (i.e., + if the signal were above the baseline and − if it were below the baseline). For the point on the section of strip chart in Figure 8-9 marked with an arrow, the deviation from the baseline would be approximately 13 millimeters. The direction of the deviation would be "negative" since the signal falls below the baseline. (Note that the readout has a 1-millimeter grid printed on it.)

The measurement of displays could involve a *frequency counting operation*. This

FIGURE 8-9   Section of a readout from a two-channel strip chart recorder.

involves determining the number of times a particular attribute, or configuration, of a signal occurs. Frequency of occurrence usually is specified with relation to a particular time interval. Thus, a frequency counting operation may also require a distance measuring operation. The frequency of occurrence of an attribute may be related to a particular time interval that would correspond to a particular distance on the readout paper strip—that is, the number of inches (or millimeters) of the readout marked by the pen or stylus during the time interval to which the frequency count is related. The frequency of a tone could be determined from an oscillographic recorder readout by counting the number of cycles that were inscribed by the stylus during a 1-second time interval. The number of inches of paper that passes under the stylus during a given time interval is estimated from information supplied by the manufacturer of the readout device concerning the speed at which the paper is moving. If 6 inches of paper passed under the stylus each second, the frequency of a tone would correspond to the number of cycles that were inscribed on a 6-inch strip of the paper.

The measurement procedures for oscilloscope screen tracings (or computer monitor simulations thereof) are essentially the same as those for oscillographic recorder readouts. The attributes of signals that can be measured from oscilloscope screen tracings include frequency and amplitude. Frequency can be estimated by counting the number of cycles displayed on the screen with the oscilloscope set to display a particular time interval. If the interval were 50 milliseconds (i.e., 50/1000 second) and 10 cycles were displayed on the screen, the frequency of the signal (e.g., tone) would be 200 cycles per second. Amplitude can be estimated by a grid inscribed on the oscilloscope screen. It can be measured in millimeter deviation from a baseline, as with an oscillographic recorder, or in volts (a measure of the electrical magnitude of a signal). Measurements can be made directly from the screen display or from photographs of the screen display.

Measurements of attributes of speech and other auditory signals from magnetic tape recordings are made in a variety of ways. In some cases, such signals are fed into an instrumentation measurement scheme before being measured. They are passed through an amplifier stage and a modification and shaping stage and then are transmitted to a readout and recording device such as a strip chart recorder, X-Y recorder, oscillographic recorder, oscilloscope, meter, or computer programmed to function as such a device. The instrumentation scheme helps to abstract the target attribute from the taped signal and thus facilitates the measurement process. A taped speech signal might be fed into a sound spectrograph (or computer simulation thereof) to analyze and display its spectral characteristics—that is, the amount of energy present at specific frequencies during given moments in time. Several characteristics of the speech spectra could be measured from the resulting spectrogram (e.g., vowel formant frequencies).

It usually is possible to make the distance and frequency measurements described in the preceding paragraphs with a computer (Silverman, 1997). However, whether doing so would be cost effective is a function of both the cost of the software and the time investment required to learn to use it. If, for example, an investigator only had to make a few measurements, it probably would be more cost effective (and faster) for him or her to make them by hand than by computer.

Attributes of communicative behavior observable in audiotape or videotape recordings can also be measured by rating techniques. Six such techniques—known as *psychological scaling methods*—are described in the final section of this chapter.

Sources of Error in Measurements from Readout Devices

There are several sources of random and systematic error that can influence the accuracy of quantitative data derived from meter dials and from strip chart recorders, X-Y recorders, oscillographic recorders, oscilloscopes, and similar types of displays (including computer simulations thereof). These can be grouped under three main headings: (1) gross errors, (2) systematic errors, and (3) random errors (Stout, 1962, pp. 21–26).

Gross errors consist of mistakes in reading meters and other readout displays and in recording numbers resulting from measurement processes. Misreading a meter would be an example of such an error. The pointer on a VU meter indicates –2 but is read as indicating –3. Perhaps the person misread the meter because the signals measured previously were –3 and he or she expected further –3 readings. It is well known that your expectations can influence your perceptions (Johnson, 1946). Gross errors also include mistakes in recording (e.g., writing down or typing) the numbers that result from a measurement process. One of the most common errors of this type is transposition. The person making and recording the measurements from a meter may read 35.2 but write down 32.5. Gross errors can be reduced by making each measurement several times, preferably with one measurement not immediately following the next. These errors usually do not bias the measurement process in any meaningful way because they occur infrequently and tend to be random.

Systematic errors can be classified as three main types: (1) instrumental errors, (2) environmental errors, and (3) observational errors. *Instrumental errors* include those that result from shortcomings of the instrument, or misuse, or loading effects of the equipment. The performances of all components of instrumentation measurement schemes probably deviate to some degree from their nominal values (i.e., those specified by their manufacturers) even when they are new. If the instruments included in such schemes are not recalibrated periodically, this deviation is likely to increase because of use and age. If the deviation is fairly small, it may not bias the measurement process in any meaningful way.

The problem of instrumental errors resulting from *shortcomings of equipment* can be illustrated by means of the pure-tone audiometer. All such audiometers, even when they are new, would not measure exactly the same thresholds at given frequencies, because of factory calibration error. Differences in threshold measurements arising from factory calibration error are likely to be too small to be significant clinically. However, if pure-tone audiometers are not recalibrated periodically, error due to use and age may increase to the point where threshold measurements will not be sufficiently accurate for at least some clinical purposes.

Instrument calibration errors can be handled in two ways. The best, but usually the most expensive, is to have the instrument recalibrated. The second is to determine the extent of the calibration error and apply a *correction factor*. If you knew, for example, that the amount of hearing loss indicated by a pure-tone audiometer at 1000 Hz was 5 dB too great, you could subtract 5 dB from the degree of hearing loss indicated by this audiometer at this frequency.

Instrumental error also can result from *misuse* of components of instrumentation measurement schemes. Failure to use or maintain an instrument according to the manufacturer's instructions can cause instrumental error. Failure to use the recommended type of earphones on an audiometer, for example, could result in an impedance mismatch that would probably cause the loudness levels of the pure tones generated by that audiometer to deviate from their nominal values. Such errors can be reduced or eliminated by following manufacturers' recommendations regarding the use of their instruments.

The *loading effects* of components of instrumentation measurement schemes is another source of instrumental error. What sometimes happens is that the measurement process influences what is being measured. The circuitry of a measuring instrument (e.g., a voltmeter) can interact with that of the instrument producing the signal being measured (e.g., a pure-tone audiometer), altering this signal and hence producing inaccurate measurements. To avoid this source of error, it is essential to "isolate" the circuitry of measurement instruments from the circuitry of the instruments producing the signals being measured.

The second subclass of systematic errors is *environmental errors*. These result from factors external to a measuring device (i.e., in the environment in which it is being used) that can influence the functioning of one or more of the components within it and thus influence the accuracy of measurements made with it. Environmental factors that can influence the functioning of the components of such schemes include temperature, humidity, barometric pressure, and stray electrical and magnetic fields. The accuracy of the calibration of many electronic instruments is dependent on their being used in an environment in which the temperature is maintained within a specified range. If such an instrument is used in a room in which the temperature is either above or below this range, measurements may be biased. It may be possible to use this instrument in such an environment if the effect of the temperature in the room where the measurements are being made on the resulting measurements is known. A correction factor can be applied to measurements made in this environment. If they are too high, a constant can be subtracted from them; and if they are too low, a constant can be added to them. The most direct way to control for the effects of environmental factors is to use instrumentation measurement schemes in environments that conform to manufacturers' recommendations.

The third subclass of systematic errors are *observational errors*. Different persons measuring the same phenomenon with the same instrumentation under identical environmental conditions will not necessarily record the same measurements. An observer may consistently record values from a VU meter that are higher or lower than they should be because of the angle at which he or she views the meter. For these values to be accurate, the meter must be read from directly in front. If it is viewed at an angle, the indicator may appear to be pointing to a different number on the scale than that which it would appear to be pointing to if it were viewed from in front. This source of error can be reduced or eliminated by having measurements made by more than one observer and by using the average of the measurements made of a particular phenomenon as the measure of that phenomenon.

The third, and final, classification of measurement error based on Stout's scheme is *random error*. The sources of this type of error were described at the beginning of this chapter and in Chapter 6.

Strategies That Utilize Instruments That Are Not Electronic or Intended for Physical Measurement

Five types of measurement strategies are described in this section that utilize instruments that are not electronic or intended for physical measurement. They are tests and structured tasks, semantic differentials, Likert-type scales, questionnaires, and structured interviews.

Tests and Structured Tasks

Communicative disorder specialists have used many types of tests and structured tasks clinically to facilitate the observation and description of attributes of communicative behavior. Doing them permits the target attribute to stand out sufficiently from other behavioral attributes and/or to occur at an appropriate time for it to be observed and described. If, for example, the target attribute were "accuracy of articulation of certain consonant phonemes in initial, medial, and final positions in words," having a child respond to the stimulus items on a picture articulation test would make it possible for the production of these phonemes to be observed in the desired contexts at an "appropriate" time and their accuracy assessed.

The numerals (i.e., scores) assigned by tests to target behavioral attributes theoretically can be on any level of measurement. However, their properties rarely exceed those necessary for ordinal measurement because the intervals between them (with regard to the attribute being measured) usually are not equal *throughout the range of possible scores*, and they are usually not related to an absolute zero. Consequently, interpretations of the magnitudes of the differences between test scores have to be made with considerable caution. Because one child's performance on an articulation test improved by 4 points while a second child's performance on the same test improved by 2 points does not necessarily mean that the first child's articulation improved twice as much as the second child's. In fact, it may not even be true that the first child's articulation improved more than the second child's. The first child's 4-point increase may have resulted from learning to produce /s/ blends in the initial positions in words, while the second child's 2-point increase may have resulted from learning to produce /s/ and /r/ correctly in the initial positions of words. Regardless of the score differences, many speech-language pathologists would look upon the second child as having improved more than the first. If this were the case, it probably would be most appropriate to interpret scores on the test as having nominal rather than ordinal properties.

The data from tests and structured tasks consists of scores and/or verbal descriptions. The former, like all numerals assigned to attributes of events, are subject both to random and to systematic measurement error. The sources of random and systematic error that influence test scores are the same as those indicated for instrumentation measurement schemes, that is, gross errors, systematic errors, and random errors.

Gross errors include mistakes in reading test and subtest scores and in recording such scores. Recording subtest scores incorrectly on a test profile summary sheet or a data sheet would be an example of such an error. Scores could be recorded incorrectly either because they are misread or because they are written down incorrectly (e.g., numbers are transposed).

Systematic errors, as previously indicated, are of three types: instrumental errors, environmental errors, and observational errors. *Instrumental errors* include those that result from shortcomings of the test instrument. Age norms developed for interpreting test scores, for example, may not be accurate. If the normative group used to standardize a language development scale was not representative of the population of which it was supposed to have been representative, scores from this scale may be consistently interpreted as indicating higher (or lower) language ages than would be the case. Consequently, language age estimates based on this scale would be biased.

Instrumental errors also include those resulting from *misuse* of test instruments. If an educational or psychological test is not administered according to the instructions in the test manual, the scores obtained may be systematically higher (or lower) than they should be.

Environmental errors include those due to factors external to the device that influence the accuracy of measurements made with it. If a test were administered in an environment that caused the testee to become anxious, this could cause his or her score to be lower than it would have been in a relatively relaxed environment.

Observational errors include those that result from differences in internal standards among test administrators. All testers would not necessarily evaluate a given test performance in the same manner. A response that one tester would consider to be "within normal limits" another may regard as "not within normal limits." One tester may classify a slightly lateralized /s/ production on an articulation test as "within normal limits," and another may classify it as "not within normal limits." Thus, one tester may consistently identify higher percentages of children as having a lateral lisp than would another.

The third, and final, source of error that can influence test scores is *random error.* While this type of error, as previously indicated, will not bias measurements (i.e., cause them to be consistently higher or lower than they should be), it will reduce their reliability. One source of random error in a test situation may be inconsistency of response by the testee to the test stimuli. It *sometimes* is possible to reduce this source of error by administering test items more than once.

These same types of errors, of course, can influence the accuracy of qualitative (verbal descriptive) data from tests and structured tasks.

The Semantic Differential Technique

The semantic differential technique (Osgood, Suci, & Tannenbaum, 1957; Snider & Osgood, 1968) was developed by Professor Charles Osgood and his associates at the University of Illinois in the 1940s. With this approach, clients are provided with a set of 7-step, bipolar adjectival scales and instructed to indicate for each scale the direction and intensity of its association to the stimulus being rated. If, for example, we wished to determine a client's attitude toward a hearing aid, one scale that might be included in the semantic differential for this purpose would be:

acceptable _:_:_:_:_:_ unacceptable

If a client's attitude toward the hearing aid was *very closely related* to one or the other of these adjectives, he or she would mark the scale in the following manner:

acceptable **X**:_:_:_:_:_ unacceptable

or

acceptable _:_:_:_:_:**X** unacceptable

If a client's attitude toward the hearing aid was *quite closely* (but not extremely) *related* to one or the other of these adjectives, he or she would mark the scale in the following manner:

acceptable _:**X**:_:_:_:_ unacceptable

or

acceptable _:_:_:_:**X**:_ unacceptable

If a client's attitude was *only slightly related* to one or the other of these adjectives, he or she would mark the scale in the following manner:

acceptable _:_:**X**:_:_:_:_ unacceptable

or

acceptable _:_:_:_:**X**:_:_ unacceptable

Finally, a client who felt that his or her attitude toward the hearing aid was either *neutral* on the scale or that both adjectives were *completely irrelevant* would mark in the following manner:

acceptable _:_:_:**X**:_:_:_ unacceptable

A semantic differential that can be used, with minor modification, for assessing attitudes toward persons who have almost any type of communicative disorder is reproduced in Figure 8-10.

An overview of the process used for constructing and analyzing semantic differentials to measure attitudes toward communicative disorders and persons who have them is presented in this section. Considerable "practical" information is available about the construction, administration, scoring, and interpretation of semantic differentials. The books by Osgood, Suci, and Tannenbaum (1957) and Snider and Osgood (1968) are particularly helpful.

One of the first considerations in constructing a semantic differential is generating the set of bipolar adjectival scales. The specific scales selected will be determined by the stimulus to which reactions are desired. The stimulus, incidentally, does not have to be a word or words. Any observable object or event (e.g., a multimedia computer presentation) could serve as the stimulus.

There are three approaches that—singly or in combination—are useful for creating a set of semantic differential scales. The first is to consult the thesaurus sample of bipolar adjectival scales that Osgood and his associates included in *The Measurement of Meaning* (pp. 53–61). The second is to conduct a brainstorming session in which the members of a group are asked to suggest scales relevant to their reactions to the stimulus. And the third is to solicit responses from a number of persons to a statement such as this: "Please list all the adjectives you can think of that describe (the stimulus)." Bipolar scales can be created for adjectives mentioned by two or more persons.

After the scales for a semantic differential scales have been selected, they should be numbered consecutively. Random numbers should then be used to determine the order in which they will be printed on the semantic differential response sheet (see Figure 8-10). Either a table of random numbers (see Appendix B) or computer-generated random numbers can be used for this purpose. Whether the positive or negative adjective in each pair appears on the left should also be determined by random numbers.

To administer a semantic differential, present a response sheet to each subject along with a set of instructions. The author has found the set included in *The Measurement of Meaning* (pp. 82–84) quite satisfactory. To maximize the probability that a subject will

THE PERSON WHO IS SPEAKING

afraid ____ : ____ : ____ : ____ : ____ : ____ : ____	not afraid
mature ____ : ____ : ____ : ____ : ____ : ____ : ____	immature
unlovable ____ : ____ : ____ : ____ : ____ : ____ : ____	lovable
speech intelligible ____ : ____ : ____ : ____ : ____ : ____ : ____	speech unintelligible
intelligent ____ : ____ : ____ : ____ : ____ : ____ : ____	unintelligent
secure ____ : ____ : ____ : ____ : ____ : ____ : ____	insecure
natural ____ : ____ : ____ : ____ : ____ : ____ : ____	unnatural
no sense of humor ____ : ____ : ____ : ____ : ____ : ____ : ____	sense of humor
speaks rapidly ____ : ____ : ____ : ____ : ____ : ____ : ____	speaks slowly
unselfish ____ : ____ : ____ : ____ : ____ : ____ : ____	selfish
dishonest ____ : ____ : ____ : ____ : ____ : ____ : ____	honest
fluent ____ : ____ : ____ : ____ : ____ : ____ : ____	disfluent
cautious ____ : ____ : ____ : ____ : ____ : ____ : ____	rash
witty ____ : ____ : ____ : ____ : ____ : ____ : ____	dull
speech monotonous ____ : ____ : ____ : ____ : ____ : ____ : ____	speech not monotonous
stable ____ : ____ : ____ : ____ : ____ : ____ : ____	unstable
employable ____ : ____ : ____ : ____ : ____ : ____ : ____	unemployable
unsociable ____ : ____ : ____ : ____ : ____ : ____ : ____	sociable
loud ____ : ____ : ____ : ____ : ____ : ____ : ____	soft
old ____ : ____ : ____ : ____ : ____ : ____ : ____	young
coordinated ____ : ____ : ____ : ____ : ____ : ____ : ____	uncoordinated
dominant ____ : ____ : ____ : ____ : ____ : ____ : ____	submissive
speech dysrhythmic ____ : ____ : ____ : ____ : ____ : ____ : ____	speech rhythmic
speech unpleasant ____ : ____ : ____ : ____ : ____ : ____ : ____	speech pleasant
hesitant ____ : ____ : ____ : ____ : ____ : ____ : ____	not hesitant
boring ____ : ____ : ____ : ____ : ____ : ____ : ____	interesting
unfriendly ____ : ____ : ____ : ____ : ____ : ____ : ____	friendly
cowardly ____ : ____ : ____ : ____ : ____ : ____ : ____	brave
confused ____ : ____ : ____ : ____ : ____ : ____ : ____	oriented
superior ____ : ____ : ____ : ____ : ____ : ____ : ____	inferior
speech slow ____ : ____ : ____ : ____ : ____ : ____ : ____	speech fast
reputable ____ : ____ : ____ : ____ : ____ : ____ : ____	disreputable
optimistic ____ : ____ : ____ : ____ : ____ : ____ : ____	pessimistic
excitable ____ : ____ : ____ : ____ : ____ : ____ : ____	calm
handicapped ____ : ____ : ____ : ____ : ____ : ____ : ____	not handicapped
untrustworthy ____ : ____ : ____ : ____ : ____ : ____ : ____	trustworthy
relaxed ____ : ____ : ____ : ____ : ____ : ____ : ____	tense
contrary ____ : ____ : ____ : ____ : ____ : ____ : ____	agreeable
reliable ____ : ____ : ____ : ____ : ____ : ____ : ____	unreliable
extrovert ____ : ____ : ____ : ____ : ____ : ____ : ____	introvert
rich ____ : ____ : ____ : ____ : ____ : ____ : ____	poor

FIGURE 8-10   A representative semantic differential task.

THE PERSON WHO IS SPEAKING

insane	___ :	___ :	___ :	___ :	___ :	___ :	___ sane
contented	___ :	___ :	___ :	___ :	___ :	___ :	___ discontented
soothing	___ :	___ :	___ :	___ :	___ :	___ :	___ aggravating
not frightened	___ :	___ :	___ :	___ :	___ :	___ :	___ frightened
not frustrating	___ :	___ :	___ :	___ :	___ :	___ :	___ frustrating
alert	___ :	___ :	___ :	___ :	___ :	___ :	___ not alert
speaks poorly	___ :	___ :	___ :	___ :	___ :	___ :	___ speaks well
discourteous	___ :	___ :	___ :	___ :	___ :	___ :	___ courteous
quarrelsome	___ :	___ :	___ :	___ :	___ :	___ :	___ congenial
lazy	___ :	___ :	___ :	___ :	___ :	___ :	___ industrious
deaf	___ :	___ :	___ :	___ :	___ :	___ :	___ not deaf
emotional	___ :	___ :	___ :	___ :	___ :	___ :	___ unemotional
realistic	___ :	___ :	___ :	___ :	___ :	___ :	___ idealistic
approachable	___ :	___ :	___ :	___ :	___ :	___ :	___ unapproachable
not talkative	___ :	___ :	___ :	___ :	___ :	___ :	___ talkative
not aggressive	___ :	___ :	___ :	___ :	___ :	___ :	___ aggressive
weak	___ :	___ :	___ :	___ :	___ :	___ :	___ strong
positive self concept	___ :	___ :	___ :	___ :	___ :	___ :	___ negative self-concept
uneducated	___ :	___ :	___ :	___ :	___ :	___ :	___ educated
deliberate	___ :	___ :	___ :	___ :	___ :	___ :	___ impulsive
nervous	___ :	___ :	___ :	___ :	___ :	___ :	___ calm
sensitive	___ :	___ :	___ :	___ :	___ :	___ :	___ insensitive
able to carry on conversation	___ :	___ :	___ :	___ :	___ :	___ :	___ unable to carry on conversation
scrupulous	___ :	___ :	___ :	___ :	___ :	___ :	___ unscrupulous
independent	___ :	___ :	___ :	___ :	___ :	___ :	___ dependent
masculine	___ :	___ :	___ :	___ :	___ :	___ :	___ feminine
confident	___ :	___ :	___ :	___ :	___ :	___ :	___ not confident
frustrated	___ :	___ :	___ :	___ :	___ :	___ :	___ not frustrated
competent	___ :	___ :	___ :	___ :	___ :	___ :	___ incompetent
inhibited	___ :	___ :	___ :	___ :	___ :	___ :	___ uninhibited
depressed	___ :	___ :	___ :	___ :	___ :	___ :	___ happy
organized	___ :	___ :	___ :	___ :	___ :	___ :	___ unorganized
accept	___ :	___ :	___ :	___ :	___ :	___ :	___ reject
isolated	___ :	___ :	___ :	___ :	___ :	___ :	___ not isolated
comfortable	___ :	___ :	___ :	___ :	___ :	___ :	___ uncomfortable
insincere	___ :	___ :	___ :	___ :	___ :	___ :	___ sincere
enthusiastic	___ :	___ :	___ :	___ :	___ :	___ :	___ unenthusiastic
soothing	___ :	___ :	___ :	___ :	___ :	___ :	___ aggravating
kind	___ :	___ :	___ :	___ :	___ :	___ :	___ cruel
naive	___ :	___ :	___ :	___ :	___ :	___ :	___ sophisticated

FIGURE 8-10 *Continued*

understand what is required, it is advisable to read the instructions aloud while the subject follows along on his or her copy.

To facilitate analysis of semantic differential ratings, the seven points between pairs of adjectives are each assigned a numeral. The set usually assigned is either

$$1, 2, 3, 4, 5, 6, 7$$
or
$$-3, -2, -1, 0, +1, +2, +3$$

If the first set is used, the numeral 4 would be assigned to the center of the scale, 1 to the lower end, and 7 to the upper end. The lower end of the scale could be associated with the negative adjective and the upper end with the positive.

The numerals in the second set are more descriptive of the bipolar nature of the adjectives than those in the first. However, they are more difficult to manipulate arithmetically because some have negative values. Since both sets lead to the same result, and since the numerals in the 1 to 7 set are easier to manipulate arithmetically than those in the -3 to $+3$ set, the 1 to 7 set is usually used.

Data concerning attitudes toward an event (e.g., a therapy program) can be abstracted from semantic differential ratings. Obviously, the ratings assigned to individual scales by persons doing the task can provide information about their reactions to, or attitude toward, the stimulus. Comparable information for the "typical" member of a group can be derived by computing the mean or median of the ratings assigned to each scale (see Chapter 9 and Appendix A). This would be its scale value. The closer a scale value is to the center of a scale, the less likely the adjectives defining that scale are to be relevant to reactions to the stimulus.

Spreadsheet software can be used to automate the calculation of scale values. The rows would be scales and the columns data. In the first column would be keyboarded the adjectives defining the scales; in columns two through eight, the numbers of subjects giving each of the seven responses to each scale; and in column nine the mean or median of the ratings assigned by the subjects to each scale. A formula for the mean or median would be placed in the cells in column nine.

Data generated by the semantic differential technique, of course, are subject to the same sources of error as were mentioned in the preceding section for tests and structured tasks.

We have found the semantic differential technique to be extremely useful for answering questions about attitudes toward communicative disorders and persons who have them. Among the attitudes that we have used it to quantify are those toward elementary-school-age children who wear hearing aids (Silverman & Klees, 1989) and teenagers who have /w/ for /r/ sound substitutions (Silverman & Paulus, 1989).

The Likert Methodology
Likert-type scales consist of a series of statements, each of which reflects either a favorable or an unfavorable attitude. Printed below each statement is a response line, similar to the following:

Strongly Agree   Agree   Undecided   Disagree   Strongly Disagree

Respondents are told to circle, or place a checkmark over, the response that best describes their reaction to the statement.

The way in which responses are analyzed is determined by whether a single subject or group design is being used. If a single subject design is being used, the responses from individual subjects are not combined. If a group design is being used, the percentage of the respondents who gave each of the five responses to each statement is determined. Because three responses—agree, undecided, and disagree—usually are easier to interpret than five, the two "agree" categories and the two "disagree" categories may be combined. If this is done, statements can be made similar to the following: 70 percent of hearing-impaired clients six months after being fitted with a particular type of hearing aid agreed with the statement, "The benefits I gained from using the aid have exceeded my expectations."

It sometimes is desirable to describe the overall reaction of respondents to the subject to which the statements refer. This can be done by assigning the scale value indicated below to each of their responses to each statement reflecting a favorable attitude:

Strongly agree	5
Agree	4
Undecided	3
Disagree	2
Strongly Disagree	1

For each statement reflecting an unfavorable attitude, the scale would be reversed (e.g., the scale value assigned for "strongly agree" would be 1). The average (mean or median) of the ratings assigned by a respondent to the various statements would indicate the degree to which his or her attitude toward the subject was favorable.

Likert-type scales have been used a great deal by speech-language pathologists and audiologists. They have been used, for example, to assess individual clients' attitudes toward their communicative disorder—for example, the *Iowa Scale of Attitude toward Stuttering* (Johnson, Darley, & Spriestersbach, 1963).

Likert-type scale responses are subject to the same types of errors as the other data-generating schemes discussed in this chapter. For further information about such scales, see Best and Kahn (1989, pp. 195–198) and Henerson, Morris, and Fitz-Gibbon (1987, Chapter 6).

Questionnaires or Structured Interviews

Questionnaires and structured interviews are among the most frequently used tools for generating data in speech and hearing research. They are used for this purpose in almost every study (e.g., for finding out the ages of subjects). Both require subjects to answer questions and/or respond to statements. Structured interviews can be looked upon as oral questionnaires—that is, instead of writing responses subjects give information orally, either face-to-face or by telephone.

Structured interviews are usually conducted by a person. However, for some purposes they can be conducted by a computer. The questions would either be "spoken" by the computer or printed on a monitor screen.

If an interview is conducted by a person, answers to questions and responses to statements are either written down by the interviewer (sometimes on a printed form) or are tape-recorded and transcribed later. If an interview is conducted by a computer, the interviewee uses an input device—for example, a keyboard or a touch screen—to answer questions and respond to statements.

Interviews for collecting research data are conducted in a manner similar to that used by clinicians for gathering case-history data. Consequently, a case-history interview is a type of a structured interview.

Questionnaires can either be administered personally or by mail. While the former is usually preferable, individuals who have the desired information cannot always be contacted personally without the expenditure of a great deal of time and money in travel. One problem that can be encountered when using mailed questionnaires is that the rate of return may be too low. This is particularly likely to occur if the questionnaire is relatively long (would take more than 5 minutes to complete) and/or those who are asked to complete it see no advantage to themselves in doing so. A questionnaire administered in this manner, therefore, should be kept as short as possible, and a strong case should be made the letter accompanying the questionnaire for why it would be advantageous to recipients to complete and return it. One way that it may be possible to make such a case is to offer to send a summary of the findings to those who do so. If the topic of a questionnaire is a "hot" one, such an offer may be sufficient to ensure a good return.

There are two types of response forms that can be used in questionnaires and structured interviews: closed-form and open-form. With the closed-form, or restricted, type you usually are asked to check items from a list of suggested responses. The following example illustrates the closed-form item:

Why did you choose to do graduate work at this university? Kindly indicate three reasons in order of importance, using the number 1 for the most important, 2 for the second most important, and 3 for the third most important.

		RANK
(a)	*ASHA accreditation*	_____
(b)	*Advice of someone*	_____
(c)	*Reputation of institution*	_____
(d)	*Expense factor*	_____
(e)	*Financial aid*	_____
(f)	*Location*	_____
(g)	*Other* _____ *(kindly indicate)*	_____

Even when using the closed-form type, it is a good idea to provide for unanticipated responses by including an "other" category.

The open-form, or unrestricted, type calls for a free response in the respondent's own words. The following item seeks the same type of information as in the previous example:

Why did you choose to do graduate work at this university?

While this type provides the possibility for greater depth of response than the closed-form one, the data it generates tend to be more difficult to interpret and summarize than those from the other. Both types, of course, can be used in the same questionnaire or structured interview.

Questionnaires and structured interviews are subject to the same sources of error as the other data-generating strategies discussed in this chapter.

Both questionnaires and structured interviews are used a great deal in educational and social science research. A number of books and articles have been written by investigators in these fields that can be helpful when designing a study in which they will be used. Three that I have found particularly helpful were written by Best and Kahn (1989), Chadwick, Bahr, and Albrecht (1984), and Henerson, Morris, and Fitz-Gibbon (1987).

Strategies That Rely Primarily on Observer Judgment: Psychological Scaling Methods

This section contains an overview of psychological scaling methods and their use for quantifying observable attributes of communicative behavior. Practical information needed to use them for this purpose is in Appendix C.

Need for Psychological Scaling Techniques in Speech, Language, and Hearing Research

Psychological scaling techniques provide a methodology for quantifying observable attributes of events with levels of validity and reliability that are sufficiently high for most purposes. An *event* is a phenomenon that occurs in a certain place during a particular interval of time. All events have attributes, or measurable properties (see Chapter 7 for a discussion of the relationship between events and attributes).

Speech can be classified as an event, since it is a "phenomenon that occurs in a certain place during a particular interval of time." Literally hundreds of attributes of speech have been delineated. (To prove this to yourself, examine the indexes of representative speech-language pathology and speech science texts.) Many have been defined on the basis of observer judgment. In fact, they *are* observer judgments. The observer is the "instrument" by which such attributes are abstracted from the speech signal.

After an attribute of speech has been identified by observers, investigators may attempt to identify the acoustical properties of the speech signal that result in observers detecting it. An example of an attribute that was studied in this manner is hypernasality. Investigators attempted to identify the acoustical properties of the speech signal that caused observers to detect hypernasality by creating speech samples that contained those that they thought contributed to it being heard. They then had groups of observers listen to the speech samples to determine whether they sounded hypernasal to them.

If you accept that at least some attributes of speech events are observer judgments, then for an instrumentation scheme for measuring, or quantifying, such attributes to have at least *face validity* (or appear intuitively to be valid), it would have to involve observer judgment. It would have to require one or more observers to indicate in some manner the amount of the target attribute present. Thus, the observer (or panel of observers) would function as a "measuring instrument" with his or her (their) judgments being the "readout." Judgments of the amount of a target attribute in a speech sample can be indicated by words, numbers, and marks on a line.

Psychological scaling techniques are methodologies that can be used for "measuring" the relative amounts of target attributes present in speech events through the use of observer judgments. With these methodologies, an observer (or panel of observers) is instructed to indicate in some manner the relative amount of a target attribute present in each of a group of stimuli (e.g., speech segments). Since they are based on observer judgment, these methodologies have *at least face validity* for measuring attributes of speech events that are observer judgments. As such, they can be quite useful to speech-language pathologists and audiologists because many of the attributes of events that are of interest to them are observer judgments.

How have psychological scaling methods been used in speech, language, and hearing research? What attributes have they been used to measure, or quantify? Due in large part to the pioneering methodological research of Professor Dorothy Sherman of the University of Iowa, psychological scaling methods have been used for quantifying numerous attributes of speech events. A partial list of such attributes is presented in Table 8-1. This list was compiled from a search of the first thirteen volumes of the *Journal of Speech and Hearing Research* for papers in which psychological scaling methods had been used. It includes most of the attributes that were scaled in the studies reported in these papers. The studies cited in Table 8-1, in addition to indicating applications that have been made of psychological scaling methods in speech, language, and hearing research, provide information that could be useful to investigators who wish to rate a set of stimuli for one or more of the attributes listed. Aspects of the scaling methodologies used by the investigators in the studies cited may be utilized by other investigators who wish to quantify these same attributes. Incidentally, most (if not all) of the papers cited were vetted by Professor Sherman and/or her students for methodological errors prior to publication.

Psychological Scaling Methods as Measuring Instruments

Psychological scaling methods are measuring instruments in the same sense that rulers and thermometers are, because they result in numerals being assigned to attributes of events that have certain characteristics (see Chapter 7). They have these characteristics because of the rules that are used to assign them. As indicated in Chapter 7, the rules used to assign numerals to attributes of events determine the meaning of the numerals—that is, the "level of measurement" of the scale that they define. A *scale* consists of a succession or progression of steps or degrees, or a graduated series of categories.

The "rules" used for assigning numerals with psychological scaling methods *theoretically* result in one of three types of scales: ordinal, interval, or ratio (the characteristics of each are described in Chapter 7). We emphasize "theoretically" to highlight the fact that psychological scaling methods do not always result in numerals, or ratings, that possess the characteristics they are supposed to possess (i.e., achieve the level of measurement they are supposed to achieve). There are several reasons why this may be the case. One of the most

TABLE 8-1   Representative Attributes of Events of Interest to Speech-Language Pathologists and Audiologists That Have Been Quantified by Means of Psychological Scaling Methods

Attribute	References
Abstraction of words, level of	II, 161
Articulation defectiveness, severity of	III, 191; III, 303
Articulation proficiency, degree of	VI, 49
Bizarreness, degree of	XII, 246
Breathiness, severity of	XII, 246; XII, 747
Difficulty of listening to compressed speech, degree of	XI, 875
Effeminate voice quality, degree of	IX, 590
Esophageal speech, acceptability of	X, 417
Favorability of description, degree of	X, 339
Force or strain while speaking, degree of	IV, 281
Foreign dialect, degree of	VIII, 43
General merit of speech sample, degree of	IX, 248; IX, 323
Harshness, severity of	I, 155; I, 344; XII, 246
Hoarseness, severity of	XII, 246
Intelligibility, degree of	XII, 246, XXIV, 441
Language development, level of	X, 41; X, 828
Language usage, intricacy of	XI, 837
Lipreading ability, level of	II, 340
Loudness, level of	XII, 103; XII, 246
Moment of nonfluency, severity of	I, 132
Nasal emission, severity of	XII, 246
Nasality, degree of	I, 383; II, 40; II, 113; IV, 381; V, 103; X, 549; XI, 553; XII, 246
Preference, degree of	1, 86; V, 370
Pitch, level of	XII, 246; XII, 747
Pitch variability, degree of	XII, 747
Quality of EDR audiometric records, level of	IV, 41
Representativeness to intended vowel, degree of	IV, 203
Rhythm pattern, normality of	IV, 281
Roughness, degree of	XII, 330
Sibilant intensity, level of	XII, 747
Similarity, degree of	VI, 239; VII, 310; VIII, 23; X, 225
Social adequacy, degree of	V, 79
Speaking rate, normality of	IV, 281; XII, 246; XII, 747
Stress, normality of	XII, 246
Stuttering severity, degree of	I, 40; I, 61; V, 256; V, 332; VI, 91; VIII, 263; VIII, 401; XIII, 360
Vowel imitation, abruptness of	I, 344

(Roman numerals refer to volumes of the *Journal of Speech and Hearing Research;* Arabic numbers to the first pages of papers in which the attributes were scaled.)

common is the inability of observers to assign numerals, or rate the stimuli, in the manner in which they are instructed.

We will use six psychological scaling methods to illustrate how numerals are assigned to attributes of events by observer judgments: paired, or pair, comparisons (Edwards, 1957); rank order, or order of merit (Guilford, 1954); equal-appearing intervals, or category scaling (Edwards, 1957); successive intervals, or successive categories, or graded dichotomies (Edwards, 1957); constant sums (Guilford, 1954); and direct magnitude-estimation (Prather, 1960). These psychological scaling methods, incidentally, are the ones that have been used most frequently in speech, language, and hearing research.

Paired (Pair) Comparisons

With this method, which theoretically results in an ordinal scale, all possible pairs of stimuli are compared to an *internally generated standard* (or scale) for the attribute being rated, or scaled, and the stimuli in each pair are ordered on the basis of the amount of the attribute that each is judged to possess. The task is performed by a group, or panel, of observers. Each observer is presented with all possible ordered pairings (i.e., permutations) of the stimuli. The number of such pairings for a set of stimuli (N) can be determined by multiplying the number of stimuli by the number of stimuli minus one, or

$$N (N - 1)$$

For a set of ten stimuli, the number of pairs rated would be

$$N (N - 1) = 10 (10 - 1) = 90$$

and for a set of 100 stimuli it would be

$$N (N - 1) = 100 (100 - 1) = 9900$$

Note how the number of pairs increases dramatically as the number of stimuli increases.

Observers are told to indicate the stimulus in each pair that possesses the greater amount of the attribute being scaled. They perform this task by comparing the amount of the target attribute they perceive in each of the two stimuli in it to their internal standard, or scale, for that attribute. For example, an observer who was presented with speech segments from two persons who have hypernasal speech and was asked to indicate which was the most hypernasal would perform this task by comparing the level of hypernasality he or she perceived in the two segments to his or her internal standard, or scale, for degree of hypernasality and, on the basis of these comparisons, would indicate which is the most hypernasal.

Rank Order (Order of Merit)

With this method, which theoretically results in an ordinal scale, sets of stimuli are compared to an internally generated standard, or scale, for the attribute being rated, and the stimuli in the set are ordered on the basis of the amount of the target attribute they are judged to possess. The task is performed by a group, or panel, of observers. Each observer is presented with the set of stimuli and is told to rank order them on the basis of the amounts of the target attribute that they possess. He or she is instructed to indicate the ordering of the stimuli by assigning the numeral to each stimulus that designates its position. The highest numeral assigned (N) is equal to the number of stimuli being ordered. Observers may be instructed to assign either 1 or N to the stimulus possessing the greatest amount of the target attribute. They rank order the stimuli by comparing the amount of the target attribute they perceive in each to their internal standard, or scale, for that attribute. For example, an observer who was presented with speech segments from five persons who have hypernasal speech and was told to order them on the basis of the amount of hypernasality they possess (with 1 designating least hypernasality and 5 designating most) would perform this task by comparing the level of hypernasality he or she perceived in the five segments to his or her internal standard, or scale, for degree of hypernasality and on the basis of these comparisons indicate the ordering of the stimuli.

This method can be viewed as an extension of the method of paired comparisons. The only real difference in the judging task is that observers are required to order N rather than two stimuli.

Equal-Appearing Intervals (Category Scaling)

With this method, which theoretically results in an interval scale, each of a set of stimuli is compared to an internally generated scale, or continuum, for the attribute being rated, which is *divided into a specified number of equal-size segments* (usually 5, 7, or 9), and the numeral is assigned to it that designates the segment of the internally generated continuum that corresponds to the amount of the attribute it is perceived to possess. The task is performed by a group, or panel, of observers. Stimuli are presented to observers one at a time. Observers are instructed to assign the numeral between 1 and the number that corresponds to the number of points on the scale (e.g., 7) to each stimulus that indicates the amount of the target attribute it possesses. They are informed that the scale is one of equal intervals—from 1 to 7 (or some other value)—with 1 representing the least possible amount of the target and 7 (or some other value) representing the greatest possible amount; 4 (or some other medial value) represents the midpoint between 1 and 7 with respect to the attribute, with the other numbers falling at *equal distances* along the scale. For example, an observer who was presented with speech segments from five persons who have hypernasal speech and was told to assign a numeral to each on the basis of the amount of hypernasality present (with 1 designating least possible hypernasality, 7 designating most possible hypernasality, and the numbers between falling at equal distances along the scale) would perform this task by comparing the amount of hypernasality he or she perceived in each speech segment to each of the seven segments of his or her internal scale for degree of hypernasality and on the basis of these comparisons assign each a numeral between 1 and 7. Observers may assign the same numeral to two or more speech segments. They would rate in such a manner if they felt the degree of hypernasality present in the segments fell within the same segment of their internal scales for hypernasality.

Equal-appearing intervals has been one of the most frequently used scaling methods for quantifying attributes of speech, language, and hearing. Recent studies that utilized it include the following: de Krom (1994), Finn and Ingham (1994), Kreiman, Gerratt, Kempster, Erman, and Berke ((1993), Martin and Haroldson (1992), Onslow, Hayes, et al. (1992), and Schiavetti, Martin, Haroldson, and Metz (1994).

Successive Intervals (Successive Categories; Graded Dichotomies)

With this method, which theoretically results in an interval scale, each of a set of stimuli is compared to an internally generated scale, or continuum, for the attribute being rated, which is divided into a specified number of segments (usually 5, 7, or 9) that are not necessarily of equal size, and the numeral is assigned to it that designates the segment of the internally generated continuum that corresponds to the amount of the attribute it is perceived to possess. The task is performed by a group, or panel, of observers. Stimuli are presented to observers one at a time. Observers are instructed to assign the numeral between 1 and the number that corresponds to the number of points on the scale (e.g., 7) to each stimulus that indicates the amount of the target attribute it possesses. They are informed that the scale contains a specified number of points, ranging from 1 to 7 (or some other value). In some instances, each point on the scale is *anchored*, or defined, and in others only the extremes are anchored. A 7-point scale (that could be used for assessing attitudes toward statements) on which each point is anchored is illustrated by the following:

_____ :	_____ :	_____ :	_____ :	_____ :	_____ :	_____
Completely Disagree (1)	Mostly Disagree (2)	Slightly Disagree (3)	Undecided (4)	Slightly Agree (5)	Mostly Agree (6)	Completely Agree (7)

On the other hand, such a scale may have only the extremes anchored:

Strongly
Disagree _____ : _____ : _____ : _____ : _____ : _____ : _____ Strongly Agree

         (1)   (2)   (3)   (4)   (5)   (6)   (7)

For example, an observer who was presented with speech segments from five persons who have hypernasal speech and was asked to assign a numeral between 1 and 7 to each on the basis of the amount of hypernasality exhibited by the speaker with the points on the scale defined as

1. No hypernasality
2. Extremely mild hypernasality
3. Mild hypernasality
4. Moderate hypernasality
5. Moderately severe hypernasality
6. Severe hypernasality
7. Extremely severe hypernasality

The observer would perform this task by comparing the amount of hypernasality he or she perceived in each speech segment to that designated by each of the seven modifiers on his or her internal scale of hypernasality and on the basis of these comparisons would assign each a numeral between 1 and 7. The observer may assign the same numeral to two or more speech segments if he or she feels the amount of hypernasality present in them is designated by the same modifier.

The main difference between the methods of equal-appearing intervals and successive intervals is the assumption made regarding the sizes of the segments of the internally generated scale for the attribute. With the method of equal-appearing intervals, these segments are assumed to be of equal size (e.g., the difference in degree of nasality between a speaker assigned the numeral 2 and a speaker assigned the numeral 3 and a speaker assigned the numeral 4, etc.). With the method of successive intervals, no assumption is made regarding the relative sizes of segment widths; the segment widths are estimated from the data.

Constant Sums

With this method, which theoretically results in a *ratio* scale, *all possible pairs* of stimuli are compared to an internally generated scale for the attribute being rated, and a judgment is made regarding the relative amount of the attribute possessed by each member of each pair. The proportion of 100 points is then assigned to each of the stimuli in each pair which reflects the relative amount of the attribute possessed by each member of each pair. The points assigned to the stimuli in each pair always total 100. To illustrate this method, suppose that one of the stimuli in a pair was judged to possess twice as much of a target attribute (e.g., nasality) as the other. The former would be assigned 67 points and the latter 33 points.

The task is performed by a group, or panel, of observers. Each observer is presented with all possible ordered pairings (i.e., permutations) of the stimuli to be scaled. The number of such pairings that will result from a set of stimuli of a given size (N) can be determined by multiplying the number of stimuli by the number of stimuli minus one, or

$$N (N - 1)$$

Note that the number of pairs of stimuli presented to observers is the same as for the method of pair comparisons.

Observers are told to indicate for each pair of stimuli both the stimulus that possesses the greater amount of the target attribute and the *ratio* of the amount of the attribute this stimulus possesses in relation to that possessed by the other stimulus through proportional point assignments to the two stimuli. (Note that the first part of the judging task is the same as for the method of pair comparisons). They perform this task by comparing the amount of the target attribute they perceive in each of the two stimuli in a pair to their internal scale for that attribute. For example, an observer who was presented with speech segments from two persons who have hypernasal speech and was asked to indicate how much more hypernasal the most hypernasal speaker was than the least hypernasal speaker (through a proportional assignment of 100 points) would perform this task by comparing the levels of hypernasality he or she perceived in the two segments to his or her internal scale for degree of hypernasality and on the basis of these comparisons would make the point assignments. Observers could make any point assignments they wished as long as the points totaled 100 and portrayed the ratio of degree of hypernasality exhibited by the two speakers.

Direct Magnitude-Estimation

With this method, which theoretically results in a ratio scale, each of a set of stimuli is compared *to a point* on an internally generated scale, or continuum, for the attribute being rated, and a numeral is assigned to each stimulus that designates the relative amount of the attribute that it possesses as compared to the amount of the attribute at that point on the internally generated scale. If the point on the internally generated scale that is serving as the standard were assigned a value of 100 points, and a stimulus to be rated were judged to possess three times the amount of the attribute as the standard, it would be assigned 300 points. If a stimulus, on the other hand, were judged to possess one-half as much of the attribute as the standard, it would be assigned 50 points.

The rating task is performed by a group, or panel, of observers. Stimuli are presented one at a time. The observers are presented with a stimulus of the type they will be rating to use as a standard, prior to beginning the rating task. The amount of the target attribute present in this stimulus (the standard stimulus) is assigned a value of 100 points. The observers are instructed to assign the number of points to each stimulus representing the relative amount of the target attribute it possesses with reference to that possessed by the standard stimulus. If, for example, the observers felt a stimulus possessed twice the amount of the target attribute as the standard stimulus, they would assign it 200 points. If, on the other hand, they felt it possessed only half the amount of the target attribute as the standard, they would assign it 50 points. They can use any point assignment they feel appropriate. They need not limit themselves to even fractions and even multiples of the 100 points assigned to the standard. They can use any point assignment they choose as long as it represents their judgment of the amount of the target attribute possessed by a stimulus in relation to that possessed by the standard. If, for example, observers were presented with speech segments from five persons who have hypernasal speech and were told to assign points to each on the basis of the amount of hypernasality each possesses in relation to that present in the speech segment of a sixth person (standard), which is assigned 100 points, they would perform this task by comparing the amount of hypernasality they perceived in each speech segment they were asked to rate and in the standard segment to their internal scale for degree of hypernasality, and on the basis of these comparisons they would assign each stimulus a number of points. The standard would serve as an *anchor* to align their internal scales of hypernasality. They can assign the same number of points to two or more speech segments if they feel the speakers in these segments exhibit the same amounts of hypernasality.

Direct magnitude-estimation has been one of the most frequently used scaling methods for quantifying attributes of speech, language, and hearing. A recent study that utilized it was Schiavetti et al. (1994).

Considerations in the Choice of a Scaling Method

Six scaling methods were described in the previous section. What factors should you consider when deciding which to use for quantifying a particular attribute of a particular set of stimuli? Ten that you should consider are the following: (1) the minimum level of measurement required, (2) the number of stimuli to be rated, (3) the maximum number of the judges available, (4) the age and intelligence level of judges, (5) computational ease, (6) the maximum length of a judging session, (7) the necessity that ratings for stimuli scaled at different times be comparable, (8) the statistical sophistication of the audience to whom the results are to be reported, (9) the duration of individual stimuli, and (10) the judges' reactions to the scaling task. In this section we will consider how each can affect the choice of a scaling method.

Minimum Level of Measurement Required

The consideration here is whether the minimum acceptable level of measurement for judges' ratings is ordinal, interval, or ratio. This level usually can be inferred from the *kinds of statements* you want to be able to make about the ratings or the *kinds of questions* you want to be able to answer using them. If, for example, you decided to rate "before and after" therapy speech samples for hypernasality and you wanted to make a judgment from these ratings on whether the clients were less hypernasal after therapy than before it, only *ordinal* measurement would be required. On the other hand, if you wanted to be able to make a judgment regarding the *amount of reduction* in hypernasality following therapy (assuming there was such a reduction), *ratio* measurement would be required.

Any of the six scaling methods can be used if only *ordinal* measurement is required. It has been demonstrated empirically that they order sets of stimuli in the same manner.

If the minimum level of measurement required is *interval*, then equal-appearing intervals, successive intervals, constant sums, or direct magnitude-estimation could be used. If observers perform the rating tasks *as instructed*, these methods should result in ratings that have properties that *approximate* (or come close to achieving) interval level measurement.

If *ratio* measurement is required, either constant sums or direct magnitude-estimation can be used. Both methods should result in ratings with properties approximating those for ratio level measurement *if* the observers perform the rating tasks as instructed.

Number of Stimuli to Be Rated

If the number of stimuli to be rated were fewer than ten, this probably would not be an important consideration. However, if this number exceeds ten, three of the scaling methods (i.e., pair comparisons, rank order, and constant sums) may not be practical. The reason for pair comparisons and constant sums is that too many stimulus pairs may have to be rated. As I have already indicated, the number of stimulus pairs that have to be rated when these methods are used is the product of the number of stimuli times this number minus one, or

$$N(N-1)$$

For twenty stimuli, the number of stimulus pairs would be

$$20(20-1)$$

or 380. Obtaining 380 ratings would probably be too time-consuming in most instances. Pair comparisons and constant sums would rarely be practical when the number of stimuli to be scaled exceeded ten.

The method of rank order may also be impractical when the number of stimuli to be scaled exceeds ten, because it may be too difficult for an observer to keep in mind the amount of the target attribute possessed by each stimulus while ordering them. This is particularly likely to be the case when the stimuli, or events, to be ordered are auditory (e.g., speech segments).

Maximum Number of Judges Available

Some scaling methods require larger panels than others to achieve scale values that possess a given level of reliability. Equal-appearing intervals, for example, tend to require fewer judges to achieve scale values that have a given level of reliability than does direct magnitude-estimation. Also, a variation of direct magnitude-estimation in which an interval rather than a point standard is used (referred to as direct interval-estimation) appears to require fewer raters than direct magnitude-estimation to achieve scale values that have a given level of reliability (Silverman & Johnston, 1975).

Age and Intelligence Level of the Judges

Some rating tasks are more difficult than others. The task associated with the method of pair comparisons probably would be easier for both children and adults with below-normal intelligence than those associated with the other scaling methods.

Computational Ease

Some scaling methods require less computation than others to derive scale values. Equal-appearing interval scale values, for example, require less computation than successive interval scale values. While computational ease probably would not be one of the first considerations in selecting a scaling method, it nevertheless would probably make sense if two or more methods would serve *equally well* to select the one that requires the least amount of computation.

Maximum Length of a Judging Session

The number of stimuli that can be rated in a given amount of time is different for different methods. Fewer stimuli can be rated in a given amount of time with pair comparisons and constant sums than with the other methods. Equal-appearing intervals, successive intervals, and direct magnitude-estimation would probably require approximately the same amount of time to rate a given number of stimuli. The time required for rank order is apt to be longer than for equal-appearing intervals, successive intervals, or direct magnitude-estimation, particularly if the number of stimuli to be ranked is relatively large or the differences in the amounts of the target attribute they possess are relatively small.

Necessity That Ratings for Stimuli Scaled at Different Times Be Comparable

With some scaling methods, the rating assigned to a stimulus to indicate the amount of the target attribute it possesses is apt to be influenced by the amount of that attribute present in the other stimuli with which it is rated. This is almost certain to be a problem when the methods of pair comparison, constant sums, and rank order are used. If it is necessary for ratings for stimuli scaled at different times to be comparable, the safest method to use probably would be direct magnitude-estimation (assuming the same standard stimulus is used for rating all stimuli).

Statistical Sophistication of the Audience to Whom the Results Are to Be Reported

Some scaling methods require a better statistical background to understand intuitively than do others. Equal-appearing intervals, for example, would not require as much statistical sophistication to understand as would successive intervals. While this would not usually be one of the main considerations in the choice of a scaling method, if two or more methods would be equally appropriate for a particular purpose, it would probably make sense to choose the one requiring the least statistical sophistication to understand, or interpret.

Duration of Individual Stimuli

The duration of individual stimuli may be a relevant consideration in the choice of a scaling method, particularly with regard to the practicality of pair comparisons and constant sums. If their duration is relatively long, the judges may not be able to remember both members of a pair well enough to make a pair comparison or constant sum rating that is adequately reliable. Also, if their duration is relatively long, the number of stimuli that could be rated in a given period of time by these methods may be too few to be practical.

Judges' Reactions to the Scaling Task

Observers' "levels of belief" in their abilities to perform rating tasks are apt not to be a constant. They would probably be more confident of their ability to make pair comparison judgments than direct magnitude-estimation judgments. If they do not believe they can perform the rating task they are asked to perform, they may not try too hard and consequently, their ratings may not be adequately reliable.

For further information about methodological considerations when designing scaling experiments, see Appendix C.

Strategies That Rely Primarily on Observer Judgment: Observation with Systematic Classification

Observation with systematic classification has been one of the main strategies used for generating data to answer questions in all research areas. It has been utilized by speech-language pathologists and audiologists for clinical as well as research purposes. A clinician, for example, who *classifies* a client's voice as "breathy" based on *observation* of his or her speech during an evaluation session is using it. So also is one who on the basis of a phonological analysis on a sample of a child's speech describes him or her as evincing certain sound substitutions and/or omissions.

Data generated in this way usually consists of "words," though the data can have a numerical component. It involves assigning attributes of an event you have observed to categories. "Stuttering severity," for example, would be an attribute of the event "speaking behavior." The category to which this attribute would be assigned would be either "mild," "moderate," or "severe." Other labels or sets of categories, of course, could be substituted—e.g., the set of seven categories that define the *Iowa Scale of Stuttering Severity* (Johnson, Darley, & Spriestersbach, 1963). If this scale were used, each category would be designated by a numeral between 1 and 7. These numerals would possess the attributes of those on a nominal scale and possibly also those on an ordinal one (see Chapter 7).

The process used here is quite similar to that described in the preceding section. Both psychological scaling techniques and those utilizing observation with systematic classification involve assigning attributes of events to categories. With the former, the categories are designated by numerals that possess ordinal, interval, or ratio scale characteristics (see Chapter 7). With the latter, on the other hand, the categories are either designated by words (or phrases) or by numerals that have nominal scale (and possibly also ordinal scale) characteristics. The mental processes involved are the same—the only difference is the manner in which categories are designated and defined.

Data derived from observation with systematic classification are subject to the same types of error as are those derived from psychological scaling techniques and the other strategies described in this chapter. They are neither more nor less likely than the others to yield "incorrect" answers!

For further information about the use of observation with systematic classification for generating data in behavioral research, see Best and Kahn (1989).

Exercises and Discussion Topics

1. You are to rate each of five utterances for "degree of syntactic complexity" by means of six psychological scaling methods: pair comparisons, rank order, equal-appearing intervals, successive intervals, constant sums, and direct magnitude-estimation. The utterances are:
   a. "David is tired."
   b. "Yes."
   c. "She ate a lot of candy."
   d. "My father really wanted to help us, but he didn't have time."
   e. "Fortunately, Ted has plenty of money."

Pair Comparisons

Instructions. Printed below are five pairs of utterances in a random order. Indicate whether you feel the first or second utterance in each pair is most *complex* syntactically.

   a. "Fortunately, Ted has plenty of money."
      "My father really wanted to help us, but he didn't have time."
   b. "David is tired."
      "Yes."
   c. "Fortunately, Ted has plenty of money."
      "David is tired."
   d. "My father really wanted to help us, but he didn't have time."
      "Yes."
   e. "She ate a lot of candy."
      "My father really wanted to help us, but he didn't have time."

Rank Order

Instructions. Printed below are five utterances in a random order. Assign a number between 1 and

5 to each that indicates its relative degree of syntactic complexity as compared to the other four utterances. Assign 1 to the utterance you feel is most complex syntactically and 5 to the utterance you feel is least complex syntactically. Do not assign the same number (or rank) to more than one utterance.

   a. "David is tired."
   b. "Yes."
   c. "My father really wanted to help us, but he didn't have time."
   d. "She ate a lot of candy."
   e. "Fortunately, Ted had plenty of money."

Equal-Appearing Intervals

Instructions. Printed below are five utterances in a random order. Assign a number to each that designates its location on a 7-point scale of "syntactic complexity." The scale is one of equal intervals—from 1 to 7—with 1 representing *least* possible syntactic complexity and 7 representing *most* possible syntactic complexity; 4 represents the midpoint between 1 and 7 with respect to complexity, with the other numbers falling at equal distances along the scale. Do not attempt to place utterances between any two of the seven points, but only at these points. You, of course, can assign the same number to two or more utterances if you feel they are equivalent with regard to syntactic complexity.

   a. "David is tired."
   b. "Yes."
   c. "My father really wanted to help us, but he didn't have time."

d. "She ate a lot of candy."

e. "Fortunately, Ted has plenty of money."

Successive Intervals

Instructions. Printed below are five utterances in a random order. Assign a number to each that designates its location on a 7-point scale of "syntactic complexity." On the scale 1 represents *least* possible syntactic complexity and 7 represents *most* possible syntactic complexity; 4 represents the midpoint between 1 and 7 with respect to complexity. Do not attempt to place utterances between any two of the seven points, but only at these points. You, of course, can assign the same number to two or more utterances if you feel they are equivalent with regard to syntactic complexity.

a. "David is tired."

b. "Yes."

c. "My father really wanted to help us, but he didn't have time."

d. "She ate a lot of candy."

e. "Fortunately, Ted has plenty of money."

Constant Sums

Instructions. Printed below are five pairs of utterances in a random order. Assign points to the two utterances in each pair so that the total number of points assigned to the utterances in a pair is 100. The proportion of 100 points assigned to each of the utterances in a pair should reflect the relative amount of syntactic complexity possessed by each member of the pair. If, for example, you felt that one utterance in a pair was twice as complex syntactically as was the other, you would assign it 67 points and the other 33 points.

a. "Fortunately, Ted has plenty of money."
   "My father really wanted to help us, but he didn't have time."

b. "David is tired."
   "Yes."

c. "Fortunately, Ted has plenty of money."
   "David is tired."

d. "Fortunately, Ted has plenty of money."
   "Yes."

e. "She ate a lot of candy."
   "David is tired."

Direct Magnitude Estimation

Instructions. Printed below are five utterances in a random order. Assign the number of points to each utterance that you believe represents its relative degree of syntactic complexity with reference to the following *standard* utterance that has been assigned a value of 100 points.

"She works hard."

The point assignment you make to each utterance should represent, with reference to the standard, its relative syntactic complexity. For example, if you feel that an utterance is *twice* as complex syntactically as the standard, you assign it *200 points*. On the other hand, if you feel that an utterance is *half* as complex syntactically as the standard, you assign it *50 points*. You may, of course, use any point assignment you wish to represent your judgment of an utterance's syntactic complexity so long as it represents your judgment of the syntactic complexity of the utterance in relation to the standard utterance.

a. "David is tired."

b. "Yes."

c. "My father really wanted to help us, but he didn't have time."

d. "She ate a lot of candy."

e. "Fortunately, Ted has plenty of money."

2. Three speech-language pathologists rated a videotaped sample of stuttered speech on a 7-point equal-appearing interval scale of stuttering severity. The first assigned it a 2 (mild); the second a 4 (moderate); and the third a 6 (severe). What factors might account for the differences in their ratings?

3. How might psychological scaling techniques be used clinically (e.g., for assessing therapy outcome)?

4. Describe an instrumentation scheme for measurement (see Figure 8-1) that is used clinically by either speech-language pathologists or audiologists.

Organizing Data for Answering Questions: I. Descriptive Techniques

Once the data have been gathered—whether qualitative or quantitative—they have to be organized, or structured, in a manner that will permit the questions that they are intended to answer to be answered. If this isn't done, the answers that they yield are less likely to be accurate than they are otherwise. You can easily be deceived if you attempt to answer questions merely by skimming through, or eyeballing, the data. You may, for example, inadvertently give too much weight or too little weight to certain aspects of your data, possibly as a function of experimenter bias (see Chapter 8). Suppose a question you were attempting to answer concerned the effectiveness of a particular therapy, and to answer it you recorded a number of observations (both qualitative and quantitative) before and after administration of the therapy to twenty persons who had a certain communicative disorder. If you skim the available data, you might tend to pay more attention to aspects of it that suggest the treatment was effective than to those that suggest it had little or no effect. Another clinician whose theoretical orientation would give him or her a set not to find the therapy effective might tend to pay more attention to aspects of the data that suggest the treatment had little or no effect. Thus, two persons skimming the same data could arrive at different answers to a question if they had different expectations, or sets (biases).

Another reason why you can be deceived easily if you attempt to answer questions merely by skimming data is that the data needed to answer a particular question may not stand out sufficiently from the other data in the set in which it is included to provide an accurate answer to the question. The problem here can be viewed as one of an inadequate separation between figure and background, or between signal and noise. To illustrate this problem, suppose you wished to answer the following question: "How was the communicative behavior of a group of aphasics different following therapy?" If you merely skimmed the pre- and post-therapy observations you had recorded in their folders rather than systematically abstracting, organizing, and summarizing these observations, you might not be able to get a sufficiently good impression of how this behavior was different to answer the question accurately. It would be difficult, if not impossible, to remember all the relevant observations recorded in the folders.

A third reason (which is related to the second) why skimming the data can be deceptive is that the number of observations that are relevant for answering a question is large. It may not be possible to integrate them sufficiently to arrive at an accurate answer without first organizing and summarizing them.

Four approaches are described in this chapter for organizing and summarizing sets of data for answering questions. They are narrative description, tabular presentation, statistical analysis, and graphical display. The first two are the ones customarily used for organizing and summarizing qualitative data. And the last three are those customarily used for organizing and summarizing quantitative data. The approaches used for organizing and summarizing qualitative data are described in the next section and those used for doing so with quantitative data in the one that follows it.

Strategies for Organizing Qualitative Data for Answering Questions

Our primary focus in this section will be on the organization of qualitative (i.e., verbal descriptive) data for clinical case studies. This is the context in which speech-language pathologists and audiologists have used such data most frequently.

Before you can summarize and organize observations to answer a question, you must first *abstract* from the available data the observations that are relevant for answering it. Suppose you administered three articulation tests to a child both before and after she received a particular program of therapy and had transcribed her responses to the test stimuli phonemically. These transcriptions, of course, would be qualitative data. If one of your questions was whether her production of /s/ at the beginnings of words was any different after the period of therapy than preceding it, to answer it you would have to abstract the data on the production of /s/ in the initial position from the remaining articulation test data.

After you abstract the data relevant for answering a question, your next task is to summarize and organize it. For example, a child's production of /s/ in the initial position in words as sampled by three articulation tests before and after a period of therapy can be summarized and organized in tabular form (see Table 9-1).

After the data have been summarized and organized, they can be used to answer the question they are intended to answer. The data in Table 9-1, for example, were intended to answer the following question: "Did the child produce /s/ correctly in the initial position of words following therapy?" These data indicate that the production of /s/ was different following therapy on all three articulation tests. Specifically, they indicate that /s/ was produced correctly in the initial positions of words following therapy (at least in the words sampled by these articulation tests and in the situation in which they were administered).

Abstracting Relevant Data

It is necessary to abstract from the available observations, or data, those that *may* be relevant for answering each of the questions posed. The word "may" is emphasized because it

TABLE 9-1   A Child's Production of /s/ in the Initial Position in Words as Sampled before and after Therapy by Three Articulation Tests

Articulation Test	Before-Therapy Production	After-Therapy Production
I	/θ/	/s/
II	/θ/	/s/
III	/θ/	/s/

is not always possible to determine at this stage of the process which will contribute to answering a particular question. If there is any reason to believe that an observation may do so, it should be abstracted.

One strategy that can facilitate the abstraction process is recording each observation on a card. To answer a question, you would then select the cards from the pile that contain data that can contribute to doing so. This is usually a better strategy than reading through a large set of data and attempting to remember those that can contribute to answering a question.

An alternative strategy to the one described in the preceding paragraph is entering each observation as a record in a computer database file. Each such record would be the computer equivalent of a card. To identify those relevant for answering a particular question, you could BROWSE through the records ("cards") in the database file and/or use the program's FIND function to locate those containing certain words. The information contained in some or all of these records could be printed "as is" or transferred electronically to a word-processing program for inclusion in a report or other document.

Organizing and Summarizing Relevant Data

After the observations that may be relevant for answering a question have been abstracted, they are organized and summarized in a manner that permits the question to be answered. Several approaches can be used here. First, the data can be organized in tabular form, that is, summarized in a table. To illustrate the possibilities for organizing and summarizing qualitative data in tabular form, Table 9-2 presents references to tables containing qualitative data from two issues of the *Journal of Speech and Hearing Research.*

A second approach for organizing and summarizing is to set down the qualitative observations in narrative form. Speech-language pathologists and audiologists typically use this approach in evaluation reports for summarizing relevant observations (both formal and informal) made on clients. They also typically use this approach for daily logs of therapy sessions.

This approach is employed in most clinical case studies for summarizing and organizing qualitative observations. The following two paragraphs from case studies illustrate this application:

Subject 1 in Condition A usually produced touch velopharyngeal closure and his port configuration was oval. . . . Openings lateral to midline palate-posterior pha-

TABLE 9-2   References to Tables That Were Used to Organize and Summarize Qualitative Data in Two Issues of the *Journal of Speech and Hearing Research*

| | Reference | | |
Data Tabulated	Volume	Year	Pages
Occurrences of verbs in language samples	38	1995	1078–1080
Parent-offspring classification comparisons	38	1995	1100
Summary of studies examining transparency of Amer-Ind	38	1995	1285
Pragmatic parameters rated inappropriate on the Pragmatic Protocol	38	1995	1310
Characteristics of four individuals with hearing loss	38	1995	1389

ryngeal wall contact often were observed in this subject. The subject elevated his palate so it usually contacted the posterior pharyngeal wall. The uvula contracted during two trials. Only one lateral pharyngeal wall or palatopharyngeus muscle could be seen at one time, and it moved toward midline only on one trial and then gag was involved. The subject reported gag on three trials. The subject frequently produced a Passavant's ridge. The ridge varied across trials from slight to marked displacement. No other forward movement of the posterior wall of the pharynx was observed. Laryngeal click was usually heard at the end of trials. (Shelton, Paesani, McClelland, Bradfield, 1975, p. 238)

Once the desired pitch had been obtained, we directed Craig to continue producing phrases. He progressed quickly and by the third therapy session was able to converse using his new voice, which tended to confirm the nonorganic basis of the voice problem. Occasional pitch breaks occurred, however, and the somewhat hoarse quality persisted. Samples of conversational speech and reading were then tape-recorded so he could identify and tabulate instances when he reverted to the old pitch. At that stage both Craig and his mother were pleased with the results of therapy and encouraged. Others had also commented on his improvement. The stabilization phase of therapy continued in the speech clinic and then in various other places where Craig was often accompanied by the clinician. During the last few sessions we observed consistently low pitch and a voice quality that was almost clear of roughness. To evaluate Craig's voice in more stressful situations, one clinician attended his English class; the voice was clear, of natural pitch, and audible to those sitting in the back of the room. With the great satisfaction of Craig and his mother and with our confidence, it was mutually agreed to terminate therapy six weeks after its initiation. An interview two months later revealed that Craig's voice had remained consistently normal. (Yairi, 1974, p. 375)

Note the degree of similarity between (1) the first paragraph and an excerpt from an evaluation report, and (2) the second paragraph and an excerpt from a progress note regarding the impact of therapy on a client.

Summarizing and organizing qualitative data involves the assignment of observations to *categories*. This is true regardless of whether the data are presented in tabular or in narrative form.

There are several types of sets of category to which observations can be assigned. Some are spatial, some are temporal, some are a combination of spatial and temporal, and some are neither of these two. An example of a set of *spatial* categories is "right ear" and "left ear." An example of a set of *temporal* categories is "status prior to receiving therapy" and "status following therapy." An example of a set of *spatial-temporal* categories is "status of left ear prior to therapy" and "status of left ear following therapy." And, finally, an example of a set of categories that is *neither temporal nor spatial* is "receptive language" and "expressive language."

The categories to which observations are assigned are determined by the data needed to answer the question or questions asked. If you wished to determine, for example, whether a client's speech articulation were any different after a period of therapy than prior to it, the two categories to which you would assign your observations would undoubtedly be "speech articulation prior to therapy" and "speech articulation following therapy." On the other hand, if your questions concerned the status of a client's speech, language, and hearing (e.g., for inclusion in an evaluation report), several of the categories to which you could assign observations would be "hearing acuity," "speech fluency," "language usage," and "voice quality."

A given observation may be assigned to more than one category and used to answer more than one question. Suppose a speech-language pathologist showed a pencil to a person who had had a stroke and asked this person to name and describe it. Further suppose that the speech-language pathologist regarded the response as appropriate and all phonemes as correctly articulated. This observation, or judgment, could be assigned to more than one category and could be used to answer more than one question. For example, it could be assigned to the category of "receptive language functioning" and could be used to answer the question: "Does the person exhibit a disturbance in receptive language functioning?" It could also be assigned to the category "dysarthria" and could be used to answer the question: "Does the person exhibit any disturbances in the functioning of the articulators for speech?" Other categories to which this observation could be assigned include "auditory acuity," "auditory perceptual functioning," "conceptual functioning," and "word-finding ability."

The discussion in this section provides only a very general introduction to the organization and analysis of qualitative data. If you wish to pursue this topic further, you may find information in the sociology literature about participant observation in field research useful. You may also find useful the paper by Hinds, Scandrett-Hibden, and McAulay (1990) and the book by Bromley (1986), which deals with this topic in the context of individual case studies.

Strategies for Organizing and Summarizing Quantitative Data for Answering Questions

The remainder of this chapter is devoted to a discussion of strategies for organizing and summarizing quantitative data by using descriptive statistics, graphical displays, and tables. For statistics, the discussion emphasizes when it is appropriate to use each and how each is interpreted, rather than the mathematical model which underlies it. To develop an intuitive understanding of what statistics are and what they can do, it is necessary to have at least a little experience computing them. A computational appendix has been included to provide such experience for descriptive as well as inferential statistics (see Appendix A). The latter are discussed in Chapter 10. This appendix contains computational formulas, worked examples, Minitab software computational procedures, and exercises (including answers).

The statistical methods in the computational appendix should be regarded as representative rather than exhaustive. This is particularly true for inferential statistical methods. While this appendix contains an appropriate test of statistical significance for almost any set of data, these tests constitute only a small sample of those that have been developed. They were selected because they are ones that have been used most often by speech-language pathologists and audiologists, judging by research reports published in the journals of the American Speech-Language-Hearing Association.

All statistics in Appendix A are computed from a single set of data, which consists of frequencies per 100 words spoken of four types of speech disfluency (i.e., interjection of sounds and syllables, part-word repetition, word repetition, and revision-incomplete phrase) for each of fifty-six elementary school children. This set of data was selected because it can be segmented in ways that make it possible to compute all of the statistics in the appendix.

Descriptive Statistics

Descriptive statistics describe an aspect, or attribute, of a set of measures, that is, of a set of quantitative data. They provide indices for specific attributes of the distribution of the data in such a set. The data tabulated in the table at the beginning of Appendix A illustrate this concept. The frequencies of interjection, part-word repetition, word repetition, and revision-incomplete phrase presented in this table for 56 children (a total of 224 measures) constitute a set of quantitative data.

If you were to skim the 224 measures in this table *without looking at the column headings,* they probably would provide little information about the disfluency production of these children. About the only question they would permit you to answer reliably about the children's disfluency production would be: "Were the children homogeneous with regard to the amount of disfluency they produced?" Merely skimming these data would be sufficient to establish that they were not homogeneous with regard to this aspect of their disfluency because their frequencies were different for example, 4.83 is not the same as 0.00.

Before these data could be used for answering other questions about these children's disfluency production, they would have to be organized and summarized. The organization and summarization of quantitative data, like qualitative data, involves the assignment of observations to *categories.* Some such categories have nominal scale characteristics. Others have ordinal, interval, ratio, or logarithmic scale characteristics (see Chapter 7 for a description of these measurement scales). The assignment of measures to a set of categories results in a *distribution.* To illustrate the concept of distribution, let us again refer to the data table in Appendix A. The categories "interjection," "part-word repetition," "word repetition," and "revision-incomplete phrase" define a nominal scale; the 56 measures that are assigned to each constitute a distribution. Furthermore, the categories "second grade," "third grade," "fourth grade," "fifth grade," and "sixth grade" define an ordinal scale and the measures that are assigned to each also constitute a distribution.

Thus far we have only considered what are referred to as *univariate* distributions. The characteristic of such distributions is that observations are assigned to categories on the basis of only a single attribute of the data. With respect to our illustration, this attribute would be either the type of disfluency or the grade level of the child producing the disfluency.

It may be advantageous in some instances to categorize observations on the basis of more than one attribute. The resulting distribution would be a *multivariate* one. The type of multivariate distribution encountered most frequently in speech and hearing research is the *bivariate* one. In such distributions, observations are assigned to categories on the basis of two of their attributes. The data table in Appendix A can be viewed as a bivariate distribution. Each of the 224 measures can be regarded as having been assigned to one of the twenty joint categories, or cells. The resulting distribution, or matrix, is illustrated in Table 9-3. The number in each cell indicates how many of the 224 measures were assigned to it.

The data table in Appendix A provides some information about the disfluency production of the children whose speech was sampled. Merely skimming these data as categorized provides the information necessary to answer at least one question: "Did the children tend to produce more revisions and incomplete phrases than interjections?" A casual inspection of these data suggests that the frequencies for revision-incomplete phrase tend to be higher than those for interjection. On the other hand, merely skimming these data would probably not be sufficient to answer the question: "How much more frequently did the children tend to produce revisions and incomplete phrases than they did interjections?" To answer this question and most others these data would be appropriate for answering, further organizing and summarizing of the data are necessary. *Descriptive statistics* can be used for this purpose.

What do descriptive statistics describe? What sorts of questions are they helpful in answering? These questions will be considered in the three sections that follow. The first deals with measures of *central tendency;* the second, measures of *variability;* and the third, measures of *association.*

TABLE 9-3   Data Table from Appendix A Viewed as a Bivariate Distribution

	I	PW	W	R-IP
Second Grade	15	15	15	15
Third Grade	11	11	11	11
Fourth Grade	9	9	9	9
Fifth Grade	11	11	11	11
Sixth Grade	10	10	10	10

Measures of Central Tendency

These indices designate the "average," "typical," or most frequently occurring number in a set of numbers. A number provided by such an index is regarded as *representative* (in some respect) of the numbers in the set from which it was computed.

When the numbers in the set from which indices of central tendency are computed are measures of attributes of persons or of behaviors, they provide information concerning the average, typical, or most frequently occurring amount of an attribute. They designate an amount, or magnitude, of an attribute that in some respect can be regarded as "representative" of that present in the set. If the numbers in a set were scores on a test of language proficiency that had been administered to a class of kindergarten children, it would be possible to designate through the use of indices of central tendency: (1) the average score earned by these children, (2) the score earned by the "typical" member of the class, and (3) the score earned most often by the children in the class. Similarly, if the numbers in a set were a particular stutterer's stuttering frequencies in fifteen situations, you could designate through the use of these indices: (1) the average rate at which he or she stuttered in these situations, (2) the rate at which he or she stuttered that was most typical, and (3) the rate at which he or she stuttered most often. The values yielded for these three types of "representativeness" will be quite similar in some instances and quite dissimilar in others.

There are three commonly used measures of central tendency: the *mean,* the *median,* and the *mode.* Each describes one of the types of representativeness referred to in the preceding paragraph. Computational formulas, Minitab commands, and worked examples for all three are in Appendix A.

The *mean* is probably the most commonly used measure of central tendency, in part because it is usually the easiest to compute. It is merely an arithmetic average: You add together the scores (or other numbers) you wish to average and divide the total by the number of them that were added.

The mean can be used to answer questions such as these:

1. How many hours of therapy did the average child receive?
2. How long, on the average, was a particular cerebral palsied child able to sustain the vowel /a/ during a series of 10 trials?
3. Did the children tend to be less "nasal" following a particular type of cleft palate surgery than before?

Note that answering the first question requires averaging a single measure (i.e., time) from a number of persons; the second, a number of measures from a single person. The mean can be used as a measure of central tendency for both intersubject and intrasubject measures. The third question was included to indicate that the mean sometimes is used to describe the performance of persons *as a group.* Other measures of central tendency also may be used for this purpose.

Strictly speaking, measures from which a mean is computed must have interval or ratio properties (see Chapter 7). If the properties of such measures do not include equal intervals between scale points, their mean may not be readily interpretable with regard to the magnitude, or amount, of an attribute it represents. Suppose you administered a language test to a group of children on three occasions—before, halfway through, and after completing a program of therapy—and the means of their scores at these three points were 80, 110, and 120, respectively. If these scores could be assumed to have interval or ratio properties and be *reliable,* the following conclusions would be possible:

1. The children performed better after participating in the therapy program.
2. They exhibited some improvement halfway through the program.
3. The amount of improvement they exhibited tended to be greater during the first than the second half of the program.

If, on the other hand, the scores could only be assumed to have ordinal properties (see Chapter 7), the third conclusion would not be possible. Without being able to assume equal intervals between scale points, you would have no way of knowing whether greater improvement occurred during the first or second half of the therapy program. That is, if the scores on this test lacked the equal interval property, a child could conceivably have to modify his or her language behavior less to go from 80 to 110 than to go from 110 to 120.

Means, as well as other statistics that require measures to have interval or ratio properties, have been used in speech, language, and hearing research (and in other behavioral science areas) with measures that have only *ordinal* properties. The argument against using such statistics with ordinal data can be summarized as follows:

> *In developing procedures, mathematical statisticians have assumed that techniques involving numerical orderings, or categorization, are to be applied when these numbers or classes are appropriate and meaningful within the experimenter's problem. If the statistical method involves the procedures of arithmetic used on numerical scores, then the numerical answer is formally correct. Even if the numbers are the purest nonsense, having no relation to real magnitudes or the properties of real things, the answers are still right* as numbers. *The difficulty comes with the* interpretation of these numbers back into statements about the real world *[emphasis added]. If nonsense is put into a mathematical system, nonsense is sure to come out. (Hays, 1973, p. 74)*

Thus, while means and other statistics that are appropriate for measures having interval or ratio properties can be computed from numbers having the properties of any measurement scale—even those with nominal properties such as numerals on the backs of football players—they may not lead to accurate answers because of the difficulty of translating them back into statements about the real world.

While the mean is an appropriate measure of central tendency for data having interval or ratio scale properties, it is not necessarily a good index of representativeness for such data. A mean value may not designate the number most representative of a set. In fact, it may designate a number that *never occurs* in the set of which it is supposed to be representative. An example would be the statement that in 1973 the average household contained 3.48 persons (Golenpaul, 1973). This, of course, would not indicate the size of any household. In instances such as this (i.e., one in which the mean is not representative because fractional amounts cannot occur), it may increase the "representativeness" of the mean to round it to a whole number.

TABLE 9-4 Language Ages Earned by Two Groups, Each Consisting of Five Children

Group I	Group II
3.5 years	3.5 years
5.0 years	5.0 years
6.0 years	6.0 years
6.5 years	6.5 years
7.0 years	14.0 years
Mean = 5.6 years	Mean = 7.0 years

A more serious problem can exist when a set of data contains one (or possibly a few) extreme scores. The mean of such a set often is not representative. Suppose the Language Ages shown in Table 9-4 were earned by two groups, each consisting of five children. The only difference between the groups is the Language Age earned by the fifth child in each. The Language Age earned by the fifth child in Group II is considerably higher than that earned by any of the other children in this group. While the mean Language Age computed for the children in Group I would appear to be representative of those earned by the children in this group, this would not appear to be the case for Group II. The mean Language Age for this group is higher than that earned by four of the five children.

Another artifact that can occur when means are used is that the relationship between the means of sets of scores for a group of persons may not be representative of those between the scores in such sets for the majority of individuals in the group. Table 9-5, for example, shows two sets of scores and their means. While it would appear from these means that the stutterers tended to be more fluent following therapy, actually *only one of the five* was more fluent following therapy.

In summary, the mean is a very useful measure of central tendency, but it does have several limitations that you should be aware of both as a user and a consumer of statistics.

The next measure of central tendency that we will consider is the *median.* Except for the mean, it is probably the most frequently used such measure. The median of a set is that measure occurring at the midpoint of the set when they are ordered from lowest to highest

TABLE 9-5 Percentages of Words Stuttered by Five Clients before and after a Period of Therapy

Stutterer	Percent before Therapy	Percent after Therapy
1	5.2	5.3
2	3.4	3.6
3	7.0	7.0
4	1.1	1.2
5	30.0	12.5
Mean	9.3	5.9

(or from highest to lowest). The median, for example, of the following set of five measures would be 50.0:

$$25 \quad 26 \quad 50 \quad 60 \quad 200$$

If a set contains an *odd* number of measures, the computation of the median is straight-forward. You merely identify the measure that occurs at the midpoint of the ordering. If a set contains an *even* number of measures, the determination of the median is a little more complex, since it involves an interpolation process. To illustrate this process, let us use the following set, which consists of six measures:

$$10 \quad 20 \quad 30 \quad 40 \quad 43 \quad 43$$

The median of this set would be 35, that is, half the distance between the third and fourth measures.

The median can be used to answer the types of questions listed in the previous section that are appropriate to answer with the mean. It can also be used to answer questions similar to the following:

1. How many hours of therapy did the "typical" child receive?
2. What score falls at the 50th percentile for six-year-olds on a particular language test?

Note that to answer the first question it is necessary to identify the measure of the child at the center of the distribution, that is, the child whose time in therapy is exceeded by that of 50 percent of the children. The second question was included to highlight the fact that *the median is the 50th percentile.*

The median can be computed from measures having ordinal, interval, or ratio proper-ties. Consequently, one difference between the mean and median is that the latter is appro-priate for ordinal data.

A possible disadvantage of the median as compared to the mean in instances where both would be appropriate concerns ease of computation without statistical software (e.g., Minitab). The mean is almost always less time-consuming to compute than the median when statistical software is not used. With such software, however, there is no difference between them in ease of computation.

Another variable on which the mean and median differ is degree of stability. The mean tends to be a more stable (hence, more reliable) measure of central tendency than the median. A sample mean typically provides a more reliable estimate of a population mean than a sample median does of a population median. Partially for this reason, significance tests for differences between means tend to be more *powerful* than comparable tests between medians, and confidence intervals for means tend to be *narrower* than those for medians (significance tests and confidence intervals are discussed in Chapter 10).

One other possible limitation of the median in comparison to the mean is that it is rel-atively insensitive to extreme measures. Note that the median of all three of the following sets of measures is the same, that is, 50:

5	19	50	75	80
15	40	50	55	60
15	25	50	75	1000

If for some reason you want your index of central tendency to be influenced by extreme measures, the mean probably would be a better choice than the median.

The final measure of central tendency that we will consider is the *mode*. The mode of a set, or distribution, is the measure that occurs most frequently. The mode of the following set of ten measures would be 7 since this is the value which occurs most often:

7   7   7   8   9   10   11   11   12   13

The mode can be used to answer such questions as the following:

1. What was the most typical (i.e., most frequently occurring) response of a person (or group) to a particular test task?
2. Is a stutterer's speech fluency most likely to improve, become worse, or stay the same after receiving a particular therapy?

While the reason the mode would be appropriate for answering the first question should be obvious, it may be less so for the second. The mode is appropriate for answering such questions as the second—that is, "probability" questions—because the category most stutterers fall into (the modal category) designates the most probable outcome.

The mode is appropriate for measures having nominal, ordinal, interval, or ratio properties. It is the only measure of central tendency that can be used with nominal data.

The mode is generally regarded as a less stable (thus, less reliable) measure of central tendency than either the median or the mean. Partially for this reason, significance tests for data treated as nominal tend to be less powerful than those for data treated as ordinal, interval, or ratio (this concept is discussed in Chapter 10).

While the mean, median, and mode are the most frequently used measures of central tendency in speech and hearing research, they are not the only such measures. Two others are the geometric mean and the harmonic mean (Campbell, 1974, pp. 73-74). Since these measures have rarely been used in speech and hearing research (or for that matter in research in any behavioral science), they will not be described here.

Measures of Variability

These indices provide information about the spread, dispersion, homogeneity, and variability of a set of numbers. They indicate how far the numbers in a set deviate from its mean or median—that is, its measure of central tendency. The more they deviate, the larger the value of the index.

When the numbers in a set are measures of attributes of persons or behaviors, they provide information about the degree of variability of such attributes. In a sense, they provide information about the degree of representativeness of indices of central tendency. The less variable the measures in a set, the more representative would be any index of central tendency. Suppose five children who had a rare neuromuscular disorder and were approximately the same age earned the following scores on a test of articulation proficiency:

$$75 \quad 77 \quad 78 \quad 78 \quad 80$$

The median score would be 78. Since the other scores deviate little from the median, it would be quite representative of them. If, however, the scores earned by these children had been the following:

$$25 \quad 40 \quad 78 \quad 90 \quad 150$$

the median (which again is 78) would have deviated considerably from several of the scores and consequently, would not have been particularly representative of them.

There are three commonly used indices of variability: the range, the interquartile (or semi-interquartile) range, and the standard deviation. Computational formulas and worked examples for all are in Appendix A.

The *range* is a frequently used measure of variability. It is relatively simple to compute, since it is merely the difference between the highest and lowest measures in a set. In some instances, the highest and lowest measures are reported rather than the difference between them. In the example above, the articulation test scores could be reported as *ranging* from 25 to 150, rather than the *range* being reported as being 125 (150 − 25 = 125).

The range can be used to answer such questions as the following:

1. What was the age range of the clients receiving a particular therapy?
2. How variable was a client's stuttering frequency during a series of ten telephone calls?

Note that the range can be used as an index of both intrasubject and intersubject variability.

The range is an appropriate index of variability for measures having ordinal, interval, or ratio properties. As such, it can provide information about the amount of deviation from either the mean or median of a set of measures.

The main advantages of the range are that it is relatively easy to compute and interpret. To compute it you only have to identify the highest and lowest measures in a set. Its interpretation is more "intuitive" (i.e., understandable to persons who are not highly trained in statistical methodology) than any of the other indices of variability.

The main disadvantage of the range is that it can make a set of measures appear more variable than they are. A single measure that is relatively large or small compared to the others can increase the magnitude of the range a great deal. Suppose a group of ten children earned the following scores on a language test:

$$75 \quad 80 \quad 80 \quad 85 \quad 85 \quad 85 \quad 90 \quad 95 \quad 95 \quad 135$$

The range of these scores would be 60 points (135 − 75 = 60). Except for one score (135) these measures are not very variable. If it were deleted, the range would only be 20 points (95 − 75 = 20). Thus, one relatively extreme score resulted in a 300 percent increase in the magnitude of the range. This limitation of the range sometimes can be partially compensated for by reporting it both with and without the extreme values. In the above example this could be done as follows: "While the children's scores on the language test ranged from 75 to 135, their performances were not as heterogeneous as this would suggest. Excluding the child who earned a score of 135, the range was from 75 to 95."

Because of the susceptibility of the range to distortion by a few extreme measures, various restricted ranges (i.e., ranges in which a certain percentage of the extreme measures are ignored) have been developed. The two such ranges most frequently used in speech and hearing research are the *interquartile range* and the *semi-interquartile range.* Both are based on the middle 50 percent of measures—that is, the highest 25 percent and the lowest 25 percent are ignored. The relationship between them is that the semi-interquartile range is equal to the interquartile range divided by two. For the ten language scores, the interquartile range would be 15 (95 – 80 = 15); the semi-interquartile range, 7.5.

The interquartile and semi-interquartile ranges can be used to answer questions such as the following:

1. How well do speech-language pathologists agree when rating speech segments from persons who have cleft palates for degree of nasality?
2. Do children's scores of Form A of a language test tend to be more variable than on Form B?
3. Within what range of scores do the 25th and 75th percentiles fall for 6-year-olds on a particular test of language performance?

Note that both ranges indicate the degree of separation between the 25th and 75th percentiles, that is, they describe the variability of the middle 50 percent of measures.

The interquartile and semi-interquartile ranges are appropriate indices of variability for measures having ordinal, interval, or ratio properties. In this regard they are similar to the range. Since they are appropriate for measures with ordinal properties, they can provide an index of the dispersion of measures around the median.

The main advantage of these indices over the range is that they are not susceptible to distortion by a few extreme measures. They are therefore more *stable* indices of variability than the range. Their main disadvantage when compared to the range is that they are not as easily interpretable. While the interpretation of the range is relatively straightforward, even for someone with little or no statistical training, both interquartile and semi-interquartile ranges may be somewhat difficult to interpret even for someone who has had statistical training. This is particularly true for the interpretation of their absolute magnitudes (e.g., What do an interquartile range of 15 or a semi-interquartile range of 7.5 "mean"?). The interpretation of their relative magnitudes, however, may be straightforward (e.g., a set of scores with an interquartile range of 15 is less variable than one with an interquartile range of 30). For an illustration and application of this strategy for interpreting these indices, see Silverman, 1967b.

Another *possible* limitation of both the interquartile and semi-interquartile ranges is that they do not reflect the variability of all measures in a set, only the middle 50 percent. This is most likely to be a limitation in instances where it is necessary to describe the absolute (as opposed to the relative) variability of the measures in a set.

The final index of variability we will describe here, the *standard deviation,* does not have this limitation. It reflects the variability of all measures in a set. It also has an advantage over the range in that its magnitude is less likely to be distorted by a few extreme measures (assuming that the number of measures is relatively large). Partially for these reasons, the standard deviation has been the most frequently used measure of variability in speech, language, and hearing research.

The *magnitude* of a standard deviation indicates the degree of variability of the measures from which it was computed. The larger the standard deviation, the more variable the measures. The smallest possible standard deviation is 0, which, of course, indicates no variability. There is no upper limit on its size, or magnitude.

If the measures in a set are *normally distributed* (which is often the case for scores on standardized tests such as intelligence tests), the percentage, or proportion, of the population that deviates a given number of *standard deviation units* from the mean of that set can be estimated. The normal distribution is a symmetrical bell-shaped curve in which certain relationships hold regarding its height at specified distances from its center (see Figure 9-1). In a normal distribution, for example, approximately 68 percent of the measures are within one standard deviation of the mean. If the scores on a test that has a mean of 100 points and a standard deviation of 15 points are normally distributed, approximately 68 percent of persons from the population on which the test was standardized will have scores between 85 and 115.

The standard deviation can be used to answer such questions as the following:

1. How variable are the scores on a particular diagnostic test?
2. What range of scores would constitute "normal limits" on a particular diagnostic test (assuming that scores on this test are normally distributed)?
3. How far, on the average, did a person's thresholds for a 100 Hz tone deviate from this mean threshold for this tone? (The assumption is made here that this threshold was measured a number of times. Another way to ask the same question would be: "How representative was a person's mean threshold for a 1000 Hz tone of those that were obtained on repeated testing?")

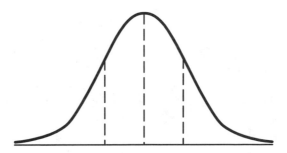

FIGURE 9-1   The normal curve, or distribution. The vertical line at the center designates the position of the mean, median, and mode, which are identical in this distribution. The other two vertical lines designate positions that are one standard deviation from the mean. Note that approximately 68 percent of the area under the curve falls between these two vertical lines.

The first question illustrates the use of the standard deviation as a measure of variability. The second illustrates its use in estimating proportions of the population whose scores (or other measures) fall within certain limits. If you defined the lower boundary of "normal limits" on a particular test as that score that is equaled or exceeded by 90 percent of 8-year-olds, you could use the standard deviation to estimate that score. The third question illustrates its use in assessing the representativeness of the mean. The smaller the standard deviation (i.e., the less the average deviation of the scores from their mean), the more representative the mean.

The standard deviation is an appropriate index of variability for measures having interval or ratio properties. It is the most frequently used such index for the dispersion of measures around the mean.

The main *advantages* of the standard deviation over other indices of variability are: (1) It reflects the dispersion of all the measures in a set, and (2) it is the most stable index of variability and thus the most reliable such index. Also, if scores (or other measures) are normally distributed, the standard deviation provides more information about them than the other indices of variability do.

The main *disadvantage* of the standard deviation as an index of variability is the same as that mentioned for the interquartile and semi-interquartile ranges. Unless measures are normally distributed, the *absolute* magnitude of their standard deviation may be difficult to interpret. To know that a set of measures that are not normally distributed has a standard deviation of 3.5 provides little information regarding their dispersion.

While the absolute magnitudes of standard deviations may be difficult to interpret, their *relative* magnitudes frequently provide useful information. If the means of the scores earned by two groups on a test of language functioning were approximately the same, but the standard deviations of their scores were quite different, this would indicate that the persons in one of the groups were more heterogeneous in their performance on this test than those in the other group.

Measures of Association

These indices are used to describe the *strength* and *direction* of the relationships between sets of measures (these attributes of relationships are described in Chapter 6). They indicate how the attributes described by such sets of measures are related to each other, that is, correlated. The numbers that are yielded by such indices are referred to as *correlation coefficients*. Computational formulas and worked examples for several types of correlation coefficients are in Appendix A.

Correlation coefficients typically provide several kinds of information about the relationships between sets of numbers. First, they provide information about the *strength* of the relationship between the attributes measured by such sets. The larger the correlation coefficient (i.e., the closer it is to +1.00 or −1.00), the stronger the relationship. The smaller the correlation coefficient (i.e., the closer it is to 0), the weaker the relationship. (If the correlation coefficient is 0, there is no relationship.)

Suppose you administered a test of auditory discrimination ability and a test of articulation proficiency to a kindergarten class and correlated the two sets of scores earned by the children on these tests. If the resulting correlation coefficient was 0.60, this would suggest that auditory discrimination ability and articulation proficiency were more closely associated, or related, for these children than would have been the case if the resulting correlation coefficient had been, for example, 0.15. The strength of this relationship, however, would *not* have been four times as great if the coefficient had been 0.60 rather than 0.15. Correlation coefficients have *ordinal* properties. Thus, a correlation coefficient of 0.50 indicates a greater degree of association than one of 0.30 and a lesser degree than one of 0.90.

Correlation coefficients may also provide information about the *direction* of the relationship between the attributes measured. The direction can be either *positive* or *negative.* If it is positive, persons who tend to exhibit relative high (or low) levels of one of the attributes tend to exhibit corresponding levels of the other. Thus, height and weight are positively correlated (i.e., the taller a person is, the more he or she tends to weigh).

If the relationship between two attributes is negative, persons who tend to exhibit relatively high (or low) levels of one of the attributes tend to exhibit opposite levels of the other. Thus, chronological age and number of articulation errors is negatively correlated for elementary-school children (i.e., the older an elementary-school child, the fewer articulation errors he or she is likely to have). If a correlation coefficient is preceded by a minus sign, the relationship between the attributes correlated is negative.

Correlation coefficients usually range between -1.00 and $+1.00$. A correlation coefficient larger than 1.00 is impossible.

The correlation coefficients that are described in detail in this section and dealt with in Appendix A (i.e., the contingency coefficient, phi coefficient, Spearman rank-order coefficient, and Pearson product-moment correlation coefficient) are for assessing the association between pairs of attributes. While the most frequently used indices of association are of this type, they are not the only ones. Several other types—including multiple correlation and partial correlation—will be dealt with briefly at the end of this section.

The first measure of association we will describe is the *contingency coefficient.* It is an index of the degree of relationship, or association, between two attributes of events that had been assigned on the basis of these attributes to the cells of a contingency table. This is a table that contains two or more rows and two or more columns. The numbers of rows and columns do *not* have to be the same. Consequently, a contingency table could have two rows and five columns, or five rows and two columns, or five rows and five columns, or two rows and two columns, and so on. (An example of a two-row and two-column contingency table is presented in Appendix A in the section on the contingency coefficient.)

The number of columns (or number of rows) in a contingency table is determined by the number of categories into which the scale for an attribute is divided, or segmented. For the attribute "biological sex," the scale would typically be divided into two categories: male and female. For the attribute "type of speech disorder," the scale could be divided into the following four categories: phonation, articulation, resonance, and fluency.

While the scales for attributes mentioned thus far have been nominal, those representing any level of measurement can be used in contingency tables. An example of an attribute with ordinal properties that could be used in such tables would be "grade level." The categories into which the scale for this attribute could be divided would include "first grade," "second grade," "third grade," and so on.

To illustrate the application of contingency tables and contingency coefficients, suppose you wished to determine whether the number of words repeated by elementary-school children tended to be related to their grade level. That is, you wished to determine whether older elementary-school children tended to repeat words less frequently than younger elementary-school children or vice versa. One approach you could use would be to determine the frequency of word repetitions per 100 words spoken by ten first graders and ten sixth graders and then compute the median word repetition frequency for the twenty first and sixth graders combined. Each of the twenty children would then be assigned to one of the four cells of a contingency table on the basis of: (1) whether he or she was a first or sixth grader, and (2) whether his or her word repetition frequency fell at or below the median or above the median. Three possible results from this assignment are depicted in Table 9-6. The configuration of *A* suggests a *strong positive* relationship between word repetition frequency and grade level; the ten sixth graders all had higher word repetition frequencies than the ten first graders. The configuration of *B* suggests *no* relationship between grade level and word repetition frequency; the sixth graders' word repetition frequencies exhibited no tendency to be systematically higher or lower than those of the first graders. The configuration of *C*, on the other hand, suggests a *strong negative* relationship between grade level and word repetition frequency; the ten first graders all had higher word repetition frequencies than the ten sixth graders. In most "real-world" research, the relationships (or lack of them) would not be as clear-cut as those depicted in Table 9-6.

The procedure for computing the contingency coefficient is outlined in Appendix A. This procedure is applicable to a contingency table of any size.

The contingency coefficient is zero when no relationship, or association, exists between the two variables. If the relationship between them is perfect (e.g., as depicted in parts A and C of Table 9-6), the value of the contingency coefficient will approach, but not equal, 1.00. How close it will come to 1.00 is a function of the size of the table; the larger the table, the closer it will come to 1.00. For a 2×2 table (which is the size of the tables in Table 9-6), the upper limit of the contingency coefficient is 0.71.

The nature of the relationship between the variables in a contingency table (i.e., positive or negative) has to be inferred from the configuration of the table, since it is impossible for a contingency coefficient to have a minus value. Thus, a contingency coefficient of 0.60 can indicate either a positive or a negative relationship between the attributes.

The contingency coefficient can be used to answer such questions as:

1. Is there a relationship between school grade and word repetition frequency for elementary-school children?
2. Is the acceptability of an electrolarynx associated with the socioeconomic level of the person who is laryngectomized?

A contingency table that could be used to answer the first question has already been described (see Table 9-6). One that could be used to answer the second question is presented in Table 9-7. Obviously, socioeconomic status could have been categorized in other ways in this table.

The contingency coefficient can be computed from measures having nominal, ordinal, interval, or ratio properties. It is the only measure of association that can be used with nominal data in contingency tables larger than 2×2.

While the contingency coefficient is a very useful index for assessing degree of association in contingency tables larger than 2×2, it does have several limitations. First, it is

TABLE 9-6   Three Possible Results from the Assignment of Twenty Children to the Cells of a Contingency Table on the Bases of Their Word Repetition Frequencies and Grade Levels

WORD REPETITION FREQUENCY

	At or Below Median	Above Median
1st Grade	10	
6th Grade		10

GRADE LEVEL

A

WORD REPETITION FREQUENCY

	At or Below Median	Above Median
1st Grade	5	5
6th Grade	5	5

GRADE LEVEL

B

WORD REPETITION FREQUENCY

	At or Below Median	Above Median
1st Grade		10
6th Grade	10	

GRADE LEVEL

C

somewhat difficult to interpret because its upper limit is less than 1.00. Consequently, a contingency coefficient of 0.70 could indicate either a perfect relationship or a fairly strong relationship between the attributes, depending on the size of the contingency table.

A second possible limitation of this index is that contingency coefficients cannot be compared unless they are yielded by tables of the same size, since the upper limits of contingency coefficients are a function of the sizes of tables on which they are computed. Thus, a contingency coefficient of 0.70 for a 2×2 table would indicate a higher degree of asso-

TABLE 9-7   A Contingency Table for Studying the Association between Acceptability of an Electrolarynx and Socioeconomic Status

ACCEPTABILITY OF ELECTROLARYNX

	Acceptable	Unacceptable	Undecided
Upper			
Middle			
Lower			

SOCIOECONOMIC STATUS

ciation between the attributes than one of 0.75 on a 3×3 table (the upper limit for a contingency coefficient on such a table would be 0.82).

A third possible limitation of the contingency coefficient as an index of association, or correlation, is that its value is not directly comparable to those yielded by other such indices including the three dealt with in the computational appendix—the phi coefficient, the Spearman rank-order coefficient, and the Pearson product-moment correlation coefficient.

In spite of these limitations, however, the contingency coefficient is a useful index of association (or correlation) for contingency tables larger than 2×2.

For contingency tables that are 2×2, an index of association that ordinarily would be preferable to the contingency coefficient is the *phi coefficient*. The phi coefficient has an upper limit of 1.00 (which would indicate a perfect relationship between the attributes), and the nature of the relationship between the attributes (positive or negative) is indicated by the sign of the coefficient. Thus, in Table 9-6, the phi coefficient for *A* would be +1.00, for *B* would be 0.00, and for *C* would be –1.00. The phi coefficient is easier to interpret than the contingency coefficient, and its value is directly comparable to those yielded by the Spearman rank-order coefficient and the Pearson product-moment correlation coefficient. The coefficients yielded by these three indices on a given set of data, however, usually are not identical (a demonstration of this is provided in Appendix A, where all three were computed from the same set of data).

The procedure for computing the phi coefficient is outlined in Appendix A.

The phi coefficient can be used to answer the same types of questions as the contingency coefficient as long as the data can be cast into a 2×2 table.

The phi coefficient (like the contingency coefficient) can be computed from measures having nominal, ordinal, interval, or ratio properties. It is a particularly useful index of correlation between dichotomous attributes. (An example of a dichotomous attribute would be biological sex, which consists of the categories "male" and "female.")

The advantages of the phi coefficient over the contingency coefficient as an index of association for 2×2 contingency tables already have been mentioned.

In summary, the phi coefficient is a useful index of association, particularly for measures having nominal properties. The phi coefficient and the contingency coefficient are the only such indices described here that are appropriate for measures having nominal properties.

If the measures of the attributes you wish to determine the relationship between have at least ordinal properties, the *Spearman rank-order coefficient* can be used as an index of association. This coefficient is an index of the extent to which two sets of measures *rank order* a group of persons in the same manner. If both rank order the persons in the identical manner, this would indicate a *perfect positive* relationship between them and the Spearman rank-order coefficient would be +1.00. On the other hand, if they rank order the persons in exactly the opposite manner, this would indicate a *perfect negative* relationship between them, and the Spearman rank-order coefficient would be –1.00. Spearman rank-order coefficients for less than perfect relationships fall between –1.00 and +1.00.

The procedure for computing the Spearman rank-order coefficient is outlined in Appendix A.

Suppose that in order to determine whether any relationship existed between the degree of recovery exhibited by receptive aphasics and their socioeconomic level, you rank ordered five receptive aphasics both on the basis of the amount of recovery they exhibited and their socioeconomic level. Three possible sets of orderings of the five aphasics on the basis of these attributes are presented in Table 9-8. The Spearman rank-order coefficient for the first set would be +1.00, for the second approximately 0.00, and for the third –1.00. Thus, the first set would suggest a *strong positive* relationship between improvement level and socio-

TABLE 9-8   Three Possible Sets of Orderings for Five Receptive Aphasics Based on Their Socioeconomic Levels and the Amount of Improvement They Exhibited (The aphasics are designated by the letters A, B, C, D, and E)

Set I		Set II		Set III	
Socioeconomic Level	Improvement Level	Socioeconomic Level	Improvement Level	Socioeconomic Level	Improvement Level
A	A	A	E	A	E
C	C	C	A	C	D
B	B	B	D	B	B
D	D	D	C	D	C
E	E	E	B	E	A

economic level, the second essentially *no* relationship between these variables, and the third a *strong negative* relationship between them.

The Spearman rank-order coefficient can be used to answer questions similar to these:

1. Is the amount of recovery exhibited by receptive aphasics related to their socioeconomic level?
2. Do the levels of children's performances of two particular tests of language functioning tend to be similar?
3. How well do two speech-language pathologists agree in their orderings of clients with regard to degree of improvement following a program of therapy?

Using the Spearman rank-order coefficient to answer the first question has already been described. Answering the second question would involve ordering the children on the basis of the two sets of language scores. And answering the third would involve ordering the clients on the basis of each speech-language pathologist's ratings of degree of improvement.

The Spearman rank-order coefficient can be computed from measures having ordinal, interval, or ratio properties. It has been one of the most frequently used indices of association for measures having ordinal properties in speech-language pathology and audiology research.

The Spearman rank-order coefficient provides a satisfactory index of the degree of correspondence (or correlation) between two rank orderings of a group of persons. Thus, it is appropriate for measures having ordinal properties. While it is also appropriate for measures having interval or ratio properties, it has a limitation when used with such measures. This limitation is that the Spearman rank-order coefficient is insensitive to the sizes, or magnitudes, of the differences between measures. It is not possible with this procedure to detect the form of the relationship between a pair of attributes—that is, whether the form is linear or nonlinear (see Figures 6.2, 6.5, and 6.6 and accompanying text for description of linear and nonlinear relationships). To answer some questions, you must be able to determine whether the relationship between a pair of attributes is linear or nonlinear; to answer others, this information is not necessary. For answering questions of the second type, the Spearman rank-order coefficient would be satisfactory.

If the measures of the attributes you wish to determine the relationship between have interval or ratio properties and the relationship between them can be assumed to be linear (see Chapter 6), an index of association you can use for assessing this relationship is the *Pearson product-moment correlation coefficient*. This coefficient, which is also known as the *Pearson r,* is probably the most frequently used index of association (or correlation) in speech-language pathology and audiology research.

The Pearson *r* can be visualized, or interpreted, in several ways. First, it can be viewed as an index of how closely two sets of measures rank order a group of persons. Its magnitude is determined in large part by the extent to which the rank orderings are similar. As long as the relationship between a pair of attributes is not grossly nonlinear, the magnitude of the Pearson *r* will be quite similar to that of the Spearman rank-order coefficient.

The Pearson *r* also can be visualized as an index of the amount of deviation of the points in a scattergram (see Chapter 6) from the straight line from which they would deviate least. The more the points deviate from this line, the smaller will be the value of the

Pearson *r*. If the points all lie on the line, the Pearson *r* would be +1.00 or −1.00. If the deviation of the points about such a line looked circular (i.e., if their deviation from this line was considerable), the Pearson *r* would be approximately 0.00. Scattergrams that depict these possibilities are presented in Figures 6.2 and 6.3.

The Pearson *r* is similar to the phi coefficient and Spearman rank-order coefficient in two ways: (1) Its possible values fall between −1.00 and +1.00, and (2) the closer its value to +1.00 or −1.00, the stronger the association between the attributes. The procedure for computing the Pearson *r* is described in Appendix A.

The Pearson *r* can be used to answer questions similar to these:

1. What is the nature of the relationship between preschoolers' auditory discrimination ability and their articulation proficiency?
2. To what extent are first graders' levels of performance on a particular test prior to participating in a therapy program *predictive* of their levels of performance on that test after completing the program?

Note that answering the first question involves assessing the relationship between performances of *different* tasks by a group of persons at the *same* point in time, and answering the second question involves assessing the relationship between performances of the *same* tasks by a group of persons at *different* points in time.

Strictly speaking, the Pearson *r* is only an appropriate index of association for measures having interval or ratio properties. Nevertheless, it has been used a great deal in speech-language pathology and audiology research with measures that appear to have ordinal properties. Examples of such measures would be scores on tests of auditory discrimination ability and articulation proficiency. In most instances, probably no great harm is done if the Pearson *r* is used with measures that have ordinal properties. When it is used with such measures, the magnitude of a Pearson *r* can be interpreted as an *approximation* of what the coefficient describing the relationship would have been if the Spearman rank-order coefficient had been used.

To estimate the relative strength of the relationship indicated by a Pearson *r*, the *square* of its value (rather than its value) should be used. Squaring a Pearson *r* results in a reduction in its magnitude (except when its value is 1.00). The extent of this reduction can be surmised from Table 9-9, in which r^2 magnitudes are presented for selected *r* values. Note that a Pearson *r* of at least 0.70 is needed before even 50 percent of the variation observed in a scattergram can be accounted for on the basis of a linear relationship between the attributes. In fact, a Pearson *r* of 0.50 is needed before even 25 percent of the variation observed in a scattergram can be accounted for on the basis of a linear relationship between the attributes.

How would you describe in words the strength of the relationship depicted by a particular Pearson *r*? While there is no universality of agreement among statisticians regarding strengths of relationships designated by particular Pearson *r* values, some rough guidelines exist, with which most statisticians probably would agree, that can be used for making such judgments, including the following:

- Pearson *r* coefficients of less than 0.30 usually indicate that for most *practical* purposes *no* linear relationship exists between the attributes.

TABLE 9-9 r^2 **Magnitudes for Selected Pearson**
r **Values**

r	r^2	r	r^2
0.05	0.00	0.55	0.30
0.10	0.01	0.60	0.36
0.15	0.02	0.65	0.42
0.20	0.04	0.70	0.49
0.25	0.06	0.75	0.56
0.30	0.09	0.80	0.64
0.35	0.12	0.85	0.72
0.40	0.16	0.90	0.81
0.45	0.20	0.95	0.90
0.50	0.25	1.00	1.00

- Pearson *r* coefficients between 0.30 and 0.50 usually indicate a *weak* linear relationship between the attributes.
- Pearson *r* coefficients between 0.51 and 0.85 usually indicate a *moderate* linear relationship between the attributes.
- Pearson *r* coefficients between 0.86 and 0.95 usually indicate a *strong* linear relationship between the attributes.
- Pearson *r* coefficients higher than 0.96 usually indicate an *extremely strong* linear relationship between the attributes.

In summary, the Pearson *r* is an extremely useful index of association between pairs of attributes when the measures of such attributes have interval or ratio properties and the relationship between them is fairly linear. It provides information concerning the strength, direction, and linearity of the relationship between pairs of attributes.

The indices of association described in this section are representative of a fairly large number of indices for assessing relationships between pairs of attributes that have been developed by mathematical statisticians. Descriptions of other such indices can be found in intermediate and advanced statistics texts intended for psychologists, sociologists, and researchers in the field of education.

Indices of association are not limited to describing the relationships between pairs of attributes when the relationship between the attributes is presumed to be linear. There are indices of association for other purposes or types of data, including the following:

1. *Indices of association between pairs of attributes where the relationships between the attributes are presumed to be nonlinear.* These indices can be used to answer the same kinds of questions that could be answered by means of a Pearson *r* if the relationship between the attributes were linear. To determine whether it would be most reasonable to assume that the relationship between two attributes were linear or nonlinear, you can plot the measures you made of them on a scattergram. If the line that best fits the configuration of the points does not appear to be a straight line, it might be safest to assume that the relationship between the attributes is nonlinear (a scattergram in which a nonlinear relationship exists between attributes is presented in Figure 6.5). These indices assess the goodness of fit of the points plotted in a scattergram to various types of curved lines.

If you feel the relationship between a pair of attributes is nonlinear, show the scattergram to a statistician. He or she should be able to recommend an appropriate nonlinear correlation coefficient.

2. *Indices of association between pairs of attributes with the effects of a third attribute held constant, or eliminated.* Indices used for this purpose are referred to as coefficients of *partial correlation.* Suppose you wished to determine whether a relationship existed between auditory discrimination ability and articulation proficiency for the children in a kindergarten classroom. It is conceivable that there could appear to be a relationship between the two because both are related to mental age. The higher the mental age of a child, the better the child is likely to do on both tasks. You may therefore wish to answer the question: "Would there be any relationship between auditory discrimination ability and articulation proficiency if the effects of mental age were eliminated (i.e., held constant)?" Coefficients of partial correlation can be used to answer this type of question. See Shriberg and Kwiatkowski (1982) for an example of how coefficients of partial correlation can be used.

3. *Indices of association between an attribute and the composite of two or more other attributes.* These indices are referred to as coefficients of *multiple correlation.* They are computed from multiple regression equations. Suppose you wanted to identify the attributes of speaking behavior that influence judgments of stuttering severity. One approach would be to have speech samples from a number of stutterers rated for "degree of stuttering severity" by the method of direct magnitude-estimation (see Chapter 8). These samples would also be analyzed to determine the amounts of various attributes each possesses that might influence listeners' impressions of stuttering severity. Such attributes would include frequency of stuttering, average duration of moments of stuttering, and speaking rate. A multiple regression equation would be computed from measures of these three attributes and the ratings of stuttering severity. From the values in this equation, a coefficient of multiple correlation would be computed. If this coefficient were quite high (i.e., larger than 0.85), it would suggest that these attributes are likely to influence listeners' judgments of stuttering severity. Programs for computing multiple regression equations and indices of multiple correlation from them are available for almost all microcomputers. For illustrations of the use of multiple correlation in speech and hearing research, see Table 10.2.

4. *Indices of association between more than two sets of measures.* To answer a question, it is sometimes necessary to assess the degree of association, or agreement, between a number of sets of measures. This need arises most often in speech and hearing research when an investigator wishes to determine how well a group of judges agree in their ratings of a set of stimuli. Suppose you wanted to determine how well three judges agreed in their ratings of the children. Several indices of association could be used for this purpose. The Kendall coefficient of concordance (Siegel, 1956) would be appropriate if the ratings were assumed to be ordinal; the intraclass correlation coefficient (Ebel, 1951) would be appropriate if they were assumed to have interval or ratio properties.

Graphical Displays

Such displays are used frequently by speech-language pathologists and audiologists for organizing quantitative data. There are several types including line graphs, bar graphs, pie graphs, and column graphs. In *line graphs,* the scale for one attribute is presented on the horizontal (*X*) axis and the scale for the second on the vertical *(Y)* axis (see Figure 9-2). Each event is plotted at the point that would correspond to its value for the attributes. If its value for the first attribute was 3 and the second was 2, it would be plotted at the point indicated in Figure 9-2.

Several types of line graphs are often used by speech-language pathologists and audiologists. One of these, the *scattergram,* already has been described in considerable detail (see Chapter 6). Another used by both speech-language pathologists and audiologists is the *pure-tone audiogram.* A third, which is frequently used by behaviorally oriented clinicians (particularly those who utilize operant conditioning), plots the frequency of occurrence of a specified behavior (or behaviors) over time. In Figure 9-2, *Attribute I* would be a time measure (e.g., seconds, minutes, hours, days, or weeks), and *Attribute II* would be frequency of occurrence (on a specified task or during a specified time period). Numerous examples of line graphs can be found in almost any volume of the *Journal of Speech and Hearing Research.*

Line graphs can be used to answer questions such as the following:

1. What is the nature of the relationship between number of articulation errors and chronological age?

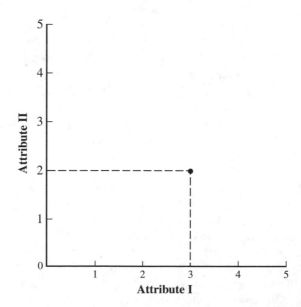

FIGURE 9-2   A line graph with one point plotted. After all the points were plotted, they would be connected.

2. What are a person's thresholds for pure tones of various frequencies?
3. What is the effect of response-contingent reinforcement on a particular behavior over a period of time?

The types of graphical displays that could be used for answering questions one through three respectively would be a scattergram, a pure-tone audiogram, and a behavior chart. Line graphs can be used for organizing measures with ordinal, interval, ratio, or logarithmic properties.

A second type of graphical display that has been used by speech-language pathologists and audiologists for organizing and summarizing data is the *bar graph* (see Figure 9-3). These are similar to line graphs in that the scale for one attribute is presented on the horizontal axis and the scale for the second on the vertical axis (see Figure 9-3). Each event is depicted by a bar the length of which indicates its value on the horizontal scale. Thus, in Figure 9-3, the mean number of interjections per 100 words was approximately 2.0 for the nonstutterers and 3.0 for the stutterers.

Bar graphs can be used for answering questions such as the following:

1. Do stutterers differ from nonstutterers with regard to how likely they are to revise (i.e., correct their speaking errors)?
2. Do stutterers tend to repeat phrases as frequently as they repeat words?

Both questions can be answered using the data in Figure 9-3.

Bar graphs, like line graphs, can be used for organizing data with ordinal, interval, ratio, or logarithmic properties. They also can be used for organizing data with nominal properties.

A third type of graphical display that has been used by speech-language pathologists and audiologists to summarize data is the *pie graph* (see Figure 9-4). These depict the per-

FIGURE 9-3   A representative bar graph.

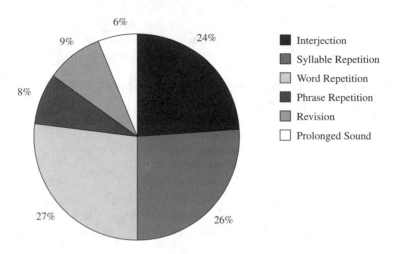

FIGURE 9-4   A representative pie graph.

centage of total events that fall into each of a series of categories (see Figure 9-4). Each category is represented by a "wedge" of pie: the higher the percentage of total events that fall into a particular category, the larger the "wedge." Thus, in Figure 9-4, the "wedge" for interjections is larger than that for revisions because a higher percentage of the total disfluencies were interjections.

Pie graphs can be used for answering questions such as the following:

1. What types of disfluency tend to occur most often?
2. Do stutterers differ from nonstutterers with regard to the relative frequency of occurrence of various disfluency types?

The first could be answered using the graph in Figure 9-4. For answering the second it would be necessary to have two such graphs, one for stutterers and one for nonstutterers. Pie graphs are used mainly for organizing data having nominal properties—for example, frequency counts.

A fourth type of graphical display, the *column graph,* is identical to the bar graph except that everything is rotated 90 degrees—that is, the bars are vertical rather than horizontal. It can be used for answering similar questions and for organizing data having the same properties. Bar graphs are preferable to column graphs when the categories on one axis are defined by words or phrases (see Figure 9-3). The reason is that it is unnecessary to rotate the graph to read them.

While these are not the only types of graphs that have been used by speech-language pathologists and audiologists, they are the ones that they have used most often. Others they have used include area charts and various types of three-dimensional displays.

Just as computers are useful tools for doing statistical analyses of numerical data, they are also useful tools for preparing graphs from such data. There are programs for most microcomputers that will draw all of the types of graphs mentioned in this section. Most sophisticated spreadsheet programs (e.g., *Microsoft Excel*) have this capability.

For further information about the analysis and interpretation of graphical displays, see the chapter by Parsonson and Baer (1978).

Tables

Quantitative data, like qualitative data, can be organized and summarized in tabular form (e.g., see the data table in Appendix A). Most articles in research journals (e.g., the *Journal of Speech and Hearing Research*) contain at least one table of quantitative data. The content of such a table may include both descriptive statistics and the data on which they are based. Furthermore, data sometimes are presented in both graphical displays and tabular form.

Just as a computer can facilitate the drawing of graphs and the computation of statistics, it can also facilitate the preparation of tables. Most sophisticated word processing programs (e.g., Microsoft Word and WordPerfect) contain table editors that can automatically set up columns and rows and align numbers within them. Tables can also be created with spreadsheet programs and statistical analysis programs.

Exercises and Discussion Topics

1. There are 23 computational exercises in Appendix A. The first 10 provide experience in computing most of the descriptive statistics mentioned in this chapter. Your instructor will tell you which to do and whether to do them with a calculator, a computer (with a statistical program package), or both.

2. The interpretation of descriptive statistics and graphical displays for answering questions is not "objective"—it is based on human judgment. Often, a set of data can be interpreted to support several different answers to a question. Justify *both* a "yes" and a "no" answer to each of the following questions using the numerical or graphical data provided.

   a. Do stutterers exhibit the adaptation effect during a series of fifteen consecutive readings of a passage? (The adaptation effect is the tendency for stutterers to become progressively more fluent during a series of consecutive readings of a passage.)

   Observational Procedures. Ten adult stutterers each read a passage fifteen times, one after the other.

   Their frequency of disfluency on each reading of the passage was determined.

   Data. The mean frequency of disfluency on each of the fifteen readings of the passage is presented graphically in Figure 9-5.

   b. Do receptive aphasics tend to benefit from the x therapy program?

   Observational Procedures. Ten receptive aphasics are administered the Peabody Picture Vocabulary Test (PPVT) both before and after participating in the x therapy program.

   Data. The "before" and "after" PPVT scores for the ten receptive aphasics are the following:

Subject Number	"Before" PPVT Score	"After" PPVT Score
1	40	39
2	79	79
3	25	20
4	50	51
5	15	12
6	15	90
7	75	73
8	65	65
9	38	36
10	48	49
Mean	45	51

FIGURE 9-5   Frequency of disfluency on each of the fifteen readings of the passage.

3. Why is knowledge of descriptive statistics important for evaluating therapy outcome research reports?

4. Which of the approaches mentioned in this chapter are usable for organizing qualitative and quantitative data in clinical evaluation reports?

Chapter 10

Organizing Data for Answering Questions: II. Inferential Techniques for Group Designs

The statistical techniques that have been discussed thus far are intended for summarizing, organizing, or describing aspects of a set of data. They convert it into a form that enables it to be used for answering questions.

Inferential statistical techniques enable you to answer several kinds of questions about a set of data that go beyond the descriptive analyses made of it. One of them pertains to the *reliability* of differences or relationships that are observed in a set of data. Suppose you found that a group of children, on the average, made fewer articulation errors after participating in an experimental therapy program than before participating in it. This finding would allow you to answer the question: "Did the children in the experimental therapy program improve?" It would not by itself, however, permit you to answer the question: "If some other children similar to these children went through this experimental program, is it likely they also would improve?" The reason you could not answer this question is that the reliability of the difference between pre- and post-therapy measures would be uncertain. These measures would be unlikely to be identical even if the program had no effect. In fact, assuming the therapy had no effect, the children would stand a 50 percent chance of having the difference between their pre- and post-therapy measures suggest that it had an effect merely on the basis of "chance," or random fluctuation. The reason for the 50 percent chance is that there are only two outcomes possible here, both of which are equally likely— that is, post-therapy measures "better" than pre-therapy ones or vice versa. Before concluding, therefore, that an observed difference between pre- and post-therapy measures could have resulted from participating in a therapy program, it would be necessary to determine the likelihood that it could have resulted from random fluctuation. *Significance tests,* which are an aspect of statistical inference, can be used to estimate the probability that observed differences between means or medians (or other descriptive statistics) resulted from chance, or random fluctuation. These tests *do not* tell you whether an observed difference arose from this source, only the probability that it did so. Significance tests are described in the next section of this chapter and computational formulas, Minitab commands, and worked examples for representative ones are in Appendix A.

Significance tests can also be used for assessing the reliability of observed *relationships.* Just as a difference between pre-therapy and post-therapy measures would be unlikely to be zero if a therapy program had no effect, a correlation coefficient would be unlikely to be zero if there was no relationship between the attributes described by the measures correlated. By chance, a correlation coefficient can have a value between 0.01 and 1.00. Significance tests can be used for estimating the probability that nonzero correlation coefficients resulted from chance, or random fluctuation.

Another type of question that inferential statistical techniques allow you to answer concerns the *generality* of differences and relationships that you observe in a set of data when a group design is used. Specifically, they allow you to answer the question: "How likely is it that the differences or relationships (or both) that I have observed in the sample of persons I've studied also are present in the *population* from which these persons were selected?" Suppose you developed a therapy program that seemed to be very effective for modifying some aspect of the communicative behavior of a group of persons in your caseload, based on differences between the means (or medians) of measures made of this aspect of their communicative behavior both before and after they participated in the program. While the difference you observed would permit you to conclude that the program appeared to be effective for the average or typical person in the group on which it was used, it would not permit you to conclude it also would be effective for persons like them who were not in this group. Significance tests provide you with a way of estimating how safe you would be in concluding that differences or relationships you observed in a *sample* of persons also are present in the *population* to which these persons belong (assuming that your sample was *randomly selected* from this population or approximates such a sample).

Significance tests only indicate the likelihood that a difference or relationship observed in a sample is present in the population from which it comes. They do *not* provide an estimate of the *magnitude* of the difference or relationship in the population. You *cannot* assume that the magnitude of a difference or relationship present in a sample is a good estimate of that in the population from which the sample comes. This magnitude in the population may be considerably smaller or larger than that in the sample.

A third type of question that inferential statistical techniques enable you to answer pertains to estimating population values, or magnitudes, of descriptive statistics and of differences between descriptive statistics. Once you have established with a significance test that a difference or relationship in your sample is likely to be present in the population from which your sample was selected, you may wish to estimate the magnitude of the difference or the strength of the relationship in this population. Also, you may wish to estimate indices of central tendency and variability for it. Confidence intervals allow you to make such estimates. They will be described in some detail later in this chapter.

A fourth type of question that inferential statistical techniques help you to answer deals with inferences that are not related to population values of descriptive statistics. These include inferences about factors that influence a particular judgment (e.g., degree of nasality) or performance on a particular task (e.g., an aphasia test) or most reliably allow us to distinguish between groups (e.g., children who are normally disfluent and children who are beginning to stutter). Inferential statistical techniques for answering such questions are described at the end of the chapter.

Significance Tests

These statistics can be used for answering the following question: "How likely is it that a difference or relationship observed in a set of data is the result of chance, or random fluctuation?" The differences referred to could be between almost any types of measures including means, medians, modes, frequencies, percentages, proportions, standard deviations, and correlation coefficients. The relationships referred to involve correlation coefficients.

What does the chance, or random fluctuation, estimated by significance tests refer to? The most direct way to answer this question is through the use of probability theory. The basic point here is that measures that are not different or related can appear to be different or related. Suppose you had a stutterer perform a speaking task in two situations, and she stuttered on 10 percent of the words she spoke in Situation I and 13 percent of those she spoke in Situation II. Would it be safe to conclude that she tends to stutter more frequently in Situation II than in Situation I? The answer to this question would be "no," because this outcome would occur by chance approximately 50 percent of the time. (We use the word *approximately* here because the two stuttering frequencies would be identical by chance a small percentage of the time.) For probability, the situation is analogous to tossing a coin. If you tossed a penny many times, approximately 50 percent of the time it would come up heads and approximately 50 percent of the time it would come up tails. A small percentage of time it may stand on edge, which would be analogous in our illustration to the two stuttering frequencies being identical.

Significance tests are the "tools" that are used most often in speech, language, and hearing research for determining whether the probability of an outcome being due to chance, or random fluctuation, is adequately small—usually either *equal to or less than* 5 percent or 1 percent. They perform this function by estimating the likelihood of a *null hypothesis* being "true."

Null hypotheses state that observed differences or relationships are due to chance, or random fluctuation. They state that if it were not for chance, or random fluctuation, the differences between the measures or the magnitudes of the correlation coefficients would have been 0.00.

All significance tests have a single function—to determine the probability that null hypotheses are true. If the probability that a null hypothesis is true is small enough, it can be *rejected*. The investigator must decide before a significance test is "run" how small this probability has to be. The levels that are used most frequently for this purpose are 0.05 (5 percent probability of a null hypothesis being true) and 0.01 (1 percent probability of a null hypothesis being true). Obviously, the 0.01 level is more conservative than the 0.05 level since it is more difficult with the 0.01 level to reject a null hypothesis. The 0.05 level is sometimes selected for a study because by making it more likely that null hypotheses will be rejected it also makes it more likely that a report of the study will be accepted for publication—i.e., journals tend to view studies in which null hypotheses are rejected as being of greater value than those in which they are not (Greenwald, 1975).

In the statistical literature, the 1 percent level is referred to as the *0.01 level of confidence,* and the 5 percent level as the *0.05 level of confidence.* Thus, if a null hypothesis were rejected at the 0.01 level of confidence, it would be approximately 99 percent certain that the observed difference or relationship was not the result of chance, or random fluctuation.

Rejection of a null hypothesis only means that an observed difference or relationship is unlikely to have resulted from chance, or random fluctuation. It does not mean that it was due to the reason suggested by the experimenter in his or her *research hypothesis.* Often there is more than one possible explanation for an observed difference or relationship other than chance, or random fluctuation. Rejection of a null hypothesis provides no information about which such explanation is most viable. It only indicates that chance, or random fluctuation, is unlikely to be the explanation.

How do you decide on an explanation for an observed difference or relationship if you reject the null hypothesis? Two approaches can be used: logical and logical-empirical. With a logical approach, you specify the possible explanations for a difference or relationship and, on the basis of the information that is available to you, decide which explanation (or combination of explanations) is most plausible. One obvious limitation of this approach is that the "real" explanation (or explanations) may not have occurred to you and hence would not have been among those you considered. Under this circumstance, the most plausible explanation would not be the most plausible explanation.

The logical-empirical approach goes one step beyond the logical approach. After the explanation for a difference or relationship that appears to be the most plausible is identified by a reasoning process, experiments are conducted to assess its viability. If the findings of the experiments are consistent with the explanation, you could have more confidence in its viability than if it were arrived at by a reasoning process alone.

Failure to reject a null hypothesis does *not* necessarily mean that the difference or relationship observed was the result of chance, or random fluctuation. There are at least two other possible explanations:

1. The difference or relationship was a real one, but because its magnitude was relatively small, the significance test was not *powerful* enough to detect it. The smaller a difference or weaker a relationship, the larger the number of subjects or observations needed to detect it, that is, cause the null hypothesis to be rejected. While a significance test on the difference between the means of two groups, each consisting of ten persons, may not lead to rejection of the null hypothesis, the same significance test on the difference between the same means could lead to this outcome if the groups consisted of twenty-five persons. For further discussion of this issue, see Lieber (1990).

2. The "real" difference or relationship (i.e., the one in the population) is larger in magnitude than the observed difference or relationship. By chance, subjects representing the extremes of the population distribution (or distributions) were not adequately represented in the sample. If the sample had been more representative, the difference between the means would have been larger, or the relationship stronger, and the null hypothesis would have been rejected.

Failure to reject a null hypothesis when it should be rejected is known as a *Type II error.* This is one of the two types of error that can occur in a decision on a null hypothesis. The other, a *Type I error,* occurs when a null hypothesis is rejected when it should not have been rejected—that is, when the observed difference or relationship really was the result of chance, or random fluctuation.

A Type I error can occur for several reasons. First, on the basis of random fluctuation you will occasionally obtain a difference large enough, or a relationship strong enough, for a null hypothesis to be rejected. Thus, if a significance test were run at a 5 percent *alpha level* (i.e., a 0.05 level of confidence), the probability of the null hypothesis being rejected on the basis of chance alone would be 5 percent. You would expect 5 percent of the null hypotheses you test to be rejected when they should not be rejected— that is, when they are true.

A Type I error may also occur because the measures on which a significance test is performed are biased. One of the most common sources of such bias is the investigator's expectations regarding the results of the research. Such expectations can consciously or unconsciously influence measurements. This is particularly apt to happen in therapy outcome research. Clinicians may feel such a strong need for their therapy to appear effective that they may unconsciously manipulate pre- and post-therapy measures so that the magnitude of the difference between them is increased. This could cause a true null hypothesis to be rejected.

Suppose that in order to assess the impact of a therapy program on a group of stutterers, you measured twenty-five aspects of their behavior both before and after participating in the program and tested the reliability of the difference between the means of each of these twenty-five pairs or measures at the 5 percent (i.e., 0.05) level of confidence. Suppose, further, that the difference between only one of these twenty-five sets of pre- and post-therapy means was *statistically significant*—that is, was large enough for the null hypothesis to be rejected. Could you conclude that the behavior this measure measured had changed? The answer to this question is no, because you would expect approximately one out of every twenty true null hypotheses tested at the 0.05 level of confidence to be rejected. The probability of a Type I error having occurred when this null hypothesis was rejected is *not* 5 percent (the probability if only one null hypothesis had been tested) but *close to 100 percent.* It is necessary to consider the *experiment-wise error rate,* then, when interpreting the results of studies in which more than one null hypothesis is tested. The level of confidence at which a given null hypothesis is tested applies only if a single null hypothesis is tested. Unless a statistical correction is made to keep the probability of a Type I error for individual tests of the null hypothesis at the appropriate level, it will be higher.

Many types of significance tests have been developed for testing null hypotheses. A representative sample of such tests is presented in Table 10-1. There is a test in this table that would be appropriate for most occasions when a speech-language pathologist or audiologist wished to assess the statistical significance of differences between sample means or medians. The formulas and Minitab commands for computing the significance tests in

TABLE 10-1   Significance Tests Categorized on the Basis of: (1) Their Level of Measurement, (2) Whether They Are Intended for Independent or Related Samples, and (3) Whether They Are Intended for the Two-Sample Case or the More Than Two-Sample Case

Level of Measurement	Two-Sample Case		More Than Two-Sample Case	
	Related Samples	Independent Samples	Related Samples	Independent Samples
Nominal		Chi square		Chi square
Ordinal	Sign test	Mann-Whitney U test	Friedman two-way analysis of variance	Kruskal-Wallis one-way analysis of variance
Interval and *Ratio*	*t*-Test for related measures	*t*-Test for independent measures	One-way analysis of variance for related measures	One-way analysis of variance for independent measures

Table 10-1 are in Appendix A. Some representative studies from the communicative disorders literature in which the tests presented in Table 10-1 were used are listed in Table 10-2.

The significance tests in Table 10-1 that are recommended for nominal and ordinal data sometimes are referred to as *nonparametric* ones (Sutor & White, 1992). They differ from those recommended for interval and ratio data—that is, parametric significance tests—in that they do not require an assumption of equal intervals between scale points and an absolute zero to be made for the data (see Chapter 7). While they are more appropriate for nominal and ordinal data than the parametric tests, they are also less powerful than them. Consequently, they require more subjects (a larger N) to keep the probability of a Type II error at an acceptable level.

How do you identify an appropriate significance test? To do this, you need the following information about the data on which the significance test is to be performed:

- The *level of measurement* of the measures
- Whether the measures are *independent or related*
- The *number of sets* of means, medians, or other measures you wish to test the differences between

TABLE 10-2   Representative Studies in the Communicative Disorders Literature in Which Certain Inferential Statistics Were Used

Statistic	Reference
Analysis of covariance (ANCOVA)	Fey et al. (1994); Gorenflo et al. (1994); Grose et al. (1994)
Analysis of variance (ANOVA)	At least one paper in every issue of the *Journal of Speech and Hearing Research*
Binomial test	Leonard et al. (1992); Tomes & Shelton (1989)

TABLE 10-2   *Continued*

Statistic	Reference
Chi-square test	Felsenfeld et al. (1994); Gutierrez-Clellen & Hofstetter (1994); Viswanath & Neel (1995)
Cluster analysis	McLeod et al. (1994); Washington & Craig (1994)
Confidence intervals	Dubno et al. (1995); Kuehn & Moon (1994); Macrae (1995)
Discriminant function analysis	Hall et al. (1993); Hillenbrand & Gayvert (1993); Liles et al. (1995);
Factor analysis	Elliott & Hammer (1993); Humes et al. (1994); Peach (1992)
Fisher exact test	Bird et al. (1995)
Friedman two-way analysis of variance	Clark & Stemple (1982); Karlsen et al. (1992)
G statistic	Elliott (1986); Macmillan et al. (1988); Sussman (1993a, 1993b)
Hotelling's statistical tests	Girolametto & Tannock (1994); Snow (1994); Wilson & Miller (1993)
Kappa statistic	Logemann et al. (1994)
Kolmogorov-Smirnov test	Ziegler et al. (1993)
Kruskal-Wallis one-way analysis of variance	Caruso et al. (1994); Langmore & Lehman (1994); Mayberry (1993)
Log-linear analysis	Perlman et al. (1992); Walden et al. (1993); Weston & Shriberg (1992)
Mann-Whitney U test	Langmore & Lehman (1994); Shriberg et al. (1994); Thal & Tobias (1992)
McNemar test	Logemann et al. (1994)
Meta-analysis	Fitz-Gibbon (1986); Wachter & Straf (1990)
Multidimensional scaling	Kempster et al. (1991); Kreiman et al. (1992); Maré et al. (1992)
Multiple comparisons following a significant F (ANOVA)	At least one paper in every issue of the *Journal of Speech and Hearing Research*
Multiple correlation and regression	de Krom (1995); Martin et al. (1995); McClean et al. (1994)
Randomization tests	Thal & Tobias (1992); Wit et al. (1993)
Resampling tests	Kaiser & Hester (1994)
Sign test	Mayberry (1993)
T-test	At least one paper in every issue of the *Journal of Speech and Hearing Research*
Test for proportional differences	Linville (1992)
Tests for homogeneity of variance	Grose et al. (1993); Stagray et al. (1992); Swanson et al. (1992)
Wilcoxon-Mann-Whitney test	Shriberg (1993)
Wilcoxon matched pair signed-ranks test	Caruso et al. (1994); Mulligan et al. (1994); Shriberg (1993)

With this information, you can enter Table 10-1 to identify an appropriate significance test.

The level of measurement of the measures refers to whether they possess nominal, ordinal, interval, or ratio properties (see Chapter 7). There are different significance tests for nominal, ordinal, and interval-ratio measures (see Table 10-1). The same significance tests are used for both interval and ratio measures.

While it is permissible to use a significance test appropriate for a lower level of measurement than that present in the data, this is usually not done, because such a test would probably be less *powerful* than one appropriate for the level of measurement present in the data. (Nominal would be a lower level of measurement than ordinal, ordinal would be a lower level of measurement than interval, and so on.) One consequence of using a less powerful test is that more subjects (i.e., larger groups) are needed to detect differences of a given size—that is, cause a false null hypothesis to be rejected at a given level of confidence. The less powerful the test you use, the more likely you are to commit a Type II error (i.e., retain a false null hypothesis).

Another piece of information you need about the data to select an appropriate significance test is whether the sets of measures that you wish to assess the difference (or differences) between are independent or related. If the sets of measures were made on the same persons, they are *related.* Consequently, if you wanted to assess the difference between measures made on a group of persons before and after participating in a therapy program, you would have to use a significance test appropriate for related measures.

If the sets of measures were made on different persons, they *usually* would be regarded as *independent.* Consequently, if you wanted to compare a group of persons who had spastic dysarthria to a group of persons who did not have spastic dysarthria on some measure, ordinarily you would have to use a significance test appropriate for independent measures. We use the qualifier *ordinarily* here because there is one circumstance when this would not be true. If the persons on whom the sets of measures were made were *very closely matched* for all relevant variables, the sets of measures could be treated as related. About the only time that you really can be quite confident that this level of matching has been achieved is when the persons in the group are identical twins and one twin from each set is in each group.

The third piece of information that you need to select an appropriate significance test is the *number* of sets of means, medians, or other measures you wish to assess differences between. If this number is *two,* one set of significance tests is appropriate; if it is *more than two,* a second set is appropriate. For "before and after" therapy measures a significance test for two sets would be appropriate, and for "before and after" therapy plus follow-up measures (three sets) a significance test for more than two sets would be appropriate.

With these three pieces of information, you may enter Table 10-1 to identify an appropriate significance test. To illustrate how to use this table, let us suppose you administered a picture vocabulary test to a group of children twice, once preceding and once following their participation in a therapy program. Most likely you would wish to determine whether a difference you observed between medians of the two sets of scores were large enough for chance or random fluctuation to be unlikely as an explanation. It would probably be safest to assume that the scores on such a vocabulary test have *ordinal* properties. The sets of measures would be *related* because they were made on the same persons, and the number of sets would be *two.* The significance test in Table 10-1 appropriate for two sets of measures having ordinal properties is the *sign test.*

Table 10-1 does not suggest any tests for sets of related measures having nominal properties. While there appear to be no commonly used tests for such measures, significance tests have been developed for them—for example, the McNemar test for the significance of change (Siegel, 1956). A statistician should be consulted to identify the most appropriate one for determining the reliability of differences between specific sets of such measures.

Table 10-1 also does not include tests appropriate for relatively complex comparisons between means or medians. Such tests would be required to answer questions similar to this one: "Was the effect of a speech improvement program that was administered to a group of kindergarten children different for boys than for girls?" If a difference did exist, it would probably be inadvisable to combine outcome data from boys and girls. A multivariate analysis-of-variance design could be used to assess the likelihood that the program affects boys and girls differently (i.e., to test the null hypothesis that the differences between boys and girls arose from chance, or random fluctuation). These are described elsewhere in this chapter.

You should consult with someone knowledgeable about significance tests if you want to follow up an analysis-of-variance in which you reject the null hypothesis. Rejecting the null hypothesis in this case indicates that at least one of the possible differences between means is unlikely to be due to chance. It does not indicate that all of the differences are likely to be "real" ones! To determine which one (or ones) is real, you would test the differences between the various pairs of means that were included in the analysis-of-variance. *T*-tests are *not* appropriate for this purpose. Appropriate tests include the Newman-Keuls post hoc tests, the Sheffe post hoc tests, and the Tukey post hoc tests. (Examples that illustrate the use of these tests can be found on the following pages in the 1989 volume of the *Journal of Speech and Hearing Research:* 36, 333, 447, 506, 629, 710, 718, 768, 819, 833, 838, and 841.) There are commands for doing tests of this type in the Minitab statistical software package as well as most other such packages.

All of the significance tests described thus far have been for *differences* between means, medians, and other descriptive statistics. As was indicated earlier, there are also significance tests for assessing the likelihood that observed *relationships* (as designated by nonzero correlation coefficients) arose from chance, or random fluctuation. A test of this type appropriate for Pearson product-moment correlation coefficients is included in Appendix A.

After the statistic for a significance test has been computed, it is necessary to determine whether the probability of its occurrence is smaller than the level of confidence selected. If the value of this statistic (e.g., x^2, x, z, t, or F) is such that the probability of its occurrence as a result of chance is less than (i.e., smaller than) this level, the null hypothesis is rejected. Otherwise, it is retained. For example, if the level of confidence selected was 0.05 and the probability for the statistic computed resulting from chance was 0.03, the null hypothesis would be rejected. On the other hand, if the level of confidence selected was 0.01 and the probability for the statistic computed resulting from chance was 0.03, the null hypothesis would be retained.

How do you determine whether the value computed for a significance test statistic has a small enough probability of occurrence under the null hypothesis to reject it? To do this, you can use a *table* that provides either: (1) the probability associated with the value for the test statistic that the difference or relationship was due to chance, or (2) the value the test statistic would have to *exceed* before you could conclude that the probability of the difference or relationship being due to chance was equal to or less than the level of confidence selected. The tables in Appendix A for the binomial distribution (Table A-3) and the normal distribution (Table A-4) provide probability values, and those for the chi square distribution (Table A-2), the *t*-distribution (Table A-5), and the *F*-distribution (Table A-6) provide values that have to be exceeded. The Minitab statistical software can generate the information in these tables.

You will need several pieces of information before you can enter a table to determine whether the results of a significance test permit the null hypothesis to be rejected. Those required most often include:

1. The appropriate distribution (table) to use
2. The alpha level, or level of confidence, at which the null hypothesis is being tested
3. The degrees of freedom *(df)*
4. Whether the test is to be one-tailed or two-tailed
5. the value computed for the test statistic

The first thing that you need to know before you can determine whether the outcome of a statistical test permits the null hypothesis to be rejected is what distribution to use. The appropriate distribution, or table, for a particular significance test usually is indicated in its description. There are distribution tables in Appendix A for the significance tests in Table 10-1.

A second piece of information that you will need is the alpha level, or level of confidence, at which the null hypothesis is to be tested. While any level 0.05 or smaller is considered acceptable by the editors of scientific and professional journals, most investigators limit themselves to the 0.05 and 0.01 levels. The tabled distributions in Appendix A can all be entered at these two alpha levels.

A third piece of information you may need to enter a table is the number of degrees of freedom *(df)* in your data. Tables that require this information to enter them (e.g., x^2, *t*, and *F*) contain a *number* of distributions, one for each *df* value designated in them. The *df* value for a set of data designates the distribution in a table that contains the *critical value* of the statistic that the one computed on the data must *exceed* before the null hypothesis can be rejected. With the exception of contingency tables, degrees of freedom for the significance tests in Appendix A are based on (but not equal to) the number of subjects. For contingency tables, *df* values are based on the numbers of rows and columns in a table rather than on the numbers of subjects contained in them.

The method for determining the *df* value for a particular test is indicated in the description of the computational procedure for that test. (This information is provided in Appendix A for all of the significance tests described in it that require *df* values.) Note that the table for the *F* distribution (Table A-6) requires two *df* values rather than one to locate critical values of the statistic.

A fourth piece of information that sometimes is necessary for determining whether the outcome of a statistical test allows the null hypothesis to be rejected is whether the test is to be *one-tailed* or *two-tailed*. If, to answer a question, you only have to be able to detect a difference in one direction, a one-tailed test can be used. The following are representative questions that can be answered with a one-tailed test:

1. Are stutterers more anxious than nonstutterers in a particular situation?
2. Do children evince fewer articulation errors after participating in a particular therapy program?

To answer the first question, it would not be necessary to determine whether nonstutterers are more anxious than stutterers. To answer the second question, it would not be necessary to determine whether children exhibit more articulation errors after participating in the therapy program.

If to answer a question you have to be able to detect a difference in either direction, you must use a two-tailed test. The following questions require a two-tailed test to answer:

1. Do stutterers and nonstutterers *differ* with regard to intelligence (IQ)?
2. Do aphasics' word-finding abilities tend to be *different* two years after they terminate a particular therapy program than when they terminated it?

To answer these questions, it would be necessary to be able to detect differences in both directions. Stutterers would differ from nonstutterers if their IQ were either higher or lower. Also, the aphasics' word-finding abilities two years following termination of treatment would be different, regardless of whether they were better or poorer than at termination.

It is advantageous to use a one-tailed test *if it is appropriate to do so* because the probability of committing a Type II error is less than for a two-tailed test. For detecting differences in a single direction using a *one-tailed* test, the 0.05 level of confidence really is the 0.05 level of confidence. However, for detecting differences in a single direction using a *two-tailed* test, the 0.05 level of confidence becomes the 0.025 level of confidence. Consequently, the probability of committing a Type II error is greater.

If you use a one-tailed test, you are required by the assumptions underlying statistical inference to decide on the direction in which you want to be able to detect a difference *before you begin collecting data*. It is not legitimate to change your mind or decide on the direction after you have seen the data. If you do so, the probability of committing a Type I error will be higher than the level of confidence at which the test was run would indicate.

Some tabled distributions list critical values for two-tailed tests. Others do not. Critical values for two-tailed tests can be obtained from tables of the latter type by adjusting the level of confidence. For a two-tailed test at the 0.05 level, you would enter the table at the 0.025 level. And for a two-tailed test at the 0.01 level, you would enter the table at the 0.005 level. Note that larger values of a test statistic are needed to reject the null hypothesis if a two-tailed rather than a one-tailed test is used.

A final piece of information that is essential for determining whether the null hypothesis can be rejected is the value computed for the test statistic.

Once you have the necessary information to enter the appropriate table for a test statistic, you can determine whether the null hypothesis should be rejected. The procedure for entering each table in Appendix A is as follows:

1. *Chi Square Distribution (Table A-2).* Enter this table with the appropriate *df* value for your data and the level of confidence at which the null hypothesis is to be tested. The *df* values are indicated in the first column and levels of confidence in the top row. To identify the critical value of chi square for testing the null hypotheses, you first locate the row containing the appropriate *df* value and then the column for the level of confidence you wish to use. The value of chi square that appears at the intersection of this row and column is the critical value for testing the null hypothesis. If the value you computed is larger, the null hypothesis can be rejected. The levels of confidence are for one-tailed tests. Two-tailed tests are rarely, if ever, used for contingency tables. Rejection of the null hypothesis permits you to conclude that the configuration of frequencies in a contingency table is unlikely to have resulted from chance, or random fluctuation.

2. *Binomial Test (Table A-3).* Enter this table with the value of *x* for your data (see sign test in Appendix A) and the number of subjects *(N)* whose data are being tested for statistical significance. Numbers of subjects are indicated in the first column and *x* values are indicated in the top row. To determine the *probability* that a value of *x* resulted from chance, or random fluctuation, you locate the row for the appropriate number of subjects and the column for the obtained *x* value. The probability value that appears at the intersection of this row and column is the probability that the obtained value of *x* resulted from chance, or random fluctuation. If this probability is smaller than the level of confidence you selected, the null hypothesis should be rejected. These probability values can be used for either one-tailed or two-tailed tests.

3. *Normal Distribution (Table A-4).* Enter this table with the value you compute for *z*. Note that *z* values to one decimal place are indicated in the first column and those to two decimal places in the top row. The numbers in the table are probabilities that given *z* values resulted from chance, or random fluctuation. For a one-tailed test at the 0.05 level, if the probability associated with a given *z* is less than 0.05, the null hypothesis is rejected. For a two-tailed test at the 0.05 level, if the probability associated with a given *z* is less than 0.025, the null hypothesis is rejected.

4. *t-Distribution (Table A-5).* Enter this table with the appropriate *df* value for your data and the level of confidence at which the null hypothesis is to be tested. The *df* values appear in the first column. The levels of significance, or confidence, for one-tailed tests appear in the top row and those for two-tailed tests in the second row. To identify the critical value of *t* for testing the null hypothesis, you locate the row containing the appropriate *df* value and the column for the level of confidence you wish to use. (Note that different columns are used for one-tailed and two-tailed tests.) The value of *t* that appears at the intersection of the row and column is the critical value for testing the null hypothesis. If the value you computed is larger, the null hypothesis should be rejected.

5. *F-Distribution (Table A-6).* Enter this table with two *df* values: df_1 is the degrees of freedom for columns (or between group or treatment variation) and df_2 is the degrees of freedom for rows (or within group or treatment variation). The set of numbers that appears at the intersection of the df_1 column and df_2 row are critical values of *F* for selected levels of confidence, including 1 percent and 5 percent levels. If the value you compute is larger than that in the table for the level of confidence you are using, the null hypothesis should be rejected.

Confidence Intervals

Thus far, we have dealt with the use of statistical inference for determining whether a difference or relationship exists. This section will describe the use of statistical inference for estimating its *magnitude* after it has been shown (by rejecting the null hypothesis) to exist. Rejecting the null hypothesis merely indicates it is likely that a difference or relationship exists—it provides no information about its magnitude. *You cannot assume that the observed magnitude is the real one!* The *confidence interval* is the inferential statistic used for estimating magnitudes. There are references in Table 10-2, incidentally, to several studies in which confidence intervals were utilized in communicative disorders research.

Why might you want to compute a confidence interval? There are several reasons. First, you may want to estimate the population value of a descriptive statistic. The following are representative of questions requiring such an estimate to answer:

1. By what age do 50 percent of children perform a particular task correctly?
2. What percentage of persons with a particular communicative disorder derive benefit from a particular therapy program?
3. How predictive is a person's score on a test before he or she participates in a therapy program of what it will be after he or she participates in the program?

To answer the first question, you have to estimate a *population median;* to answer the second, a *population percentage;* and to answer the third, a *population correlation coefficient* (between the scores of a group of persons before and after participating in the program).

A second reason you may want to use a confidence interval is to estimate the population value of a difference between descriptive statistics. Once a null hypothesis has been rejected, indicating that an observed difference is likely to be a real one, it *may* be important to estimate the magnitude of the difference. Such an estimate may be helpful for judging its importance—that is, for deciding whether it is likely to be a large enough difference to make a difference in the "real world" (Gardner & Altman, 1990; Murray, 1989). Aphasics may make gains if they participate in a particular intensive therapy program (judging by the results of a significance test on the difference between pre- and post-therapy scores), but the magnitudes of these gains may not be sufficient to effect any real improvement in their ability to communicate. To determine if this were likely to be the case, the magnitude of the difference between pre- and post-therapy scores could be estimated by means of a confidence interval (assuming that the results of a test of the difference between pre- and post-therapy measures resulted in rejection of the null hypothesis). Unless the null hypothesis were rejected, indicating that the observed difference is likely to be a real one, it would make no sense to estimate its magnitude!

The following are representative of questions about differences between descriptive statistics that could be answered by computing a confidence interval:

1. How much of a reduction in the severity of a particular communicative disorder could be expected to result from participation in a particular therapy program?

2. How much of a difference is there apt to be between persons who have a particular communicative disorder and those who do not have it in the performance of a particular task?

Both questions can be answered by a confidence interval for the difference between the mean (or median) performances of the groups.

What are confidence intervals? These are intervals designated by two values—a lower limit and an upper limit—between which we can be a particular percent certain (usually 95 percent or 99 percent) that the magnitude of a descriptive statistic or a difference between descriptive statistics falls. Thus, based on confidence intervals, we might conclude it is 95 percent certain that the mean IQ for a population falls between 90 and 105, or that it is 99 percent certain that the mean amount sixth-grade children who stutter are behind their peers in academic achievement is between 5 and 12 months. In the second example, the difference between two means is being estimated—that is, the difference between the mean of the scores of sixth-grade stutterers on a test of academic achievement and that of their peers.

The two most frequently used certainty levels for confidence intervals are 95 percent and 99 percent. With the first, you can be 95 percent certain that the population value falls between the specified limits, and with the second, you can be 99 percent certain that it falls between these limits. These interpretations, of course, would only be valid if the subjects in the sample from whose data the confidence interval was computed were representative of those in the population to which the interpretations referred—that is, if they at least approximated a random sample from this population.

A 95 percent confidence interval always would be *narrower* than a 99 percent confidence interval. The *higher* the degree of confidence that the population value of the descriptive statistic (or difference between descriptive statistics) computed lies within the confidence interval (i.e., between its upper and lower limits), the *wider* it will be.

Another factor that influences the widths of confidence intervals is *sample size*. The larger the number of subjects in the sample, the narrower the confidence level.

Relatively narrow confidence intervals provide more useful information than relatively wide ones. Knowing that the mean IQ for children in a population (e.g., those who have cleft palates) is probably somewhere between 90 and 95 is likely to provide more useful information than knowing it is somewhere between 80 and 105.

In summary, you can maximize the probability that the width of a confidence interval will be adequately narrow by using a 95 rather than a 99 percent confidence level and as many subjects (i.e., as large an N) as possible.

Confidence intervals can be computed for descriptive statistics and the differences between them regardless of whether they have ordinal, interval, or ratio properties. The confidence interval for the median (see Appendix A) is one that can be computed from measures having ordinal, interval, or ratio properties. Those for the mean and differences between means (see Appendix A) can be computed from measures having interval or ratio properties.

Other Inferential Statistical Techniques

Nine sophisticated inferential statistical techniques that have been used for answering questions about communicative disorders are briefly described in this section. They are multivariate analysis of variance, multiple regression, multivariate analysis of covariance, factor analysis, discriminant function analysis, multidimensional scaling, cluster analysis, meta-analysis, and control charts. You can make the necessary calculations with the Minitab program and most other sophisticated statistical software packages.

Multivariate Analysis of Variance (MANOVA)

Univariate versions of this significance test for independent and related sets of measures are dealt with elsewhere in this chapter (see Table 10-1) and there are computational formulas for both in Appendix A. Investigators sometimes want to determine whether subjects differ on variables other than the one in which they are primarily interested. For example, in a study of the effect of an intervention on children who have a particular type of language disorder the investigator may want to determine whether the intervention is likely to improve the language functioning of both boys and girls and if it does appear to do so, whether the magnitude of the improvement is likely to be the same for both sexes. Let's assume that he or she administered a language test to a group of boys and a group of girls both prior to and after receiving the intervention and the means of the scores for the two groups were those plotted in Figure 10-1. These data could be used to partially answer the following questions:

- Is the difference between pre- and post-intervention scores for the total group of children (boys and girls combined) likely to have resulted from random sampling error?
- Is the difference between boys and girls when both conditions are combined likely to have resulted from random sampling error?
- Is the difference in the average amount of post-intervention increase in test scores for the boys and the girls likely to have resulted from random sampling error?

Note that in Figure 10-1 post-intervention mean scores tended to be higher than the pre-intervention ones, girls tended to have higher mean scores than boys, and girls' mean scores

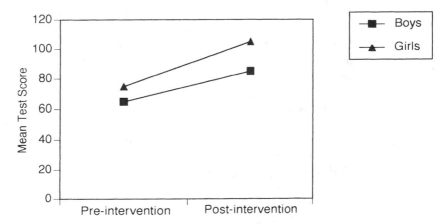

FIGURE 10-1   Mean pre-intervention and post-intervention scores on a language test for a group of boys and a group of girls.

tended to increase more than did boys'. Multivariate analysis of variance can be used to estimate the probability that these differences are real ones. That is, it can be used to test the null hypothesis that each of them resulted from random sampling error.

Multivariate analysis of variance can be used to test null hypothesis about both the *main effects* and the *interaction effects* of a "treatment." Main effects pertain to mean differences between variables. In our example (see Figure 10-1) there are two variables—sex (boys vs. girls) and intervention (pre- vs. post-intervention). Consequently, there can be two tests of main effects.

Interaction effects pertain to differences between variables other than the mean ones. If the interaction is between two variables and there is an interaction effect, their lines in a plot would not be parallel. In our example, there is a possibility of an interaction effect between sex and intervention because the lines aren't parallel (see Figure 10-1).

The *F-distribution* is used—as it is with univariate analyses of variance—to test null hypotheses. An *F* statistic is computed for each effect. Three *F*-statistics would be computed for our example (see Figure 10-1)—one for sex, one for intervention, and one for sex x intervention interaction.

Sets of measures from which *F* statistics are computed with a multivariate analysis of variance can be independent and/or related. In our example (Figure 10-1) there are both. Those for "sex" are independent and those for "intervention" are related.

Theoretically, any number of variables can be included in a multivariate analysis of variance. However, the number used is rarely more than three. One reason is that making meaningful interpretations of interactions involving more than three variables can be extremely difficult because such interactions cannot be visualized graphically.

If the value of *F* for a variable leads to the rejection of the null hypothesis, it could mean that only one of the differences between the means of measures of that variable is unlikely to have resulted from random sampling error. Let's assume that in the example in Figure 10-1 the language test had been administered to each child three times rather than two (e.g., pre-intervention, at termination of intervention, and two months following intervention) and that the *F* for the main effect for intervention was statistically significant. There are three possible comparisons between means that can be made here, any one or combination of which could have yielded this result. They are pre-intervention vs. termination, pre-intervention vs. follow-up, and termination vs. follow-up. Statisticians have developed significance tests for making *multiple comparisons* to follow up a significant *F*—that is, to determine which of the differences between means are statistically significant (see Rosenthal & Rosnow, 1985). They are regard as being more appropriate than t-tests for making such comparisons.

The interpretation of a significant *F* for a main effect or interaction is exactly the same as it is for a similar univariate significance test result. That is, while it provides evidence that a difference is unlikely to been due to random sampling error, it provides *no* information about the size or "meaningfulness" of the difference. The same is true for "significant" results from multiple-comparison follow-up tests.

Sophisticated statistical computer programs—including Minitab (see Appendix A)—can do multivariate analyses of variance. And almost all—including Minitab—can make multiple comparisons to follow-up a significant *F*.

Multivariate analysis of variance is one of the most frequently used techniques for analyzing data in speech, language, and hearing research. Almost every issue of the *Journal of Speech and Hearing Research* contains at least one paper in which it is used. The same is true for the multiple comparison significance tests used to follow up a significant *F*.

There are many books from which you can obtain further information about multivariate analysis of variance. Several that you may find helpful are Bogartz (1994), Edwards (1985), Fisher (1960), Harris (1994), Hays (1973), Lindquist (1953), and Rosenthal and Rosnow (1985).

Multiple Regression

This technique can yield calculations that can assist in answering two types of questions. The first are ones that a multiple correlation coefficient can be helpful in answering (see Chapter 9). For these, multiple regression is merely a means to an end—that is, multiple correlation coefficients are computed from the calculations yielded by it. For the second type of question—which is discussed here—multiple regression is used for estimating (predicting) test scores and other types of measures.

The following questions are representative of ones that estimates yielded by multiple regression can help to answer:

- Judging by a student's undergraduate GPA and GRE scores, what is his or her GPA in graduate school likely to be?
- What score is a child likely to earn on a language test post-intervention judging by his or her score on that test pre-intervention plus other information?
- What score is an aphasic likely to earn on a diagnostic test based on his or her responses to a sample of the items in it?

For answering the first two questions, multiple regression is used to "objectively" predict a person's future performance. Consequently, it can yield the type of documentation for a prognosis that is likely to be accepted by third-party payers and others. And for answering the third question, it is being used to make administration of a test more cost-effective. If an aphasic's score on a test can be estimated accurately by administering only a part of it, then administering it in this way should be regarded as desirable in a managed care environment (Vekovius, 1995).

The multiple regression equations that are used to estimate test scores and other measures in most cases are linear ones that have a structure similar to the following:

$$X_1 = a + b_2X_2 + b_3X_3 + \ldots \; b_mX_m$$

Here X_1 represents the dependent variable—the measure being estimated—and X_2, $X_3, \ldots X_m$ represent the independent variables that are being used to estimate X_1. The symbolism $\ldots X_m$ indicates that there can be any number of independent variables. The other entities in the equation—a and b_2, $b_3, \ldots b_m$—are constants that are generated by the multiple regression analysis.

To illustrate the use this multiple regression equation to estimate the value of a dependent variable (X_1), we will use undergraduate GPA (U-GPA) and overall GRE scores to estimate graduate GPA (G-GPA). The multiple regression equation for doing so would be:

$$X_{\text{G-GPA}} = a + b_2X_{\text{U-GPA}} + b_3X_{\text{GRE}}$$

The constant *a* probably would be the lowest possible graduate GPA. The constants b_2 and b_3 would be weights by which a student's U-GPA and GRE score would be multiplied. The three constants would be generated by the multiple regression analysis.

It is being assumed in the above example that the relationship between the two independent variables and the dependent variable is a *linear* one. That is, particular amounts of increase in undergraduate GPAs and GREs yield the same amount of increase in graduate GPAs throughout the entire range of possible graduate GPAs. If this assumption is not viable, a more complex regression equation would have to be used (Ezekiel & Fox, 1963).

Multivariate Analysis of Covariance (MANCOVA)

This is the same as multivariate analysis of variance except that subjects are matched *statistically* on a variable after the data are gathered rather than by a *selection criterion* before the data are gathered. This variable—referred to as a concomitant variable—would be one we are not studying that might cause the null hypothesis to be rejected. If we do not match groups of subjects for the concomitant variable and we reject the null hypothesis, we can not be certain whether the difference that resulted in it being rejected was one between groups for it or for the variable in which we are interested.

Suppose that we want to determine whether there is a difference in the amount of improvement that is likely to be yielded by two language stimulation programs. We have two groups of children available to us, the membership of which cannot be changed. Unfortunately, the children in one group are a little older than those in the other. Consequently, we could not be certain if the difference between groups in amount of improvement was statistically significant whether it resulted from one intervention being more effective than the other or the children in one group being older than those in the other. Using analysis of covariance, we could eliminate difference between pre- and post-intervention test scores (our criterion measures) that age differences could have caused. We would do this by adjusting the scores for such differences before performing an analysis of variance on them. Multivariate analysis of covariance, therefore, is simply an extension of multivariate analysis of variance in which criterion measures are "adjusted" to control for a concomitant variable.

For representative studies in which multivariate analysis of covariance was used in communicative disorder research, see Table 10-2.

Factor Analysis

Factor analysis is a technique for identifying general factors, or abilities, that influence performance on a series of tasks (e.g., psychological or language tests). Suppose, for example, you *told* an aphasic to do the following tasks: (1) point to the objects named, (2) name the objects shown, and (3) protrude his or her tongue. A general factor, or ability, that underlies the performance of all three can be labeled "language comprehension." To be successful in performing them it is necessary to understand the instructions you are given.

Factor analysis can be used for answering questions about: (1) general abilities, or factors, that underlie the performance of a series of tasks, and (2) tasks that can be used to evaluate (test) for each such factor.

Suppose you wanted to develop a comprehensive test for evaluating aphasics. This test would consist of a series of tasks, and there would be a great many tasks that could be included. To help you decide which to include, you would want to know: (1) the aspects, or dimensions, of speech and language that are apt to be impaired as a result of the condition, and (2) the task, or tasks, best suited to evaluate for each. This information could be obtained with factor analysis as follows:

1. A large number of possible tasks for such a test would be administered to a fairly large group of aphasics. All of the various types of tasks that have been used to evaluate aphasics would be represented.

2. The scores earned by the aphasics on all possible pairs of tasks would be correlated and displayed in a *correlation matrix*. A correlation matrix for five such tasks is depicted in Table 10-3. A correlation coefficient would appear in each square marked with an *X*. The type of correlation coefficient most often used for this purpose is the Pearson *r* (see Chapter 9 and Appendix A).

TABLE 10-3   A Correlation Matrix for Five Tasks (Each square marked with an *X* would contain a correlation coefficient.)

	Task I	Task II	Task III	Task IV	Task V
Task I		X	X	X	X
Task II			X	X	X
Task III				X	X
Task IV					X
Task V					

3. The correlation matrix would be factor analyzed, using a sophisticated statistical program, such as Minitab.

The printout from the computer will contain information about: (1) the number of general factors, or abilities, identified by the program that presumably influenced the aphasics' performances of the tasks, and (2) the specific tasks that had relatively "high loadings" and "low loadings" for each. A task with a "high loading" for a particular factor, or ability, would be good for assessing that factor, or ability. Conversely, a task with a "low loading" for a particular factor, or ability, would not be very good for assessing that factor, or ability. You would probably want to include at least one task in your aphasia test that had a relatively high loading for each factor.

How can you identify the ability that each factor represents? The computer does not label the factors. It does provide information, however, that can be used for inferring the ability each represents. Suppose two tasks had relatively high loadings and three had relatively low loadings for a particular factor. To determine what it represented, you would attempt to identify the ability that successful completion of the two tasks with high loadings required that was not required of the three with low loadings. Obviously, labels assigned to factors by such a reasoning process have to be regarded as tentative because tasks with relatively high loadings may require *more than one* ability that is not required of those with relatively low loadings.

In summary, factor analysis can be a useful exploratory procedure for identifying general abilities that underlie the performance of a series of tasks. For further information on this technique, you may find books by Basilevsky (1994), Comrey and Lee (1992), and Kline (1994) helpful.

For illustrations of the use of factor analysis in speech, language, and hearing research, see Table 10-2.

Discriminant Function Analysis

Discriminant function analysis is a statistical procedure used to assign people to categories, usually dichotomous categories. The following are examples of pairs of categories to which discriminant function analysis might be used for assigning persons:

- "Beginning stuttering" versus "normally disfluent speech"
- "Adequate velopharyngeal closure" versus "inadequate velopharyngeal closure" for speech

Programs for performing a discriminant function analysis (e.g., Minitab) are available for both Macintosh and IBM-compatible computers.

The types of questions that discriminant function analysis may be useful for answering include:

1. Is a given 4-year-old exhibiting "beginning stuttering" or "normally disfluent speech"?
2. What variables best differentiate "beginning stuttering" from "normally disfluent speech" for 4-year-olds?

3. Is the velopharyngeal closure of a given child who has a cleft palate "adequate" or "inadequate" to support speech that has normal nasal resonance?

4. What measures best differentiate "adequate" from "inadequate" velopharyngeal closure?

While these questions all involve discriminating between two categories, discriminant function analysis is not limited to the two-category situation.

The approach used for doing a two-category discriminant function analysis can be summarized as follows:

1. A series of tasks (e.g., tests), that there is some reason to believe might discriminate between persons who fall into the two categories, are administered to two groups. Each consists of persons who fall into one of the categories. For the first question, one group would consist of 4-year-olds who are known to be beginning to stutter and the other would consist of 4-year-olds who have no history of a stuttering problem.

2. A discriminant function analysis is performed on the measures (e.g., test scores). The results of this analysis indicate which task, or combination of tasks, best discriminates between the groups (assuming that both groups did not perform essentially the same on the tasks).

3. The task, or combination of tasks, identified by the analysis can be used for determining the category, or group, to assign a person when the group to which he or she should be assigned is unknown. The analysis provides an equation for this purpose. In this equation, the person's score on each task (S) is multiplied by a weight (W) that is determined by the program and the products of these multiplications are summed algebraically. The form of a typical such equation would be similar to:

$$X = S_1 W_1 + S_2 W_2$$

In words, you would multiply the person's score on task one by the weight assigned to that task and add this to his or her score on task two multiplied by the weight assigned to task two.

The value of X would indicate the category to which the person should be assigned. If it was larger than the value computed for X, the person would be assigned to one category; if it was smaller than this value, the person would be assigned to the other category.

The procedure for a discriminant function analysis involving more than two categories is essentially the same as that outlined here.

In summary, discriminant function analysis can be a useful procedure for: (1) identifying the way, or ways, in which the members of a group differ and (2) identifying the categories, or groups, to which people belong.

For illustrations of the use of discriminant function analysis in speech, language, and hearing research, see Table 10-2.

Multidimensional Scaling

Multidimensional scaling is a procedure for identifying the attributes of stimuli (or events) to which people attend, that is, the attributes that they abstract. Suppose you wanted to identify the attributes of moments of stuttering to which people attend. To do this, you could collect "moments of stuttering" from a number of stutterers on videotape. You would then have these taped moments of stuttering rated for *degree of similarity* by a fairly large number of observers. The similarity ratings could be made in several ways. One that appears to be used most often is called the "method of triads." With this method, all possible combinations of the moments of stuttering taken *three* at a time would be formed. Observers would be asked to indicate the two moments of stuttering in each group of three that are most similar. The resulting similarity ratings would be subjected to several computer analyses, including a factor analysis. The attributes of the stimuli to which the observers consciously or unconsciously attended while making their similarity ratings can be inferred from the factors identified by the factor analysis.

Multidimensional scaling has been used by speech-language pathologists and audiologists (see Table 10-2). Further information about it can be obtained from a number of sources, including books by Davison (1992), Green, Carmone, Jr., and Smith (1989), and Young (1987).

Cluster Analysis

Cluster analysis is an exploratory procedure for identifying possible subgroups, or groupings, of subjects. Groupings are based on calculations of the distances between measures of the subjects' behavior during the performance of one or more tasks (Everitt, 1993; Kaufman & Rousseeuw, 1990). A grouping identified by a cluster analysis would consist of subjects who performed similarly to each other and dissimilarly to the others on the task(s). That is, a grouping would consist of subjects whose criterion measures for one or more tasks *differed little* from each other. After a subgroup of subjects is identified by a cluster analysis, a hypothesis usually is formulated to explain how the subjects in it differ from the others. One or more experiments may be conducted to test this hypothesis. Some statistical program packages, including SYSTAT (Wilkinson, 1988) and Minitab (see Appendix A), can do the necessary calculations.

Investigators in our field have used cluster analysis to answer the following questions:

- Are there different types of phonological disorders (see McLeod, Hand, Rosenthal, & Hayes, 1994)?
- Are there subgroups of African American English users (see Washington & Craig, 1994)?

The groupings identified by a cluster analysis should be interpreted with caution. There are several reasons. First, the explanation for some subjects performing similarly enough to be assigned to the same group could be random sampling error. Second, there are several distance measures and subject linkage methods that an investigator can use for a cluster analysis. The distance measure and subject linkage method that he or she decides to use can influence the composition of the groupings. And third, the final partition of the subjects into groupings, or clusters, is somewhat arbitrary. Decisions concerning where one cluster ends and another begins and the number of clusters in the data are somewhat subjective. Consequently, cluster analysis should be regarded as an exploratory procedure—not a confirmatory one.

Meta-Analysis

Meta-analysis (Durlak, 1995; Fitz-Gibbon, 1986; Glass, McGaw, & Smith, 1981; Hedges & Olkin, 1985; Hunter, 1990; Hunter & Schmidt, 1990; Laird & Mosteller, 1990; Matt, 1989; Petitti, 1994; Wachter & Straf, 1990) is a statistical approach, of relatively recent origin, for combining data from separate studies for the purpose of obtaining information that cannot be derived from the individual studies. It is used to integrate information from different studies of a given problem. Consequently, it differs from the other statistical methods described in this chapter in that it is not used for analyzing the data from a single study. It has been used extensively in psychology and medicine for integrating and interpreting the results of outcome studies on specific intervention strategies (Hsu, 1989; Matt, 1989; Simes, 1990; Wachter & Straf, 1990).

Why is a methodology like meta-analysis needed? The reason is that questions, particularly those pertaining to therapy outcome, can rarely be answered unequivocally with a single set of data (i.e., by a single study). There are several reasons. First, the subjects used in a particular study may not constitute a truly random sample from the population to which the question refers, and the sample size may be relatively small. Second, if a group design was used, rejection of the null hypothesis may have resulted from a Type I error or its retention from a Type II one. Third, if a single subject design was used, the generality of the findings would be uncertain. Finally, an effect (or a lack of one) could have resulted from experimenter or subject bias (see Chapter 13) or from extraneous variables that were not adequately controlled for and biased the data.

The approach used with meta-analysis for summarizing research findings can be summarized as follows:

> *To investigate the effects of an experimental treatment . . .* all *studies concerned with that treatment—published and unpublished studies, statistically significant or not, well-designed or not—are collected for analysis. Each study is regarded as providing a sample estimate for the population parameter of interest, the Effect Size. . . . The Effect Size is an index of how much difference the treatment made. . . . In addition to obtaining Effect Sizes from studies, each study is coded for all variables that might affect the reported outcome of the treatment, such as the site, year of publication, the adequacy of the design, reliability of instruments, treatment characteristics, personnel involved, etc. The obtained Effect Sizes are then related to the characteristics of the experiments from which they arose. The aim is not to say that a treatment has an effect with a certain probability that a Type I error has been avoided, but to provide estimates of the size of effects in various circumstances, with various subjects. (Fitz-Gibbon, 1986, p. 118)*

Statistical procedures for computing Effect Sizes and combining them—that is, for performing a meta-analysis—are described in publications by Glass, McGaw, and Smith (1981), Hedges and Olkin (1985), and Laird and Mosteller (1990).

Meta-analysis can be used for the same purpose as a confidence interval—to estimate the magnitude of a difference (an Effect Size). Hence, it can be used for answering the same types of questions. In some cases, confidence intervals are used in conjunction with Effect Size estimates.

While meta-analysis is a popular methodology for combining the results of independent studies, it is not the only one that can be used for doing so. For descriptions of several others, see Rosenthal (1978).

Meta-analysis did not appear to have been utilized a great deal in speech-language pathology and audiology research when this chapter was written. The only references I was able to find to it pertained to its use in aphasia therapy outcome research (Fitz-Gibbon, 1986; Robey, 1994; Wachter & Straf, 1990), research on child language development (van Ijzendoorn, Dijkstra, & Bus, 1995), phoneme identification research (Pitt & Samuel, 1993), research on the self-esteem of persons who are hearing impaired (Bat-Chava, 1993), and research on neurophysiological aspects of language functioning (Zaidel, Aboitiz, Clarke, Kaiser, & Matteson, 1995). One reason undoubtedly is that the technique is relatively new. Nevertheless, judging by the literature pertaining to its utilization in psychotherapy and medical intervention research (in 1996 there were more than 2,000 papers reporting its utilization in such research in the PsycINFO and Medline databases), it should be a useful tool for investigators in our field who are attempting to answer questions concerning treatment efficacy.

Control Charts

This technique differs from the others discussed in this chapter in two ways. First, it is likely to be used mainly for answering "administrative" questions rather than ones about management approaches per se. And second, it is not widely used in the behavioral sciences. In fact, it is used mainly for monitoring product quality on production lines in factories.

Why describe a statistical technique that has been used little, if at all, by practitioners and researchers in our field? The reason is that a control chart can be used to "objectively" document for employers, government agencies, and others the impact of marketing and/or other variables on the size and composition of a caseload. Because of the origins of this "medium" (in quality control), its use is likely to enhance the credibility of the "message."

Figure 10-2 is a representative control chart for documenting weekly fluctuations in a daily caseload. The middle line indicates the mean for the period charted (4.75 cases). The upper and lower lines (UCL and LCL) indicate points that are three standard deviations above and below the mean. The probability of an average daily caseload falling outside of these lines by chance is less than 1 percent. Consequently, if the average daily caseload for a week exceeded 8.4, this would suggest that something other than chance (random fluctuation) caused it to increase. This outcome would be equivalent to rejecting a null hypothesis at the 0.01 level of confidence.

Daily caseload isn't the only measure that it may be worthwhile to plot on a control chart. Another would be the average proportion of the clients in a clinician's daily caseload who share something—for example, a type of disorder, a chronological age, or a third-party payer.

You can compute the values for a control chart and plot it with some statistical programs by issuing a single command. The control chart in Figure 10-2 was generated by the Minitab program (see Appendix A) in this manner.

For further information about control charts, see Hart and Hart (1989).

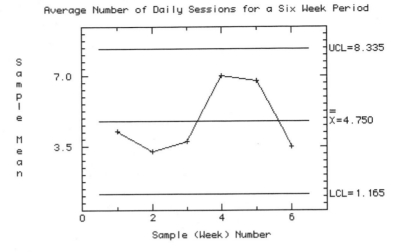

FIGURE 10-2   Control chart for documenting a caseload.

Exercises and Discussion Topics

1. There are thirteen computational exercises in Appendix A that provide experience in computing significance tests and confidence intervals. Your instructor will tell you which to do and whether to do them with a calculator, a computer (using a statistical program package), or both.

2. The interpretation of inferential statistics for answering questions is not "objective"—it is based on human judgment. Often a set of data can be interpreted to support several different answers to a question. Justify *both* a "yes" and a "no" answer to the following question using the data provided.

Do persons who have a sensorineural hearing loss understand speech better if they use an X-type hearing aid?

Observational Procedures. Three persons who had sensorineural hearing losses were administered a different 50-item PB word list while wearing an X-type hearing aid and without it.

Data. Of the 50 PB words on a list, the numbers accurately repeated by each subject under each condition were the following:

Subject Number	Number Correct without Aid	Number Correct with Aid
1	15	38
2	25	43
3	20	35
Mean	20	39

A *t*-test for two related samples (see Appendix A) was performed in these data. The value of *t* computed was not large enough to reject the null hypothesis at the 0.01 level of confidence (alpha level).

3. Why is knowledge of inferential statistics important for evaluating therapy outcome research reports?

Chapter 11

Organizing Data for Answering Questions: III. Inferential Techniques for Single Subject Designs

Our focus in the previous chapter was on the use of inferential statistical techniques for assessing the likelihood that observed differences and relationships between sets of scores and other criterion measures that had been generated by *groups of subjects* were not due to chance—that is, random fluctuation. Their use for this purpose is almost universally accepted in behavioral science research as being appropriate—it is not controversial. Our focus in this chapter will be on assessing the likelihood that observed differences and relationships between sets of scores and other criterion measures that had been generated by *a single subject* were not due to chance. The use of the inferential statistical techniques—particularly those that were described in the Chapter 10—with single subject data is considered by a number of statisticians to be inappropriate and furthermore, there is no consensus among statisticians and other research methodologists about how to assess the likelihood that an observed difference or relationship in such data is due to chance (see Levin, Marascuilo & Hubert, 1978).

Before discussing approaches that have been suggested for assessing the reliability of differences and relationships observed in data from single subjects, we will briefly consider why many statisticians believe that the use of at least some significance tests intended for data generated by group designs is inappropriate for data generated by single subject designs. The bottom line is that their use can result in vastly inflated Type I error probabilities (Levin et al., 1978). That is, if you use them, you may conclude that a difference or relationship is a real one far more often than you should at the level of confidence at which you are running your test. While the level of confidence that you use is 0.05, the actual level of confidence at which you are running your test may be 0.10 or larger (see Table 4-1 in Gottman & Glass, 1978). For an explanation of the reason, see Gottman and Glass (1978) and/or Levin et al. (1978). And for further discussion of the controversy concerning the use of group significance tests with data from single-subject designs see Cohen & Reese (1994), Edgington (1967, 1972, 1984), Gentile, Roden & Klein (1972), Gottman (1981), Gottman & Glass (1978), Kratochwill (1978), Kratochwill and Brody (1978), Kratochwill and Levin (1980, 1992), Levin et al. (1978), Revusky (1967), and Rochon (1990).

There is a difference between how inferential statistical techniques are used with single subject designs and group designs. With the latter they are used to generalize to the population from which the subjects were selected as well as assess the likelihood that an observed difference or relationship was due to chance. With the former they are used solely to assess the likelihood that a difference or relationship observed in the data was due to chance—that is, random fluctuation. They cannot be used to generalize to the population from which a subject was selected.

Four approaches are described in this chapter that have been used for assessing the likelihood that differences and relationships observed in single-subject data are due to chance. They are visual analysis ("eyeballing") of graphic data, time-series analysis, sequential analysis using Markov chains, and randomization tests. Be aware, however, that no one of them is even close to being universally accepted as appropriate.

Visual Analysis ("Eyeballing") of Graphic Data

This is the method that has been used most often in behavioral research to determine whether an experimental condition or other manipulation has produced a change in a behavior. One or more behaviors are measured repeatedly over time and the measures are plotted—usually in the form of a line graph. Measures of a behavior that were made while there was no manipulation (baseline measures) are compared to ones that were made while some type of manipulation was occurring and/or after it occurred. If there is an observable *difference* in the graph between the baseline measures and the others that appears to be too large to be attributable to chance (see Figure 11-1), it is likely to be attributed to the manipulation. Small observed differences (see Figure 11-2) are likely to be ignored. And if more than one behavior is measured and plotted and there appears to be a *relationship* between how the behaviors increase and decrease that seems too close to be attributable to chance, it is likely to be attributed to the manipulation. Such a relationship may be either positive (see Figure 11-3) or negative (see Figure 11-4).

The use of eyeballing to detect differences and relationships is subject to errors that are equivalent to Type I and Type II statistical ones. A Type I error would be declaring differences in the values of measures observed on a graph to be real ones when they were due to random fluctuation. And a Type II error would be failing to detect a real difference or relationship. The smaller a difference and the weaker a relationship, the higher the probability of making a Type II error. This also is the case when statistics are used.

Some advocates of eyeballing believe that they can keep the likelihood of a Type I error within acceptable limits by only identifying differences and relationships that are both "clearly evident" (Parsonson & Baer, 1978) and have been confirmed by a number of direct

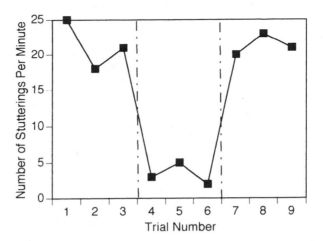

FIGURE 11-1 **Line graph depicting an obvious difference—that is, treatment effect. The experimental trials were 4, 5, and 6.**

and/or systematic replications (Sidman, 1960). While such a strategy would be likely to keep the probability of a Type I error within acceptable limits, it is also likely to increase the probability of a Type II error—perhaps to a point where it is too large to be acceptable. This is particularly likely to be the case if the differences or relationships for which you are searching could be relatively small ones. Consequently, this strategy would tend to be most useful when there is reason to believe that differences will be relatively large or relationships relatively close or when you are only interested in detecting large differences or close relationships. In therapy outcome research, for example, small differences between pre- and

FIGURE 11-2 **Line graph that may be depicting a small difference—that is, treatment effect. The experimental trials were 4, 5, and 6.**

FIGURE 11-3   Line graph depicting a positive relationship between the frequencies of two behaviors.

post-therapy test scores may not be regarded as being "clinically significant" and consequently, not particularly important to be able to detect.

Whether visual analysis of graphic data is likely to provide the information you need for answering a question depends on the magnitude of a difference in a behavior between no manipulation (baseline) and manipulation or the closeness of the relationship between changes in several behaviors that you have to be able to detect to answer it. If you only have to be able to detect relatively large differences or relatively close relationships to do so (see

FIGURE 11-4   Line graph depicting a negative relationship between the frequencies of two behaviors.

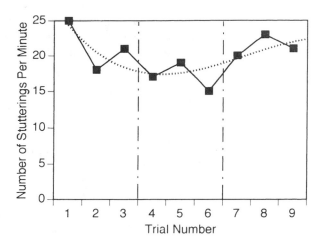

FIGURE 11-5 **Figure 11-2 with a trend line added that was plotted by the method of least squares.**

Figures 11-1, 11-3, and 11-4), then this method is likely to be adequate. On the other hand, if your question pertains to any effect of a manipulation or any relationship between behaviors resulting from a manipulation, one of the other analysis methods described in this chapter may be less likely to yield a Type II error. Of course, there is no reason why you couldn't combine a graphical analysis with one or more of the others.

Accuracy of detection of differences and relationships in data that is plotted in line graphs can sometimes be increased by fitting trend lines (curves) to the data, rather than merely connecting the data points. There are several computational procedures that can be used for doing this. The one that appears to be used most often in the *method of least squares* (see Parsonson & Baer, 1978). The trend line in Figure 11-5—which was fitted to the data in Figure 11-2 by this method—makes it appear even less likely that there is a treatment effect.

While graphical analyses for differences and relationships are less sensitive than statistical ones, they are superior to them in at least one way—they require less sophistication to understand. Almost anyone can detect a difference or relationship in a line graph, particularly if it is a relatively large one. However, a person has to know something about statistics to be able to interpret the results of a randomization test or a sequential analysis using Markov chains.

For further information about the graphical analysis of single-subject data, see McReynolds and Kearns (1983), Parsonson and Baer (1978), and Sidman (1960).

Time-Series Analysis

Time-series designs were described in Chapter 6. As I indicated there, they are characterized by:

> *The presence of a periodic measurement process on some . . . individual and the*
> *introduction of an experimental change into this time series of measurement, the*
> *results of which are indicated by a discontinuity in the measurements recorded in*
> *the time series. (Campbell & Stanley, 1966, p. 37)*

There are numerous time-series designs (see Chapter 6, Kratochwill, 1978; and Mc-
Reynolds & Kearns, 1983). The plots in Figures 11-1, 11-2, and 11-5 were yielded by one
of them—the ABA design (see Chapter 6).

The data from time-series designs are usually plotted on a line graph and interpreted by
visual inspection (eyeballing). Four configurations of trend lines that could indicate an
intervention had an effect are illustrated in Figure 11-6. The change depicted in Figure

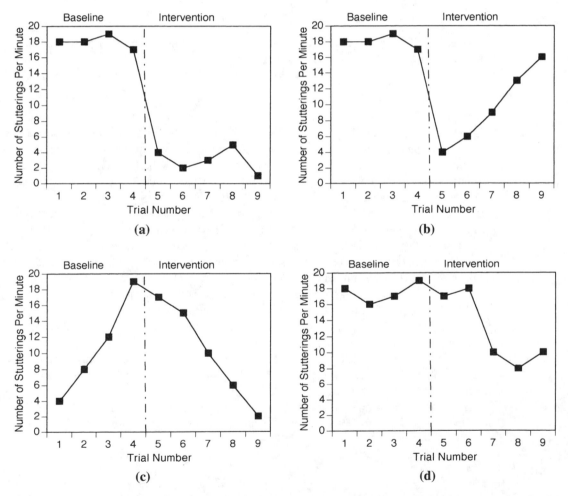

**FIGURE 11-6   Four configurations of trend lines that could indicate that an intervention had
an effect.**

11-6a is an immediate stable reduction in frequency of stuttering following the intervention. The change depicted in Figure 11-6b is an immediate reduction in frequency of stuttering after intervention followed by "relapse." The change depicted in Figure 11-6c is a progressive increase in stuttering frequency during baseline with a progressive decrease following intervention. And the change depicted in Figure 11-6d is the same as that depicted in Figure 11-6a, except that the reduction in frequency of stuttering following the intervention is not immediate.

If an experimental treatment was introduce more than once (i.e., if the experiment was *replicated*), a consistent deviation from the baseline while it was occurring would provide additional support for the conclusion that the treatment had an effect (see Figure 11-7). You can use a randomization test (discussed elsewhere in this chapter) when a time series contains replication to estimate the probability of a Type I error. If, for example, there are five replications and they all result in a deviation from the baseline in the same direction, the probability of the deviations being due to chance—of there being a Type I error—is less than 0.05.

While most of the significance tests described in Chapter 10 have been used for analyzing data from single-subject time-series designs, a number of writers (e.g., Kratochwill, 1978; McReynolds & Kearns, 1983) have expressed several concerns about the appropriateness and practicality of using them. One of their main concerns appears to be the failure to meet certain assumptions that must be met before it is safe to assume that the probability of a Type I error is equal to the level of confidence at which a test is run (see Kratochwill, 1978). Another concern appears to be the need to collect more data than necessary to keep the probability of a Type I error adequately small. The magnitude of the deviation from a baseline while a treatment is occurring may be so huge that only one or two replications are needed to establish by "eyeballing" that the treatment has an effect—not the larger number needed to do so statistically.

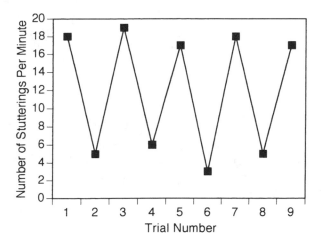

FIGURE 11-7 Line graph depicting the results of an ABABABABA design. The odd trial numbers are baseline conditions and the even trial numbers are treatment conditions.

FIGURE 11-8   Segment of a *time line* on which is recorded both the accuracy of each production of /s/ by the client (*1* for accurate and *0* for inaccurate) and the presentation of each instance of positive reinforcement by the clinician (x).

Sequential Analysis Using Markov Chains

Some of the questions that speech-language pathologists and audiologists seek to answer with single-subject designs pertain to the impact that one person's behavior has on another. This situation is somewhat different than the ones we have discussed thus far since the behavior being studied is not conceptualized as that of a person but of a *dyad*—a relationship involving two persons. Target behaviors of both persons are recorded in a time sequence and an attempt is made to relate the behavior of one to that of the other.

An example of such a question would be the following: "What effect does a clinician's positive reinforcement of correct productions of /s/ have on a client's subsequent productions of /s/?" This question could be made more "answerable" (see Chapter 4) by rephrasing it as follows: "Is the probability of a correct production of /s/ greater immediately following a clinician reinforcement of a correct production than otherwise?" To answer this question, we would record on a *time line* both the accuracy of each production of /s/ (*1* for accurate and *0* for inaccurate) and each instance of reinforcement by the clinician (see Figure 11-8). The segment of the time line depicted in Figure 11-8 suggests that the answer to our question is yes. However, such an outcome could occur by chance. Sequential analysis using Markov chains can be used for estimating the probability of the outcome being due to chance—that is, the probability of a Type I error (see Gottman & Notarius, 1978, for computational formulas).

Randomization Tests

As I have indicated elsewhere in this chapter, the appropriateness of using the types of significance tests developed for group designs (see Chapter 10) with single subject data has been questioned by a number of statisticians. The reason is that doing so would violate one or more of the underlying assumptions of such tests. This could result in their yielding an estimate of the probability of a Type I error that is inaccurate. Fortunately, there are tests that can yield an accurate estimate of a Type I error with single-subject data. They are known as randomization tests because they compare an outcome with what would be expected if the outcome was due to *random sampling error.* If the probability of an outcome being due to random sampling error were less than 0.05 or 0.01, the null hypothesis would be rejected.

Randomization tests are not a recent development. In fact, Sir Ronald Fisher, the "father" of statistical inference, included the following example in his classic text, *The Design of Experiments:*

> *A lady declares that by tasting a cup of tea made with milk she can discriminate whether the milk or the tea infusion was first added to the cup. We will consider the problem of designing an experiment by means of which this assertion can be tested. . . . Our experiment consists of mixing eight cups of tea, four in one way and four in the other, and presenting them to the subject for judgment in a random order. The subject has been told in advance of what the test will consist, namely that she will be asked to taste eight cups, that these shall be four of each kind, and that they shall be presented to her in a random order. . . . Her task is to divide the eight cups into two sets of four, agreeing, if possible, with the treatments received. . . . There are seventy ways of choosing a group of four objects out of eight. . . . At best, the subject can judge rightly with every cup and, knowing there are four of each kind, this amounts to choosing, out of the seventy sets of four which might be chosen, that particular one which is correct. A subject without any faculty of discrimination would in fact divide the eight cups correctly into two sets of four in one trial out of seventy, or, more properly, with a frequency which would approach one in seventy more and more nearly the more often the test were repeated. (Fisher, 1960, pp. 11–12)*

An outcome of eight correct identifications here would be significant at the 0.05 level of confidence, but not at the 0.01 level of confidence. This is because one trial in seventy is greater than one trial in twenty—the amount needed for significance at 0.05, but less than one trial in 100—the amount needed for significance at 0.01. If the level of confidence desired were 0.01, the number of cups would have to be increased from two sets of four to two sets of five.

The first step with any randomization test is to estimate the probability of a particular outcome being due to random sampling error. There are two basic approaches for doing so—reasoning and generating a distribution of random outcomes using a computer.

Reasoning is the approach that is used most often when all possible outcomes can be specified and it is reasonable to assume that, by chance, they all would be equally likely to occur. Suppose that a person claimed to have the ability to predict the side of a coin that would be face up after it was tossed. Here, it would be reasonable to assume that there are two possible outcomes and each would be equally likely to occur by chance. We are ignoring here a third possible outcome—the coin "standing" on its edge—because we are assuming that it would be an extremely rare event and we could always repeat the toss if it occurred. The probability of someone correctly guessing a single coin toss by chance would be 50 percent, since both outcomes would be equally likely. Consequently, the probability of a single correct guess being due to chance—the probability of a Type I error—would be too large for us to conclude that the person has the ability to predict the outcomes of coin tosses with greater than chance accuracy. How many correct tosses would the person have to predict correctly, without error, for us to reject the null hypothesis and conclude that he or she appears to have this ability? We can estimate this through the application of the *mul-*

tiplication rule. This rule states that the probability of successive correct guesses occurring by chance is the product of their individual probabilities. Consequently, the probability of two correct guesses occurring by chance would be:

$$(0.5)(0.5) = 0.25$$

This number—one chance in four—is too large to enable us to reject the null hypothesis at the 0.05 level of confidence. The person would have to guess five successive tosses correctly for the probability of the outcome being due to chance to be this small. The probability of five correct guesses in a row by chance would be:

$$(0.5)(0.5)(0.5)(0.5)(0.5) = 0.03$$

Since 0.03 is smaller than 0.05, the null hypothesis would be rejected at the 0.05 level of confidence.

Suppose that the person guessed 66 percent of the tosses correctly in a series of trials. What is the probability that this outcome was due to chance? The answer would depend on the length of the series—the longer the series, the smaller this probability. To estimate it, we would have to specify all possible outcomes and the frequency with which this *combination* of successes and failures occurs by chance. We can do so by calculating the number of *permutations* of outcomes and transforming this number into the proportion of *combinations* of outcomes that contain this particular combination of correct and incorrect guesses. If there were three trials, the number of permutations would be:

$$K^N = 2^3 = 8$$

where K = the number of possible outcomes
     N = the number of trials

These eight permutations would be:

    (correct, correct, correct)
    (wrong, wrong, wrong)
    (wrong, correct, correct)
    (wrong, wrong, correct)
    (correct, wrong, wrong)
    (correct, correct, wrong)
    (wrong, correct, wrong)
    (correct, wrong, correct)

Since in three of the eight permutations there are two correct guesses, the proportion of the total permutations in which there were two correct guesses (0.38) is larger that 0.05 and consequently, the null hypothesis would not be rejected.

While the procedure described in the preceding paragraph for determining the proportion of the permutations that contain a particular number of correct guesses is practical for a small number of trials (e.g., three), it becomes less practical as the number of trials increases. The number of permutations that would have to be listed and screened for six trials, for example, would be $K^N = 2^6 = 64$. Fortunately, a table for the binomial distribution (see Table A-3) can be used to determine the probability of a particular number of correct guesses occurring by chance for numbers of trials (values of N) between 5 and 25, when there are two equally likely outcomes ($K = 2$). To find the probability for a certain number of correct guesses occurring by chance using Table A-3, x would be the number of errors (assuming you wanted to determine whether a subject performed better than chance) and N would be the number of trials. With six trials, for example, it would only be possible for a person to demonstrate better-than-chance accuracy in guessing at the 0.05 level of confidence if he or she made no errors. While it wouldn't be possible to affirm an ability to predict at the 0.01 level of confidence with six trials, it would be possible to do so with seven trials if there are no errors.

When the number of trials (value of N) exceeds 25, the probability of a particular number of correct guesses occurring by chance can be estimated using the Z statistic and the normal distribution (see Table A-4). The computational formula for Z and the instructions for using Table A-4 are in the section of Appendix A dealing with the sign test.

The computational procedures described above can be used for any single-subject experiment or diagnostic task in which there are only two possible outcomes for each trial and the outcomes can be assumed to be equally likely. They could be used, for example, as an adjunct to visual analysis (eyeballing) for determining whether a particular manipulation can change a particular behavior. For each replication (trial), the baseline measurement of the behavior would be compared to the one in the "manipulation" condition and it would be determined by eyeballing whether there was a difference between them in a particular direction (e.g., a reduction). The number of differences observed in a series of replications would be treated similarly to the number of correct guesses of a coin in a series of trials to test the null hypothesis—that is, to estimate the probability of a Type I error.

The computational procedures for estimating the probability of an outcome being due to chance that we have considered thus far are for the situation in which there are only two possible outcomes and each is equally likely. There, of course, are situations in which there are more than two possible outcomes and/or all of the possible outcomes are not equally likely. Space limitations preclude describing appropriate statistical procedures for these situations here. However, a statistician should be able to recommend an appropriate one for most such situations.

The second approach for estimating the probability of a particular outcome being due to random sampling error is generating a distribution of random outcomes using a computer. There are at least two ways that a computer can be used for this purpose. The simplest is to use its random digit generator to provide you with data that you can plot or use for calculations. Suppose, for example, we want to determine the proportion of times that a dice when tossed would be likely to come up *3*. Since there are six possible outcomes and they should all be equally likely, you would program the computer to output *1*s through *6*s in a random order. If you had the computer print a large number of these digits (e.g., 500), you would find that approximately 17 percent would be *3*s. Chance, then, for *3*s (or any of the other numbers on the dice) would be approximately 17 percent. The computer could be programmed to output random digits for any number of outcomes, including ones that are *not* assumed to be equally likely.

The second way that a computer can be used to determine "chance" probabilities is to program it to simulate an experiment thousands of times with random digit responses and generate a distribution table from the resulting data. The layout and information needed to enter the table would, in at least some instances, be similar to that in Table A-3. Any number of possible outcomes could be accommodated and it would not be necessary to assume that they all are equally likely.

For further information about randomization tests, see Fisher (1960), Hays (1973), and Levin et al. (1978).

Generalizations from Answers

Inferential statistical techniques for group designs enable you to directly generalize conclusions (answers) derived from observations made on samples of persons to the populations from which they were selected so long as they approximate a random sample from them (see Chapter 10). Inferential statistical techniques used with single subject designs do not enable you to do so directly. However, if you are willing to assume that it is highly unlikely that your subject is the only one from the population who would respond in the ways that he or she did to a task, then it would be safe to conclude that his or her responses are representative of those of a segment of the population. It would not be possible, however, to specify the size of this segment. This view is discussed further in Chapter 6.

Exercises and Discussion Topics

1. A child who substitutes /w/ for /r/ is asked to listen to a number of CV syllables and indicate for each whether it contains a /w/ or an /r/. Half of the syllables contain each phoneme and the order in which the syllables are presented is random. The child identifies the first five syllables correctly. Is this outcome significant at the 0.05 level of confidence? Why or why not?

2. Locate a single-subject study in an ASHA journal in which an author used visual analysis ("eyeballing") of graphic data to answer a question. How likely is he or she to have made a Type I error?

$Chapter$ 12

Evaluating Answers to Questions and Interpretations Made of Them

You should always evaluate the adequacy of the answers to questions you read in journal articles as well as the cogency of the interpretations and generalizations that are made from them. It is not safe to assume that data reported in a journal article allow a question to be answered in the way it was answered, or the answer to be interpreted in the way it was interpreted, merely because the article was published. Even though most journals subject submitted manuscripts to a careful peer review process that results in many being rejected, papers nevertheless are published in which the answers to the questions asked or the interpretations made of these answers are either not appropriate or are not the only possible answers or interpretations.

Sometimes when readers detect errors in the authors' answers or interpretations, they write letters to the editor in which they indicate alternative ones. Letters to the editor about research papers are published in the *American Journal of Audiology,* the *American Journal of Speech-Language Pathology, Asha,* the *Journal of Speech and Hearing Research,* and *Language, Speech, and Hearing Services in Schools.* This, unfortunately, is not always done. One reason is that most journals permit an author to reply to a letter critical of his or her paper, and this rebuttal is printed along with it. In his or her rebuttal, the author can answer the points raised in a manner that makes it appear the criticisms are not valid when in fact they are. Unfortunately, the writer of the letter to the editor usually is not given an opportunity to respond to the author's rebuttal. This situation discourages some persons who come across "errors" and inappropriate interpretations from writing letters to the editor. Consequently, you should approach published research with an attitude of *healthy skep-*

ticism. Doing so is particularly important for answers and interpretations that could affect your clinical functioning.

Criteria for evaluating answers to questions—for deciding how much confidence you can have in their accuracy—are also needed for questions that you answer. This includes ones that you answer while you are functioning as a clinician (e.g., when you are doing a differential diagnosis).

Factors to Consider When Evaluating Answers

What factors should you consider when evaluating answers to determine the interpretations and generalizations that can legitimately be made from them? The three most important are the *validity, reliability,* and *generality* of the data on which they are based. These constructs are defined in this section.

Validity

The validity of observations refers to their *appropriateness* for answering the questions they are used to answer. If they are not appropriate, the answers they yield *may* be inaccurate.

Because the observations used to answer a question are inappropriate does not necessarily mean that the answer is wrong. An investigator will occasionally answer a question correctly using observations that are not appropriate for the purpose. A classic example previously mentioned (see Chapter 3) was Gall's conclusion that the anterior portion of the brain is important for motor speech because a friend's eyes who spoke exceptionally well were widely separated (Head, 1963). Consequently, if the observations used to answer a question appear to be invalid, it is *not* appropriate to regard the question as having been answered incorrectly because a certain percentage of the time an investigator will derive a correct answer from such observations. In fact, if a question can only be answered in two ways (e.g., yes or no) and the likelihood of each being correct is approximately equal, you can arrive at a correct answer *without even knowing the question* approximately 50 percent of the time.

The probability of answering a question correctly by chance if the likelihood of all answers being correct is approximately equal is the reciprocal of the number of ways a question can be answered. If a question can be answered in five ways, the probability of a correct answer by chance is 1/5 or 0.20. This, incidentally, is the probability of answering correctly by chance a five-choice, multiple-choice question.

In summary, if the observations used for answering a question are appropriate, the odds will be *greater than chance* that the answer reported is correct. On the other hand, if the observations used for answering a question are inappropriate, the odds will be approximately *equal to chance* that the answer reported is correct.

Reliability

The reliability of the observations used for answering questions refers to their *repeatability*. The more repeatable (or replicable) a set of observations, the greater will be their reliability.

The extent to which observations can be repeated, or *replicated,* is a function of how similarly a *given observer* would describe them on *different* occasions, or how similarly a *group of observers* would describe them on the *same occasion* (or occasions). Descriptions can consist of words, numbers, or a combination of the two. The more similar the descriptions, the more reliable the observations.

The level of reliability of the observations used for answering a question influences the odds that the answer will be correct. How reliable the observations have to be for these odds to be acceptable depends on the question. For questions concerning *differences* (e.g., "Were the language formulation abilities of a group of children better on the average after participating in a particular therapy program than prior to participating in it?"), more reliable observations are required if a difference is relatively small than if it is relatively large. Similarly, for questions concerning *relationships* (e.g., "Is there a relationship between the scores earned by a group of persons who have a particular type of communicative disorder on two tests of auditory functioning?"), more reliable observations are required if a relationship is relatively weak than if it is relatively strong.

Because the observations used for answering a question do not appear to be adequately reliable does not necessarily mean that the answer is incorrect. The answer can be correct by chance alone. As I indicated in the discussion of validity, the probability of an answer being correct by chance is the reciprocal of the number of ways the question can be answered if the likelihood that alternative answers are correct is approximately equal. Also, the observations may be more reliable than they appear to be. Some types of observations typically tend to be viewed as less reliable than they actually are. An example would be ratings obtained through the application of psychological scaling methods (see Chapter 8).

One consequence of observations not being adequately reliable is a relatively high probability of a Type II error (see Chapter 10). Briefly, this means concluding that there is no real difference or relationship when there is. Usually, when an investigator fails to reject a null hypothesis, he or she does not indicate the probability that this failure was due to the measures used not being sufficiently reliable to detect the difference or relationship present. It is quite likely there are some instances in the speech-language pathology and audiology literature when the null hypothesis was not rejected that the reason was a Type II error arising from the use of measures that were not adequately reliable.

Regardless of the reason for a null hypothesis not being rejected, it is inappropriate to interpret failure to do so as *proving* there is no difference (see the discussion of the null hypothesis in Chapter 10). Studies by speech-language pathologists and audiologists have been criticized on this basis (e.g., Finn & Glow, 1990; Meyers, 1990). Of course, if there is no difference between the means or medians (or only a minute one), it is more likely that there really is none than that there is a Type II error. But failure to reject the null hypothesis does not prove it!

In summary, the impact of the reliability of the observations used for answering a question on the accuracy of the answer obtained may not be clear-cut. Observations that do not appear to be adequately reliable can yield both correct and incorrect answers. Judgments concerning the accuracy of answers to questions, therefore, should be regarded as tentative until the data used to answer them have been *replicated*—preferably by other investigators at other institutions.

Generality

A third factor that you have to consider when evaluating the answer to a question and interpretations of it is the *generality* of the observations used to answer the question. This refers to the extent to which the persons or events observed are representative of those in the population designated by the question. The more representative they are of this population, the more viable will be any generalizations made from observations on them.

The persons or events observed to answer a question are most likely to be representative of those in the designated population if they constitute a *random sample* from that population. The only way you can be reasonably certain that they do so is if they were selected from this population by a table of random numbers (see Appendix B) or computer-generated random digits. If they were not selected in one of these manners, their generality would be uncertain. Of course, even if they were selected by a random sampling process, they may still not be representative because of sampling error.

The persons and events observed in speech-language pathology and audiology research often do not constitute a random sample from the population to which the investigator(s) want to generalize. While this population consists of *all persons* who have a particular communicative disorder, the population sampled may consist of *all persons available to the investigator* who have that communicative disorder.

If an investigator is willing to limit generalizations to the *subpopulation* of persons who have a particular communicative disorder from which he or she sampled (e.g., a caseload), then so long as the sample were randomly selected from this subpopulation, the generalizations made should be viable. There are instances, of course, when it would be meaningful to generalize to such a subpopulation. One such instance would be when you wished to assess the impact of participation in a treatment program on a group of persons at your own institution. Rather than assessing the impact of the program on all participants, it may be more economical and efficient to limit the assessment to a random sample. Inferences could be made about the impact of the program on all participants from observations made on this sample. With the probable continuing interest of administrators of clinical speech, language, and hearing programs in "accountability," such inferences could be quite useful.

If investigators are not willing to limit their generalizations to the subpopulations from which their samples were drawn, or if their samples were not randomly selected from the populations to which they wish to generalize, the cogency of their generalizations will be uncertain. To have a reasonable degree of confidence in the viability of such generalizations, it is necessary to assume that the persons observed approximate a *representative,* or random, sample from the population to which they are being made. In some instances, this assumption will seem reasonable; in others, it will not seem reasonable; in still others, insufficient information will be presented in the report about the persons observed for any judgment to be made regarding its reasonableness. Knowing, for example, that they were all receiving therapy at a particular rehabilitation center without knowing the characteristics (i.e., physical, intellectual, emotional, socioeconomic, etc.) of those who do so is likely to leave you uncertain about the reasonableness of this assumption.

Can generalizations legitimately be made from observations of persons who were not randomly selected from the population to which it was desired to generalize? The answer to this question would be yes if: (1) a single subject design were used, and (2) you were willing to assume it is highly unlikely that the only persons in the population who would perform as these subjects did under the experimental condition (or conditions) are these subjects. If you are willing to make this assumption, it would seem reasonable to conclude that the performance of the subjects is representative of that of a *segment* of the population from which they were selected. It wouldn't be possible, however, to specify the size of this segment on the basis of a single sample.

Because the interpretations and generalizations made by an author from his or her data seem inappropriate does not necessarily mean they are incorrect. As I indicated in the discussions of validity and reliability, an author can arrive at a correct conclusion for the wrong reason(s) or by chance alone.

Criteria for Evaluating Validity, Reliability, and Generality

In the preceding section we considered the implications of validity, reliability, and generality for assessing the accuracy of answers to questions. In this section an approach is described for evaluating validity, reliability, and generality that involves answering a series of questions. The answers to these questions provide a basis for making judgments about the accuracy of answers to clinical and research questions as well as the cogency of interpretations and generalizations made from them. Figure 12-1 is a checklist for recording the results of such an evaluation.

Validity

A necessary question to answer when you want to assess the validity of the observations used for answering a question is: "Were the observations made appropriate for answering the question asked?" That is, were the attribute (or attributes) of the events observed and described that were appropriate to observe and describe to answer the question? If they were appropriate ones, the observations will be valid to some degree. And if they were not appropriate ones, they will be invalid.

The attribute (or attributes) that it was necessary to describe to answer a question may not have been described because the filter used to isolate it (or them) did not do so (see Chapter 1). This could have resulted from using an inappropriate or inaccurately calibrated instrument to observe it or from failing to take on an appropriate perceptual set to do so. An inappropriate instrument in this context would be one that does not permit a target attribute to be observed and described. Such an instrument could be a part of an electronic instrumentation measurement scheme, or it could be a psychological or educational performance test or task (see Chapter 8). An example of using inappropriate electronic instrumentation to isolate a target attribute would be using an electromyographic (EMG) recorder with *surface electrodes* to study the differential activity of the internal and external intercostal muscles during breathing for speech. (*Needle electrodes* would be needed at least at some sites to study the differential activity of these muscles.) An example of an inappropriate application of educational or psychological tests for isolating and describing a target attribute would be using articulation test performance to infer intelligence level. (While both are

Indicate beside each statement whether it appears to be true. If insufficient information is presented to judge whether a statement is true, place a check mark in the ? column.

Yes	No	?	Statement
____	____	____	1. The question, or questions, that an attempt was made to answer are stated clearly enough to be "answerable" (see Chapter 5).
____	____	____	2. The appropriate type of design—single subject and/or group—was used to answer the question or questions (see Chapter 6).
____	____	____	3. The attributes of events that were selected for observation are appropriate ones for answering the question, or questions (see Chapters 1, 7, and 12).
____	____	____	4. The observations made were of the attribute(s) referred to in Statement 3, rather than some other attribute(s) (see Chapters 1, 7, and 12).
____	____	____	5. The person(s) on whom the observations were made—that is, the subject(s) or client(s)—were appropriate ones for answering the question or questions (see Chapters 1, 7, and 12).
____	____	____	6. If the design used was a group one, the subjects were selected by a method that is likely to have made them *representative* of persons in the population referred to in the question, or questions—that is, one that at least approximates random sampling (see Chapters 6 and 12).
____	____	____	7. It seems unlikely that theoretical or clinical biases consciously or unconsciously influenced the methodology used (i.e., persons observed, the choice of target attributes, and/or how the observations were made) in a manner that would have been likely to bias the data (see Chapter 12).
____	____	____	8. Electronic instrumentation used for measuring attributes of events was properly calibrated (see Chapter 8).
____	____	____	9. The observations possess an adequate level of reliability (see Chapter 12).
____	____	____	10. The observations are unlikely to have been biased by order and/or sequence effects (see Chapter 6).
____	____	____	11. It appears unlikely that the observations were biased by how the persons observed thought they were expected to respond (see Chapter 8).
____	____	____	12. The descriptive statistics, tables, narratives, and/or graphical displays used were appropriate for *organizing* the data to answer the question or questions (see Chapter 9).

FIGURE 12-1   Evaluation checklist for validity, reliability, and generality.

13. The manner in which the descriptive statistics, tables, narratives, and/or graphical displays used were *interpreted* was appropriate for answering the question or questions (see Chapter 9)

14. The *conclusions* that were drawn from the descriptive statistics, tables, narratives, graphical displays, and/or other data appear to be the most plausible ones (see Chapter 9).

15. The inferential statistical procedures that were used were appropriate (see Chapters 10 and 11).

16. A failure to reject the null hypothesis does not appear to have been due to a Type II error (see Chapter 10).

17. A failure to reject the null hypothesis is interpreted as indicating there is no *evidence* for concluding that a difference or relationship exists—not that there is no difference or relationship (see Chapter 10).

18. The magnitude of the difference between descriptive statistics (e.g., between means or medians) is not interpreted as being the magnitude of the difference in the population unless a confidence interval has been computed that indicates it is (see Chapter 10).

19. The population to which generalizations are made is an appropriate one (see Chapter 12).

20. Observed relationships are not interpreted as being clinically or theoretically meaningful just because they are "statistically significant" (see Chapter 12).

21. Theoretical, clinical, and/or cultural biases do not appear to have influenced how findings ("answers") are interpreted (see Chapters 12 and 17).

FIGURE 12-1   *Continued*

related in a general way to overall development, articulation test performance does not appear to be a particularly valid index of intelligence level.)

An *inaccurately calibrated* instrument in this context would be one that when properly adjusted, or calibrated, would isolate the target attribute to be observed and described. If the target attribute was "thresholds for pure tones" and the audiometer used was not properly calibrated, the investigator would be unable to describe this attribute validly on the basis of the thresholds obtained. The investigator would, of course, be able to describe the attribute with this type of instrumentation if it were properly calibrated.

An *inappropriate set* in this context would be one an observer assumes that does not isolate the attribute(s) that he or she wants to observe and describe. On psychological scaling tasks (see Chapter 8), for example, where observers are asked to rate a series of speech segments for two attributes *separately* (e.g., degree of "articulation defectiveness" and degree of "nasality"), they may be unable to assume the appropriate sets. That is, they may be unable to ignore one of them (e.g., nasality) while rating the speech segments for the other (e.g., articulation defectiveness).

Reliability

The question that it is necessary to answer when assessing the reliability of observations is: "Were the observations made sufficiently free from random and systematic measurement error (including experimenter bias) to reliably answer the question they were used to answer?" The sources from which both types of error arise have already been discussed (see Chapter 8). If the answer to this question is yes, the observations are likely to be sufficiently free of error to yield an answer that is likely to be correct. If, on the other hand, it appears to be no, the accuracy of the answer will be uncertain.

Impact of Random Measurement Error on Reliability

Random measurement error can influence the accuracy of answers to questions on differences and relationships (and consequently the interpretations made of them) by increasing the probability of a Type II error—that is, the probability of not rejecting the null hypothesis when it should be rejected (see Chapter 10). Obviously, if the null hypothesis is rejected, this source of error could not have influenced the accuracy of the answer. If the null hypothesis is retained, however, random measurement error could have been responsible. That is, rather than retaining the null hypothesis, which indicates that an observed difference or relationship probably resulted from chance, or random fluctuation, it merely may indicate that the level of random error was too high to detect a difference or relationship of the magnitude present with the number of subjects used. If more subjects had been used, the null hypothesis might have been rejected. (The larger the sample size, the less likely you are to retain a false null hypothesis because of random error.) For this reason, whenever you are interpreting an answer to a question that was based on failure to reject the null hypothesis, one possibility you must always consider is a Type II error. Unfortunately, most journals don't require authors to specify the probability of a Type II error when they fail to reject a null hypothesis.

A Type II error is particularly likely to explain retaining a null hypothesis if at least two of the following three statements apply:

1. The sample size was relatively small.
2. The observed difference or correlation was relatively small.
3. The alpha level (i.e., level of confidence) used was relatively small (e.g., 0.01).

In summary, unless it was possible to demonstrate the probability of a Type II error was acceptably small (i.e., 0.05 or smaller), it would be inappropriate to interpret failure to reject the null hypothesis as indicating that an observed difference or relationship is not a "real" one.

Impact of Systematic Measurement Error on Reliability

Systematic measurement error can influence the accuracy of answers to questions (and consequently the interpretations made of them) by biasing the observations used to answer them. It can make it appear that a difference or relationship exists where there is none, or that no difference or relationship exists where there is one.

Therapy outcome research is particularly vulnerable to systematic measurement error (e.g., Beasley & Manning, 1973; Meitus, Ringel, House, & Hotchkiss, 1973). It is especially likely to occur if the person or persons doing the research have an ego investment in the therapy being proven effective (e.g., Rosenthal, 1976). The bias may be subtle, and the person or persons may not be conscious of it.

In what ways can the results of therapy outcome research be biased? One way is by selecting criterion measures that are likely to make a therapy program appear successful and avoiding those that aren't likely to do so. If, for example, the therapy program was a stuttering one and it was thought that it would be more likely to improve clients' attitudes than their fluency, the criterion measure selected would be an attitude rather than a fluency one.

Another way that such research can be biased is by design-related decisions. If the therapy being evaluated was a stuttering one and it was uncertain whether clients would relapse following termination of the therapy, a design could be used that had no followups or only very short-term ones.

Therapy outcome research can be biased in other ways as well. If a clinician attempted to evaluate retrospectively the effectiveness of a therapy program, several types of distortion could bias the evaluation. He or she may be more successful, for example, in remembering factors that suggest the therapy was effective than factors that suggest it was ineffective, or vice versa. Or the clinician could conclude that a reduction in the severity of a client's communicative disorder has occurred because he or she has "adapted" to it. A person with a severe phonological disorder could seem more intelligible to his or her clinician following a period of therapy because the clinician has learned the lawful ways in which the person's language usage differs from the standard. And a stutterer's stuttering could seem less severe to his clinician because the clinician has grown accustomed to it (Trotter & Kools, 1955).

Another way that the results of therapy outcome research can be biased is by not reporting the effects of the therapy on all of the clients on whom it was tried. While it sometimes is justifiable (and indeed necessary) to exclude clients because the therapy being evaluated was not administered to them in the prescribed manner, such exclusion should be done only when absolutely necessary—that is, when not excluding them would *almost certainly* lead to a biased evaluation. Unfortunately, it is usually relatively easy to rationalize the elimination of a client from such a study who does not respond to a therapy as desired and consequently, would have to be classified as a "failure."

Therapy outcome research findings can also be biased when they are interpreted. Data pertaining to the effectiveness of a program can often be interpreted in more than one way. In fact, a given finding can often be interpreted *both* to support the conclusion that a therapy was effective and to support the opposite conclusion. It depends on whether one wishes to view the proverbial cup as half full or half empty. Suppose that a particular stuttering therapy was found to reduce stuttering frequency by 3 percent. This could be used both to support the conclusion that the therapy was effective (i.e., it reduced stuttering frequency) and to support the conclusion that it was ineffective (i.e., it didn't produce enough of a reduction in stuttering frequency to make a meaningful difference in how clients are likely to be perceived and reacted to). Both interpretations are defensible. Consequently, when you are reading and evaluating therapy outcome research, it is important that you seek out the data on which conclusions and interpretations are based so that you can decide for yourself whether they are reasonable.

Generality

The question that you have to answer to assess the generality of data yielded by a *group design* is: "Did the subjects observed at least approximate a random sample from the population to which the question refers—that is, the one to which generalizations are being made?" If the subjects observed were chosen by a random process (e.g., by a table of random numbers—see Appendix B) from the population to which a question refers, they constitute a random sample from that population and generalizations to it are appropriate.

If subjects were not randomly selected from the population to which a question refers, it would be *uncertain* whether they constitute a random sample from that population. Any inferences, conclusions, and generalizations made about the population from observations of such subjects would have to be regarded as *quite tentative.*

The question that you have to answer to assess the generality of data yielded by a *single subject design* is: "Is it reasonable to assume that the aspect of the person's behavior that was observed during the performance of the experimental task is representative of that aspect of his or her behavior on such tasks?" If the answer to this question is *no,* generalizations are not appropriate. If the answer to this question is *yes,* generalizations may be appropriate. And if the answer to this question is *uncertain,* any generalizations should be regarded as being quite tentative.

Concerns about appropriate generalizations from data yielded by a single subject design pertain to judging the cogency of conclusions drawn from clinical data—for example, that from observations made during a client's initial evaluation. For such generalizations to be appropriate, you must be willing to assume that behavior observed in the "therapy room" is representative of that in the "real world." You must be willing to assume, for example, that the amount and type of syllable repetition that a preschooler evinces in the therapy room is representative of that which has caused his or her parents to become concerned. The extent to which such "therapy room" behavior is representative of that in the "real world" is often uncertain. This is certainly the case for preschooler's syllable repetition (see Silverman, 1996).

Checklist for Evaluating the Validity, Reliability, and Generality of Observations

A number of considerations are mentioned in this chapter and elsewhere in the book for evaluating the validity, reliability, and generality of the observations used to answer a question. A checklist is presented in Figure 12-1 that can be helpful when doing such an evaluation.

The checklist consists of a series of statements that if true suggest that the observations being evaluated are adequate for answering the question.

Exercises and Discussion Topics

1. Use the Evaluation Checklist to assess the validity, reliability, and generality of answers to questions (i.e., findings) in *three* research reports published in the *Journal of Speech and Hearing Research*. At least one of these reports should deal with clinical research.

2. John's mother was asked the age at which he said his first word. She looked in his baby book and found that the age she had recorded for his first word was 18 months. Based on this evidence, the clinician stated in his report that John said his first word at 18 months. Assess both the validity and reliability of this conclusion, using the criteria presented in this chapter.

3. A clinician wishes to determine whether Mr. Smith, a stroke patient, is having any difficulty understanding speech. She asks him to point to a series of objects that she names. He does so without error. She concludes that he is having no difficulty understanding speech. Assess both the validity and generality of this conclusion using the criteria presented in this chapter.

Chapter 13

Communicating Questions, Answers, and Interpretations

Once a question has been formulated and answered and the answer has been interpreted, the next step is to communicate the question, answer, and interpretation to potential consumers of the information. This is the final step in the process. If you do clinical (e.g., therapy outcome) research and do not formally disseminate your questions, answers, and interpretations, their potential to help persons who are communicatively impaired is likely to be restricted to your caseload and those of colleagues to whom you communicate them informally.

Modes for Disseminating Research Findings

Written reports and convention presentations are the media that speech-language pathologists and audiologists use most often for formally communicating questions, answers, and interpretations to other clinicians. Written reports usually are published in professional journals. Convention presentations consist of talks and exhibits (including poster sessions) at local, state, national, and international meetings. Other media used for communication include audiotapes, motion picture films, videotapes, self-published reports, and computer networks.

Written Reports

Written reports are the medium used most often by speech-language pathologists and audiologists for communicating clinical questions, answers, and interpretations to practitioners with whom they do not communicate informally. Their reports are published in a variety of journals, including those of state speech, language, and hearing associations; the American

Speech-Language-Hearing Association; international speech, language, and hearing associations (e.g., the International Society for Logopedics and Phoniatrics); specialty speech, language, and hearing associations (e.g., the American Academy of Audiologists and the International Society for Augmentative and Alternative Communication); as well as those published by educational, psychological, sociological, medical, physics, speech communication, and linguistics associations. To identify journals that have published, and presumably will continue to publish, papers dealing with certain aspects of communicative disorders, search for them in a relevant computer database (e.g., MEDLINE and PsycINFO) or look them up in the indexes of several recent volumes of a relevant abstracts journal, such as *Linguistics and Language Behavior Abstracts,* and note the journals in which papers concerned with them have been published. A 1991 ASHA publication, *Journals in Communication Sciences and Disorders,* can also be helpful here.

Written reports in journals range in length from less than a page to more than 100 pages. Most are between four and twelve pages. They may be classified as articles, reports, clinical exchange reports, case reports, points of view, or letters to the editor.

Journals that classify papers as articles and reports may distinguish between these two categories, at least partially, on the basis of length—they may tend to classify longer papers as articles. The amount of research reported also may be a consideration. Papers that report a single study may tend to be classified as reports and those that report a series of related studies as articles.

Clinical exchange contributions tend to be relatively short reports that are clinically relevant—that is, dealing with diagnostic or therapy procedures. They are published by several journals, including the *American Journal of Audiology,* the *American Journal of Speech-Language Pathology,* and *Language, Speech, and Hearing Services in the Schools.*

Case reports (i.e., case studies) are descriptions of clients who are noteworthy for some reason. The symptomatology or etiology of their communicative disorder may be unusual in some respect; they may have responded in an unexpected way to a diagnostic or therapeutic procedure; or a diagnostic or therapeutic procedure may have been used whose value is not well established. Such papers may report a single case or several related cases.

Point-of-view papers are not intended primarily for communicating unpublished data. They are sometimes included, however, as support for the contentions, or points of view, presented.

Letters to the editor occasionally are used to communicate unpublished data. They are particularly likely to be used for this purpose when an investigator has data to report that are relevant to a question answered in a published paper. The investigator may write a letter to the editor of the journal that published the paper reporting data that either replicate those used to answer the question or suggest a different answer to the question. Letters to the editor are sometimes also used to communicate questions, answers, and interpretations that are not relevant to ones that were reported in the journal in which they appear when such information can be communicated in a few paragraphs.

Convention Presentations

Convention presentations are another medium used frequently by speech-language pathologists and audiologists for communicating questions, answers, and interpretations. There are many professional organizations at whose conventions they make such presentations, including state speech and hearing associations and American Speech-Language-Hearing Association. The three most common types are oral platform presentations (including miniseminars), poster presentations, and exhibits.

The typical platform presentation consists of a ten- or fifteen-minute talk followed by a question-and-answer period (usually five minutes or less). The organization of this kind of talk is similar to that of a journal article; however, the language is usually less formal and more conversational, and the presentation is usually less detailed and more redundant than that of a journal article.

While most miniseminars are tutorials, they can be used for reporting unpublished data. Proposals for them are most likely to be accepted by a program committee if the results of a long-term program of research, rather than that of a single study, will be reported.

The poster presentation is a relatively recent addition to convention programs. Each presenter is assigned a poster board for at least an hour. The presenter attaches sheets of paper to the board that contain questions, answers, and interpretations. These may be communicated in graphical, tabular, photographic, and/or narrative form. The presenter stands beside the "poster" and answers questions about it during the time period for which the presentation is scheduled (see Figure 13-1).

Scientific exhibits, such as those at American Speech-Language-Hearing Association conventions, can be used communicating questions, answers, and interpretations. They are similar to poster presentations, except that they usually are larger and more elaborate and are displayed for the entire convention.

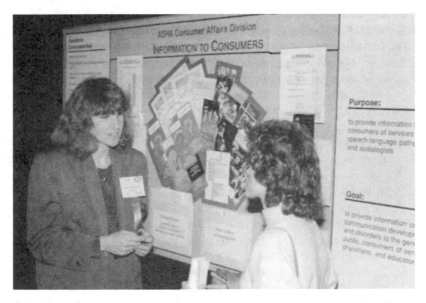

FIGURE 13-1 A poster session at an American Speech-Language-Hearing Association Convention.

Other Approaches to Communicating Questions, Answers, and Interpretations

While written reports and convention presentations are the media by which speech-language pathologists and audiologists have communicated questions, answers, and interpretations most often, they are not the only media that they have used for doing so. Others include motion picture films, videotapes, audiotapes, self-published reports, and computer networks.

Speech-language pathologists and audiologists began using motion picture film for communicating questions, answers, and interpretations before World War II. They are now using videotape more frequently for doing so than motion picture film because the technology is less expensive and more accessible.

Audiotapes have been used for communicating questions, answers, and interpretations. Presentations at state and national speech, language, and hearing conventions (including ASHA conventions) have been audiotaped and copies made available to interested persons at relatively low cost. This medium is particularly useful for reports in which speech or spoken language samples would be helpful in documenting answers to questions and interpretations of them.

Some individuals and institutions communicate research findings in reports that they publish themselves. A university speech and hearing program, for example, may periodically publish reports of research by its students and faculty. Or investigators who have written final reports for agencies that have funded their research may make them available, in whole or part, to interested persons. Because of easy access to microcomputers with desktop publishing software and copy machines, reports of this type can be produced relatively inexpensively and distributed by mail (see Silverman, 1997). Such reports can also be distributed as downloadable files on a computer network such as the Internet (see Silverman, 1997). Research reports that are distributed in one of these two ways may eventually be published in a journal and/or presented at a convention.

Research reported at conventions may also be distributed in one of these two ways. This happens, for example, when the research is regarded as "preliminary" and consequently, not yet ready to report in a journal article. Copies of convention papers, incidentally, can often be obtained from their authors. A postcard form that can be used for requesting them, as well as reprints of published articles, is reproduced in Figure 13-2.

Computer networks are a relatively new medium for communicating questions, answers, and interpretations. Persons interested in a particular disorder (e.g., stuttering) or a particular intervention approach (e.g., augmentative communication) can communicate with each other by linking their personal microcomputers, via modem, to minicomputers (e.g., Vax computers) or mainframe ones that provide access to the *Internet,* which is a network that links computer networks around the world. They can communicate questions, answers, and interpretations on the Internet in several ways, including e-mail (see Silverman, 1997). The advantage of disseminating information in this manner is that it can be done quickly. Data-based answers to questions that pertain to clinical management, for example, can be communicated to clinicians within hours after being formulated (rather than months or years), thereby possibly enabling them to immediately be more helpful to a client or clients. Findings and interpretations disseminated in this manner can later be

---

MARQUETTE UNIVERSITY

Department of Speech Pathology and Audiology
Milwaukee, Wisconsin 53233

Dear

I would appreciate receiving . . . .

. . . .

. . . .

and any related papers if available.

Cordially,

FIGURE 13-2   A form for requesting copies of convention papers and reprints of journal articles.

communicated by more traditional media—including journal articles and/or convention presentations.

Objectives of Scientific Communication

It is important for both clinical and research purposes that questions, answers, and interpretations be communicated in a manner that is consistent with the characteristics of the scientific method (see Chapter 3), regardless of the medium used. The reasons are dealt with in this section.

Overall Purpose

Before discussing the specific objectives of scientific communication, let's briefly consider its overall purpose—*communication*. Questions, answers, and interpretations should be communicated as unambiguously as possible. Anything that facilitates doing so is desirable; anything that impedes it is undesirable.

What factors can affect the adequacy of scientific communication? The answer to this question is partially dependent on the medium used. Factors likely to impede communication in oral presentations, for example, differ somewhat from those likely to do so in written reports or videotapes.

While some factors that affect the adequacy of scientific communication are specific to the medium used, there are two that tend to do so in all of them. The first is *organization*.

If specific information cannot be easily located, the adequacy of the communication will be reduced. For this reason, the organization (or structure) of research reports has been standardized to a degree. (This organization is described elsewhere in the chapter.)

A second factor that tends to affect the adequacy of scientific communication in all media is *language usage*. Accurate, detailed verbal "maps" facilitate communication, and inaccurate or vague ones impede it (see Chapter 7 for a discussion of map-territory relationships).

Specific Objectives

Scientific communication requires the following if it is to be consistent with the characteristics of the scientific method (see Chapter 3):

- Each question to be answered must be stated as unambiguously as possible.
- The importance of answering each question must be communicated, thereby establishing *scientific justification*.
- The manner in which the observations were made to answer each question must be described as clearly as possible.
- The observations made that are relevant for answering each question must be reported (i.e., each question be answered).
- At least some of the implications (clinical, theoretical, or both) of the answer to each question must be indicated.

We will now consider the contribution of these to effective communication.

One of the most important requirements for effective scientific communication, regardless of the medium used, is that a question be stated clearly before it is answered. If potential consumers of information that is being reported do not understand the question it is intended to answer, they are less likely than otherwise to understand the answer and to be able to evaluate the cogency of conclusions and generalizations drawn from it.

A second requirement is that the importance of answering a question be made explicit, preferably before it is answered. This involves providing cogent answers for the "so what" or "who cares" questions—that is, establishing *scientific justification*. If potential consumers of the information feel, rightly or wrongly, that an answer to a particular question does not affect them (i.e., is not relevant), they will probably pay little, if any, attention to the answer. It is risky to assume that they will see the relevance of an answer without it being pointed out to them. The more explicitly scientific justification is established, the more likely the information presented will be attended to and utilized.

A third requirement is a description of how the observations were made to answer each question that is sufficiently detailed to enable someone else to replicate the process. Basic to the scientific method is *intersubjective testability* (see Chapter 3), the requirement that the observations used to answer questions be verifiable by others. For this to be possible, there must be adequate descriptions of the subjects or clients who were observed and the procedures used to observe them. A detailed description of methodology also is needed to allow potential consumers of the observations reported to estimate their levels of validity, reliability, and generality for the purpose of answering the questions they were used to answer (see Chapter 11).

A fourth requirement is reporting the observations made to answer each question as clearly (unambiguously) as possible. They should be organized and presented in a manner that is likely to be understood easily (see Chapters 9, 10, and 11).

Finally, a fifth requirement is an indication of possible implications of the answer to each question. It is usually not safe to assume that consumers of the information reported will understand its implications without their being pointed out.

Organization of Written Research Reports

We will now consider in some detail the scheme that is usually used for organizing information to facilitate communication in written research reports. This scheme tends to facilitate communication for several reasons. First, the sequence in which topics are presented is a logical one. It begins with the questions and the reasons for wanting to answer them. The sequence then moves to a description of how the observations were made to answer each question. Next is the presentation of the observations that answer each question. Last, possible theoretical and clinical implications of the answers are suggested.

There is another reason why the use of this scheme facilitates communication. With it, a reader knows where within a report to locate desired information. Information about the subjects observed, for example, is almost always presented in the *Methods* section.

The traditional research report contains most, if not all, of the following elements.

- A title
- An abstract (and/or summary)
- A short list of key words
- An introduction section
- A methodology section
- A results section
- A discussion section
- Acknowledgements
- References
- Appendixes

The purpose and content of each is described below.

Title

A title is very important. If the information presented in a research report is not indicated by its title, the report may not reach potential consumers, for at least two reasons. First, the title is one of the main sources of information used by abstract journals and computer databases (see Chapter 4) to index articles for retrieval. If the title does not clearly indicate the content of an article, it is less likely than otherwise to be indexed properly.

A title is also important because people scan titles (in bibliographies, tables of contents, and so forth) to identify papers they wish to read. If the content of a paper is not evident from its title, the paper may not be read by persons who could utilize the information presented in it.

What should you keep in mind when writing a title for a paper? First, you should use wording that indicates as unambiguously as possible the content of the paper—that is, the questions dealt with. It should mention both the specific population or populations studied (e.g., adults over the age of 50 who have cerebellar ataxia) and what was studied (e.g., the outcome of a particular therapy.) Both types of information can be combined to form a title such as:

Therapy X: Impact on Adults over the Age of 50 with Cerebellar Ataxia

Second, be as concise as possible. All unnecessary words should be eliminated. Consider this title:

A Study of the Impact of Therapy X on Adults over the Age of 50 with Cerebellar Ataxia

The first four words ("A Study of the . . .") can probably be deleted without altering what the title is intended to communicate.

Third, order the words appropriately. The first word (or words) in a title should at least partially define the topic. Consider the two titles suggested in this section for a study of the impact of a therapy on persons over the age of 50 who have cerebellar ataxia. Even if the first four words of the second were eliminated, the first would still be better than the second because it begins with a word that is more important for communicating the content of the paper—the name of the therapy.

Abstract

The abstract (or summary) should provide the reader (usually in less than 150 words) with concise information about the question or questions asked, the procedures used to answer them, the answers obtained, and how the answers were interpreted. In most journals, it appears below the title. One of its most important functions is to indicate—in conjunction with the title—the content of the article to users of abstracts journals and computer literature-search databases (see Chapter 4). The titles and abstracts of almost all recent papers dealing with communicative disorders (as well as some not-so-recent ones) are in at least one of these journals and databases. An investigator doing a search of the communicative disorders literature usually uses more than one because there are none that are likely to include all literature relevant to a topic. For example, he or she may use both the Medline and PsycINFO databases (see Chapter 4). If the title and abstract of a paper do not accurately and unambiguously indicate its content, the information in it is likely to be lost to at least some potential users.

There are two basic types of abstracts. The first (and most commonly used) *summa-*

rizes the content of the paper—the question or questions asked, the observational procedures, the observations made, the answers to the questions, and the interpretations made. Here is a representative abstract of this type:

> *The effect of adaptation on the masking of tinnitus was investigated. Six patients with tinnitus performed two 5-min tracking tasks, each replicated six times. The first task investigated the masking of tinnitus by tracking the intensity of a pure tone required to mask the tinnitus. The second task examined adaptation of a suprathreshold tone by tracking the intensity of a pure tone required for constant loudness. For three patients, the change required for constant loudness did not differ from the change required for constant maskability. For three patients, however, these two changes were different. Possible implications of these results for determining the locus of tinnitus and for the use of tinnitus maskers are discussed. (Penner & Bilger, 1989, p. 339)*

The second type of abstract, which is used less often than the first, *describes* the content of the paper. It indicates the topics that were dealt with. This type of abstract frequently is used for relatively long papers where the content cannot be summarized in the number of words allowed. It also sometimes is used for one- or two-page papers because a long abstract could look ridiculous when printed in one this short. Here is a representative abstract of this type:

> *This paper describes a dimension of the stuttering problem of elementary-school children—less frequent revision of reading errors than their nonstuttering peers. (Silverman & Williams, 1973, p. 584)*

What should you keep in mind when writing an abstract (or summary)? The main thing is that it must indicate the content of the paper as accurately and completely as possible within the length (i.e., word) limit imposed by the journal. Also, the writing should be as concise as possible. The most appropriate (e.g., descriptive, concrete) words for conveying what you want to convey should be used. All unnecessary words should be eliminated. You may find it helpful to read a number of abstracts (e.g., all those in several issues of the *Journal of Speech and Hearing Research* or *Language, Speech, and Hearing Services in Schools*) one after the other. This intensive reading should help you develop an intuitive feeling for how they are written.

Key Words

These are short lists of words that some journals include in articles (usually under the abstract) to supplement, for indexing purposes, the information presented in their titles and abstracts. They are intended to assist persons who index articles for computer databases— such as Medline and PsycINFO (see Chapter 4)—to do so appropriately. It is assumed that authors probably are more knowledgeable about the search terms (i.e., words) that are likely to be used for locating information in their articles than are professional indexers.

Introduction

In the introduction to a paper, you indicate *what* you were trying to do and *why* you were trying to do it. That is, you indicate the questions you were attempting to answer and why you felt it important to attempt to answer each. Doing the latter establishes a *scientific justification* for the study. Your reasons—that is, your scientific justification—may not be the only possible ones.

It is important to demonstrate as explicitly as possible the relevance of the research you are reporting—that is, the questions you are answering. You should indicate as many *cogent* theoretical and clinical implications of possible answers to your questions as you can. Lead your readers to the point where they would agree that the questions you sought to answer were worth answering. As mentioned previously, it is not safe to assume that readers will understand the implications of answers to questions without having these implications pointed out to them.

In the introduction you also review the literature that is *relevant to the questions you were attempting to answer.* Specifically, you indicate any data you are aware of that directly or indirectly suggest an answer to these questions. These data, of course, may suggest different answers to specific questions (which would make any answer to them equivocal). An investigator usually attempts to indicate in the literature review why the available data only permit the questions asked to be partially answered and/or why it is important to gather additional data so that they can be answered more completely. If, based on a careful review of relevant literature, it appears that no data have been reported that suggest an answer to the questions asked, this should be indicated.

Before you attempt to write an introduction, you might find it helpful to read a number of them, one after the other, in articles published in an issue of the *American Journal of Audiology,* the *American Journal of Speech-Language Pathology, Language, Speech, and Hearing Services in Schools,* or the *Journal of Speech and Hearing Research.* Doing so could help you develop a "tacit knowledge" (see Chapter 3) of how they are structured.

Methodology

In the methods section of a research report, you indicate *who* you observed and *how* you observed them. You should describe both in enough detail that another investigator could replicate your observations. In cases when sufficient detail cannot be provided within the space limits imposed by the journal, an address can be included from which a more detailed description of the methodology that was used can be obtained. The address may be that of the author or of the American Documentation Institute.

How do you decide what information to include in a methods section? The sole criterion for any bit of information is whether it is necessary to replicate your observations. If you feel that a given piece of information is likely to be necessary to do so, it should be included. If you are uncertain, it would be better to make the "error" of including information that is not essential than doing the opposite. Some of the problems in interpreting research findings that can result from inadequate information being available about subjects have been described by Brookshire (1983).

Before you attempt to write a methods section, you may find it helpful to scan a number of them in an issue of the *Journal of Speech and Hearing Research,* one after the other, paying particular attention to how they are organized.

Results

In the results section of a research report, you describe *what* was observed—that is, the observations that were made to answer each question. The observations should be organized and presented in a manner that should make the answer to each question fairly obvious to most readers.

In this section, you answer each question and report the data on which each answer was based. You usually do not interpret your answers here but in the discussion section. There are instances, however, when it is desirable to interpret answers while they are being presented. A combined results and discussion section can be used in such instances.

Discussion

In the discussion section of a research report, you indicate *possible implications*—both theoretical and clinical—of the answers you obtained. You indicate both the ways in which your answers appear to be consistent with existing theory and clinical practice and the ways in which they raise questions concerning the validity of aspects of them. It is particularly important that you refer again to the implications that you mentioned in the introduction section to establish scientific justification.

Questions for future research are sometimes suggested in the discussion section. A study often raises more questions than it answers. By mentioning such questions and indicating why each would be important to answer, you can help an investigator who wishes to answer them establish scientific justification for doing so. That is, he or she can at least partially establish scientific justification by referring to the questions in your discussion section.

Acknowledgments

The primary purpose of an acknowledgments section is to credit and recognize the financial and other support of individuals and organizations you received while doing the research and preparing the research report. Any financial assistance should be acknowledged, as should any persons who significantly contributed to the research by performing such functions as locating subjects, administering the experimental treatments, or assisting in the process of data analysis. Other persons you may wish to acknowledge are consultants, investigators who provided you with unpublished data, administrators who in some manner facilitated the research process, and persons who read the manuscript critically and offered suggestions for improvement.

Another type of information that may be presented in an acknowledgment section is the author's current institutional affiliation if it differs from that given at the beginning of the article. Some journals also include in this section the name and address of the person to whom requests for reprints should be directed.

References

All papers and books mentioned in the paper should be listed here. Since there is no standard reference style, you should acquaint yourself with the style used by the journal to which you plan to submit the paper before preparing this section. ASHA journals use that of the American Psychological Association (*Publications Manual of the American Psychological Association*, 1994).

Appendixes

Appendixes usually contain unpublished documents pertaining to the methodology used for gathering data. An example would be an unpublished test or other assessment instrument.

Organization of Oral Presentations

The organization used for structuring oral reports is similar to that used for structuring written ones. The two main ways that they are likely to differ are *length* and *degree of formality*. Methodology and results in oral research reports may be summarized rather than described in detail because there is not adequate time to do so. A handout may be distributed to "fill in the gaps" when they have to be presented in summary form.

A second difference is that the style of oral reports is usually less formal and more redundant than that of written ones. It is desirable that the language used in oral reports be conversational, because otherwise many of the persons who are present will not pay adequate attention to what is being said. You are particularly likely to lose your audience if the paper you are reading aloud is a formal research report written in the passive voice.

To communicate effectively, an oral report must be more redundant than a written one. If you do not understand something in a written report, you can reread it. This is not possible with an oral presentation, unless it is on audiotape or videotape. One way to inject redundancy into oral reports is beginning by summarizing what you are going to say, then saying it, and ending by summarizing what you have said.

Preparation of Written and Oral Reports

A number of books and articles contain information you are likely to find helpful when drafting a written or oral research report. The *Publications Manual for the American Psychological Association* (1994) is a highly useful source of such information. So are *A Style Manual for Writers in Communicative Disorders* (Shipley, 1982), "Guidelines for Nonsexist Language in Journals of ASHA" (1979), and *The Publication Process: A Guide for Authors* (1991). Other publications that you may find helpful are Booth (1993), Day (1992, 1994), Jerger (1962), Moore (1969), and Sternberg (1993).

Before preparing a written report that you intend to submit for publication, you should read the "information to contributors" document for the journal to which you plan to submit it. Some journals publish it in every issue; others publish it at regular intervals (e.g., one issue a year); still others do not publish it but send copies on request. The information provided usually includes the following:

- The types of papers the journal prints (e.g., research review papers) and their topics (e.g., hearing problems, cleft lip and palate)
- Instructions for preparing tables and figures and for typing the manuscript
- The maximum length for the abstract
- The reference style
- The number of copies that should be submitted
- The name and address of the editor to whom the copies should be submitted

Locating Journals and Meetings for Disseminating Your Questions, Answers, and Interpretations

Your final task in the clinical research process is disseminating your questions, answers, and interpretations to clinicians who can use the information "to promote the welfare of the persons whom they serve professionally." Doing so usually involves either locating an appropriate journal to which to submit a report or an appropriate professional meeting (e.g., a convention of an organization) at which to present a report (or both, since many papers presented at professional meetings are later published).

The publications and convention programs that speech-language pathologists and audiologists appear to use most often to disseminate their clinical research are those of the American Speech-Language-Hearing Association (ASHA). The ASHA journals include:

American Journal of Audiology
American Journal of Speech-Language Pathology
Journal of Speech and Hearing Disorders (Combined with the *Journal of Speech and Hearing Research* in 1991)
Journal of Speech and Hearing Research
Language, Speech, and Hearing Services in Schools
Asha
ASHA Monographs
ASHA Reports

Most issues of these journals contain a statement of the types of reports they will publish. One advantage of publishing information of interest to speech-language pathologists and audiologists in ASHA journals is that you are quite likely to reach most potential consumers of the information that is presented.

More than 500 presentations dealing with all aspects of speech-language pathology and audiology are usually included in the program of the annual convention of the American Speech-Language-Hearing Association (ASHA). For a presentation to be considered for inclusion in the convention program, a proposal consisting of a cover page, summary, and abstract has to be submitted to the program committee. Additional information can be found in the annual "Call for Papers," which ASHA distributes to its members.

State speech and hearing association publications and convention programs can also be used for disseminating clinical research. However, fewer practitioners are reached through them than through ASHA convention programs and publications.

A number of other associations publish research in their journals of interest to speech-language pathologists and audiologists and include presentations of interest to them in their convention programs. The following is a representative—not an inclusive—list of such organizations:

Academy of Aphasia
Academy of Cerebral Palsy
Acoustical Society of America
Alexander Graham Bell Association
American Academy of Audiology
American Cleft Palate Association
American Psychological Association
Canadian Speech and Hearing Association
College of Speech Therapists (London)
Council of Exceptional Children
International Association of Logopedics and Phoniatrics
International Fluency Association
International Society for Augmentative and Alternative Communication
Societa Italiana di Foniatria e Logopedia

Finally, many journals that are not distributed by scientific and professional associations publish clinical research of interest to speech-language pathologists and audiologists. Two examples are the *Journal of Communication Disorders* and *Perceptual and Motor Skill*. Perhaps the best strategy for identifying possible journals to which to submit a particular report is to scan papers dealing with the same general topic in the Medline or PsycINFO computer databases (see Chapter 4) and note the journals in which they are published.

Editorial Processing of Manuscripts

How are manuscripts processed after being submitted to a journal? After the editor receives a manuscript, he or she usually sends a form letter to the author acknowledging its receipt. Next, the editor either sends copies of the manuscript to the associate editor who is responsible for processing manuscripts in the area (e.g., audiometric testing or child language disorders) or to at least two editorial consultants, or reviewers, whom the editor feels are competent to assess the suitability of the manuscript for publication. If the manuscript is sent to an associate editor for processing, he or she usually solicits the reviews.

The editor or associate editor asks the reviewers for a recommendation on the disposition of the manuscript (accept as is, accept if revised according to instructions, reject, etc.), the reason or reasons for their recommendation, and suggestions for revising the manuscript. After receiving the reviewers' recommendations and reading the manuscript, the editor or associate editor decides on its disposition and informs the author of the decision and the reason or reasons for it.

If the editor or associate editor feels that parts of the manuscript have to be rewritten before it is suitable for publication, he or she will communicate this to the author and may offer some suggestions for rewriting them. Almost all manuscripts require some rewriting. The review process can take anywhere from a few weeks to more than a year; in most cases it takes between two and six months.

What should you do if a manuscript that you submit to a journal is rejected? Few people enjoy being rejected; because of the amount of ego investment that an author usually has in a manuscript, its rejection can hurt him or her as much as would the rejection of his or her child by others. Since many journals have rejection rates of more than 75 percent, most (if not all) persons who author papers for publication are going to have manuscripts rejected sooner or later. The appropriate way to deal with a manuscript being rejected depends on the reason or reasons given in the editor's and reviewers' comments for its rejection. Your manuscript could have been rejected for any of a number of reasons, including the following reasons:

- You failed to establish adequate scientific justification for the study (i.e., the reviewers regarded it as trivial).
- The observational procedures that you used do not permit the question or questions to be answered with an adequate level of validity, reliability, and generality.
- The data analyses procedures were inappropriate.
- The writing did not meet minimum standards for publication.
- The content of the manuscript was inappropriate for the journal.
- The reviewers did not like the question or questions that you asked and/or how you interpreted your findings.

If your manuscript was rejected because you failed to establish adequate scientific justification for the study reported in it, you should rewrite the introduction to better demonstrate the relevance of the information you report. Assuming that this was the *only* reason for the manuscript being rejected, you may want to resubmit the manuscript to the journal with a note to the editor or associate editor indicating how it has been revised. Or you may decide to submit it to another journal.

If your manuscript was rejected because it was claimed that there was something wrong with the methodology you used for making observations, and you agree that the reviewers' criticisms are valid, you may want to rerun the study using appropriate observational procedures. However, if you feel that the reviewers' criticisms are not valid, you may want to send a rebuttal to the editor indicating why you feel that your methodology was adequate and ask the editor to reconsider the manuscript. Or you may decide to forgo the hassle and submit the manuscript to another journal.

If your manuscript was rejected because the reviewers felt that there was something wrong with how the data were analyzed and you agree that they were analyzed incorrectly, you should reanalyze the data and either resubmit the corrected manuscript or submit it to some other journal. If you believe that the data were analyzed appropriately and you decide to resubmit the manuscript, you should include a note indicating why you feel the analyses were appropriate. Include, if possible, supporting statements from several statisticians.

If your manuscript was rejected because it is poorly written, it should be rewritten (with particular consideration given to relevant comments by reviewers) and either resubmitted to the journal or submitted to some other journal. Hopefully, there will someone at your institution who has written and/or edited journal articles who can help you rewrite it.

If your manuscript was rejected because the content was inappropriate for the journal to which it was submitted, it should be submitted to a journal for which the content is appropriate. You may be able to identify one by searching for papers on the same topic in a computer database (see Chapter 4).

Occasionally, a manuscript is rejected because the reviewers didn't like a question the author(s) asked or an interpretation that was made of an answer. This is particularly likely to happen when an answer or interpretation challenges accepted theory or clinical practice. If you believe that a manuscript was really rejected for this reason, you should submit it to another journal. Hopefully, you will be able to locate a journal that has an editor who is "willing to be confused by facts."

For further information about why articles are rejected, see the paper by Culatta (1984).

Indicate beside each statement whether or not it appears to be true.

Yes	No	Statement
____	____	1. The need (i.e., scientific justification) for answering the question, or questions, is explained clearly before it, or they, are answered.
____	____	2. The question, or questions, that are answered are stated clearly.
____	____	3. The relationship between this attempt to answer the question(s) and previous ones is clearly explained.
____	____	4. The observational procedures that were used for answering the question, or questions, are described clearly.
____	____	5. The population from which the subjects were sampled is described clearly.
____	____	6. The data that were generated by the observational procedures are described clearly.
____	____	7. The answer, or answers, are stated clearly and it is clear how the answers were derived from the data.
____	____	8. Clinical and/or theoretical implications are clearly stated, even ones that seem obvious.
____	____	9. The language used is appropriate for the type of presentation. It is intended to communicate rather than impress.

FIGURE 13-3   Evaluation checklist for quality of communication.

Evaluation Checklist for Quality of Communication

The quality of the communication in a journal article or convention paper can profoundly influence the impact that the information in it will have on consumers. If it is poor, the clinical implications of the data may be unclear, which will significantly reduce the likelihood that clients will benefit from them.

There are a number of things that you can do to maximize the quality of the communication in written reports and oral presentations. Some of them are mentioned in the evaluation checklist (see Figure 13-3). You can use it as a guide when *preparing* written reports (including journal articles) and oral presentations (including convention papers). You can also use it as a guide for *evaluating* journal articles and convention papers in conjunction with the checklist in Chapter 12.

Exercises and Discussion Topics

1. Use the Evaluation Checklist to assess the quality of the communication in three papers from a recent issue of the *Journal of Speech and Hearing Research.*

2. Listen to tape recordings of two convention papers and assess the quality of the communication in them, using the Evaluation Checklist.

3. What statements in the Evaluation Checklist can be used for assessing the quality of the communication in clinical evaluation reports?

Part III

Clinical Issues

Chapter 14

Documenting Intervention

To continue to grow as a clinician, you must continually assess the impacts of your intervention strategies—both positive and negative—on your clients. Without the information that you gain from such an assessment, you are likely to use either a small number over and over again or continuously seek out the "newest" ones. Your reason for using or rejecting a particular strategy is likely to be its acceptance or rejection by an "authority"—such as the author of a textbook you are familiar with—rather than its impacts on your clients' behavior, particularly their communicative behavior.

You can make one of two assumptions about the impact of an intervention strategy on behaviors contributing to a client's communicative disorder: (1) You can consider it effective until it is proven ineffective, or (2) you can consider it ineffective until it has been proven effective. The choice between them is somewhat analogous to that in law between considering a person innocent until proven guilty and considering him or her guilty until proven innocent.

What are the consequences of each assumption? There are two types of consequences. The first is *clinical*. Each assumption has associated with it a type of treatment error. That is, considering an intervention strategy effective until there is reasonable evidence that it is ineffective exposes a client to an intervention strategy that could have no effect, or an undesirable effect, on him or her. On the other hand, considering an intervention strategy ineffective until there is reasonable evidence that it is effective could result in a client who could be helped by it not being so.

The assumption that is most likely to lead to undesirable consequences for a client would not be the same in all instances. To illustrate this point, let's consider two instances in which we might be tempted to try an intervention strategy that seems sound theoretically, but has not yet been proven effective. In instance A, there is at least one other intervention strategy that has been proven effective; in instance B, there are no intervention strategies that have been proven effective. The consequences of *using* the new approach in instance A and finding it ineffective are likely to be more undesirable than not using it when it would have been effective. On the other hand, the consequences of *not using* this approach in instance B are likely to be less desirable than using it and finding it ineffective.

The second type of consequence can be referred to as *logical*. A logical consequence is one related to the appropriateness of using statistical inference. If our presumption is that an intervention strategy is ineffective until it is proven effective, we can use traditional statistical hypothesis testing procedures to determine the likelihood that it has been effective (see Chapters 10 and 11). Recall that the null hypothesis—the hypothesis tested by all traditional statistical significance tests—states that a treatment has produced no difference, that is, has had no effect. For determining whether an intervention strategy has influenced behavior, the null hypothesis would state that any impacts the intervention strategy appears to have had are not real but the result of random fluctuation or sampling error. In other words, differences in behavior following intervention are not sufficiently *reliable* to be attributed to it.

Rejecting the null hypothesis provides some support for the alternative, or research hypothesis, that intervention has been effective—that is, has resulted in behavioral change. However, it is necessary to keep constantly in mind that rejecting a null hypothesis only indicates that any behavioral changes observed following intervention are unlikely to have resulted from random fluctuation or sampling error (see Chapter 10). It does not establish that such changes resulted from intervention. Other events that occurred while a client was in therapy could have been at least partially responsible for the observed behavioral changes. Examples would be: (1) maturation (particularly of concern when evaluating intervention strategies for children who have a language disorder), (2) improved self-concept (particularly of concern when evaluating intervention strategies for stuttering), and (3) spontaneous recovery (particularly of concern when evaluating intervention strategies for aphasia, agnosia, apraxia, and dysarthria).

We will now consider the logical consequences of the alternative presumption—considering an intervention strategy effective until it is proven ineffective. This is comparable to interpreting failure to reject a null hypothesis as support for a strategy's effectiveness. As you may recall from our previous discussion of the null hypothesis, it is inappropriate to interpret failure to reject a null hypothesis as support for a research hypothesis (in this case, an intervention strategy being effective).

In most instances considering an intervention strategy ineffective until there is considerable evidence that it is effective would probably be more defensible than the alternative assumption—considering it effective until there is considerable evidence to the contrary.

Questions for Assessing an Intervention Strategy

A basic premise of this book is that research can be viewed as a process of answering "answerable" questions. To assess the impacts of an intervention strategy upon persons who have a communicative disorder, it is necessary to answer to a number of such questions, including the following:

1. What are the impacts of the intervention strategy on specific behaviors that contribute to a client's communicative disorder at given points in space-time? Here "specific behaviors" include what are traditionally called "attitudes" and "feelings." We become aware of attitudes and feelings by observing behavior—that is, attitudes and feelings are *explanations* for behavior. "Points in space-time" refers to how the impacts of an intervention strategy on specific behaviors vary, over a period of time and according to situation. Space-time is hyphenated to indicate (as Einstein and others have pointed out) that time cannot be separated from space but provides the fourth dimension necessary to specify the location, or coordinates, of an event.

2. What are the impacts of the intervention strategy on other attributes of a client's communicative behavior at given points in space-time? An intervention strategy that has a desirable impact on behaviors that contribute to a client's communicative disorder can affect other attributes of his or her communicative behavior in undesirable and/or desirable ways—that is, it can have good and/or bad *side effects*. Other attributes affected might include: (1) speaking rate, (2) auditory acuity, (3) speech rhythm, (4) speech articulation, (5) voice intensity, (6) voice quality, (7) language formulation, (8) verbal output, (9) spontaneity, and (10) credibility as a communicator. If, for example, a stutterer is taught to monitor his speech for moments of stuttering and voluntarily reduce their severity, this may not only result in a reduction in his stuttering severity but in his speaking rate, spontaneity, and inflection as well. If a client's communicative behavior after intervention with a particular strategy called more adverse attention to itself than before receiving it, this would be an undesirable side effect. On the other hand, if a mentally retarded child who had little or no speech was taught to communicate manually (e.g., with American Sign Language) and as a consequence significantly increased his or her verbal output—which happens in approximately one-third of cases (Silverman, 1995a)—this side effect would be highly desirable.

3. What are the impacts of the intervention strategy on a client other than those directly related to communicative behavior at given points in space-time? The intent of this question is similar to the second, because it is concerned with identifying undesirable and desirable side effects of the strategy. The side effects we are concerned with here would include impacts on: (1) self-concept, (2) peer acceptance, and (3) anxiety. A client given an instrumental aid (such as an electrolarynx or miniature metronome with which to pace his or her speech) might be able to communicate better with the device, but might also feel there is something wrong with him or her for having to rely on it rather than being able to overcome the problem by "force of will." On the other hand, a severely motor handicapped client who cannot speak but learns to do so using a laptop microcomputer with a speech synthesizer is likely to be more accepted by peers than previously and, as a consequence, develop a better self-concept (Silverman, 1995a).

4. What are the client's attitudes toward the intervention strategy and its impacts on his or her communicative and other behaviors at given points in space-time? A client's attitude toward an intervention strategy and its impacts on his or her behavior can influence (reduce or enhance) the effectiveness of the strategy. If, for example, a person with a hearing loss refused to wear a hearing aid, the use of this strategy could not be effective in reducing the severity of the communicative disorder (unless, of course, the person's attitude could be changed). On the other hand, a client with a strong belief that an intervention strategy could benefit him or her would invest more time and energy in the program, which, in turn, would tend to enhance its effectiveness.

5. What are the attitudes of a client's clinician, family, friends, and others toward the intervention strategy and toward its impacts on the client's communicative behavior and other attributes of behavior at given points in a space-time? The attitudes of persons with whom a client interacts toward an intervention strategy being used with a client and toward its effects on his or her behavior can influence the probable success of that strategy. A clinician who does not believe that an intervention strategy will be effective is likely to communicate this attitude to the client and thereby reduce the likelihood that the client will benefit from it. If, for example, a clinician were directly or indirectly to communicate to a client who is severely communicatively impaired and could benefit from using a conversation board that he or she considered the use of such a device a last resort, this might reduce the likelihood that the client would use the device and thereby benefit from it. On the other hand, if such a client's family and friends were to spend more time with him or her after he or she has begun using a conversation board, this would increase the likelihood that the client would continue using the device and thereby benefit from it.

6. What investment is required of client and clinician at given points in space-time? Several types of investment can be required, including: (1) financial, (2) time and energy, and (3) willingness to be uncomfortable, that is, to do things one does not want to do (things that tend to make a client uncomfortable or increase his or her anxiety level). An intervention strategy may be effective but may be too demanding in cost or time to be practical for many clients. An example of such a strategy would be traditional psychoanalysis, in which the client may be required to be seen by the psychoanalyst daily for a period of several years. Also, a strategy may be effective but may cause clients to be so uncomfortable that few would be willing to make the necessary investment. One such strategy would be voluntary stuttering—"fake stuttering"—outside the clinic situation. Many stutterers find this activity extremely noxious and refuse to do it when asked by their clinician.

7. What is the probability of relapse following termination of therapy? Persons with communicative disorders, particularly stutterers, may relapse to some degree when they stop seeing their clinicians on a regular basis. While a person exposed to almost any intervention approach can relapse, the probability of relapse tends to be higher for some approaches than for others. If the positive impacts of an intervention approach were quite likely to wear off after termination of therapy, it would be of questionable value. It is important, then, when evaluating an intervention strategy to take the probability of relapse into consideration.

Methodologies for Assessing Intervention Strategies and Outcomes

Methodologies are described in this section that can be used for answering the seven questions that were discussed in the preceding one. Most of the methodologies described in previous chapters—particularly descriptive statistical, inferential statistical, and measurement-related ones—are relevant for answering these questions. The methodologies described in this section are mostly ones that have not been discussed previously.

While very few methodologies have been developed specifically for assessing the impacts of intervention strategies on persons who have communicative disorders, many have been developed for documenting intervention outcomes in education, clinical psychology, and psychiatry. Since the problems involved in assessing the impacts of teaching methods and psychotherapies are much the same as those involved in assessing the impacts of intervention on communicative disorders, some of these methodologies are described here.

What Are the Impacts of the Intervention Strategy on Specific Behaviors That Contribute to a Client's Communicative Disorder at Given Points in Space-Time?

There are a number of tasks that you have to do to systematically assess the impacts of an intervention strategy on behaviors contributing to a client's communicative disorder, including the following:

- Choosing a criterion measure or measures
- Establishing a baseline
- Establishing a measurement interval
- Selecting criteria for deciding whether an intervention strategy has been effective
- Identifying viable alternatives to the hypothesis that an intervention strategy was responsible for an effect, if an effect is observed
- Reducing the effects of the experimenter's expectations and theoretical biases on the data
- Identifying relevant organismic variables
- Identifying relevant therapist variables
- Controlling positive and negative placebo effect contamination

Some aspects of each of them are discussed below.

Choosing a Criterion Measure or Measures
The choice of a criterion measure or measures is one of the most important considerations when designing research to assess the impacts of intervention strategies on persons who have communicative disorders. If you select a criterion measure that is not sufficiently valid and reliable, it can make an effective strategy appear to be ineffective.

One way that you can increase the likelihood that you will be able to provide documentation for a therapy being effective if it is effective is to use more than one criterion measure. If, for example, we wanted to determine whether an intervention strategy for ameliorating an articulation error is effective, we might use as criterion measures the percent correct production of the "error" phoneme on several types of speaking tasks.

Establishing a Baseline
To document an impact of a therapy program on a client, a description (quantitative and/or qualitative) of an attribute of his or her post-therapy behavior is compared to what it was either prior to beginning therapy or at an earlier point—or points—while therapy was ongoing (e.g., at the beginning of the semester). A description of an attribute to which later descriptions are compared is referred to as a baseline. An example of a simple baseline would be a single criterion measure made once before beginning intervention. A more complex (and presumably more reliable) baseline could consist of: (1) a single criterion measure made several times, (2) multiple criterion measures made once, or (3) multiple criterion measures made several times. For further information about these, see Chapter 6.

Establishing a Measurement Interval

One decision that you have to make when developing a plan for documenting therapy outcome is the frequently at which to make observations (e.g., measures) of the attribute(s) of the client's behavior that you are attempting to modify. The measurement interval that has probably been used most often is twice—once preceding a period of intervention and once following it. This is the traditional *pretest-posttest* design. This design is not a particularly good one for several reasons. First, it is more likely than most designs to result in a Type II error (see Chapter 10) because random fluctuation can easily cause a pre-therapy measure to be too high and/or a post-therapy measure to be too low. Second, the use of data from this design to document therapy outcome is more questionable than that from most others because it does not allow you to control for the effects of extraneous variables. If a client's communicative disorder is less severe in the posttest than in the pretest, there may be plausible explanations for this difference other than the intervention. Among the classes of extraneous variables that could account for such a difference, according to Campbell, are the following:

- **History**: Other significant events occurring between the first and the second measurement in addition to the experimental variable (i.e., the intervention strategy).
- **Maturation:** Processes within the respondents (clients) operating as a function of the passage of time per se (not specific to the particular events), including growing older, growing hungrier, growing more tired, and the like.
- **Testing:** The effects of taking a test upon the scores of a second testing.
- **Instrumentation:** Changes in the calibration of a measuring instrument or changes in the observers or scorers that may produce changes in the obtained measurements.
- **Statistical regression:** Regression operating when groups have been selected on the basis of their extreme scores.
- **The reactive or interactive effect of testing**, in which a pretest might increase or decrease the respondent's sensitivity or responsiveness to the experimental variable and thus make the results obtained for a pretested population unrepresentative of the effects of the experimental variable for the unpretested universe from which the experimental respondents were selected. (Campbell, 1963, p. 215)

The effects of three of these causes—maturation, testing, and statistical regression—can be at least partially controlled by substituting a *time series* design such as the one illustrated for a pretest-posttest design (the notation used here is the same as that used in Chapter 6):

$$A_1 \quad A_2 \quad A_3 \quad A_4 \quad B \quad A_5 \quad A_6 \quad A_7 \quad A_8$$

With this design, a baseline measurement is made a predetermined number of times (in the above example, eight) at a set time interval. The duration of the interval between measures would be approximately equal to the duration of the intervention approach being evaluated. The clients receive the intervention (B) during the interval between two measures (in the example, they would receive it between measures of 4 and 5). The criterion measures are then plotted, and the pattern of the resulting trend line is interpreted to indicate whether the intervention has had an impact (see Figure 14-1). This design is most practical for intervention approaches of relatively short duration.

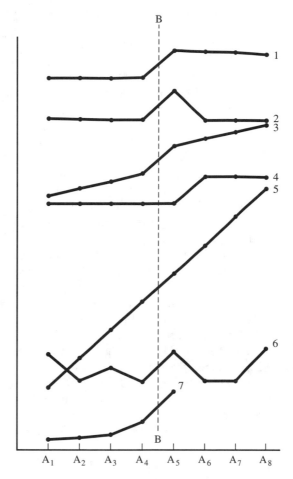

FIGURE   14-1   Some possible outcome patterns from the introduction of an experimental variable at point B into a time series of measurements, $A_1 - A_8$. Except for 4, the $A_4 - A_5$ gain is the same for all time series, while the legitimacy of inferring an effect varies widely, being strongest in 1 and 2 and totally unjustified in 5, 6, and 7. *(Adapted from Campbell, 1963, and reproduced with permission of the publisher.)*

A treatment does not have to occur at the midpoint of a time series. It could occur toward the beginning:

$$A_1 \quad A_2 \quad B \quad A_3 \quad A_4 \quad A_5 \quad A_6 \quad A_7 \quad A_8$$

Such a design could be useful for assessing the long-term impacts of an intervention strategy.

A variation of the time series design, the *multiple time series* (Campbell, 1963, p. 232), is even more effective in controlling for the effects of extraneous variables. Such a design is illustrated graphically by the following:

GROUP 1	A_1	A_2	A_3	A_4	B	A_5	A_6	A_7	A_8
GROUP 2	A_1	A_2	A_3	A_4		A_5	A_6	A_7	A_8

This design controls at least partially for five of the six classes of extraneous variables to which the pretest-posttest design is sensitive—history, maturation, testing, instrumentation, and statistical regression.

With a multiple time series design, the measures made on the members of a group with whom a particular intervention approach is used (in the example, Group 1) are compared to those made on the members of a comparable group who do not receive that type of intervention (in the example, Group 2). The measures are made on both groups at the same time intervals. The measures made on the control group provide a secondary baseline against which to assess those made on the experimental group. The primary baseline is the same as for the pretest-posttest and single time series designs, that is, the measures made prior to intervention.

The control, or secondary, baseline can be helpful in interpreting several of the outcome patterns in Figure 14-1. If, for example, the eight measures made on the members of a control group were approximately equal (i.e., the control baseline was relatively flat), pattern 4 would indicate that the intervention strategy had been effective.

One limitation of the multiple time series design is the need for a control group. You would probably have reservations about withholding therapy from a group of clients who needed it. There are circumstances, however, when this design would not require you to withhold therapy. One would be when there are sufficient people on your waiting list who: (1) have the same type of communicative disorder as the members of the experimental group, and (2) do not differ systematically from them in relevant organismic variables such as age and intellectual level. A second circumstance would be when intervention is of relatively short duration and delaying its start should do no harm.

For further information about these and other time series designs, see Chapter 6.

Selecting Criteria for Deciding Whether an Intervention Strategy Has Been Effective

Before concluding that an intervention strategy has been effective, it is necessary to demonstrate a difference between pre- and post-intervention measures that is unlikely to have resulted from random, or chance, fluctuation, and is unlikely to have resulted from extraneous variables. Demonstrating the first with quantitative data from a group design can usually be done with a significance test, provided that the probability of a Type II error can be kept low enough to make it likely that the test could detect a difference as small as the smallest one that would be meaningful in the "real world" (see Chapter 10). The size of the experimental group (and of the control group, if one is used) in therapy outcome research is apt to be relatively small, and consequently, the probability of a Type II error is apt to be relatively high.

If the null hypothesis is rejected, the next step is to demonstrate that the observed difference between pre- and post-intervention measures is more likely to have been due to the intervention than to extraneous variables. The ease with which this can be done is partially a function of the measurement interval used. It would be easier to accomplish, for example, with a time series design than with a pretest-posttest one.

Identifying Viable Alternatives to the Hypothesis That Intervention Was Responsible for an Impact, if One Was Observed

Identifying viable alternative hypotheses is not, strictly speaking, a problem of research design or statistics. It is accomplished, at least in part, by a systematic search of relevant literature (see Chapter 4).

Reducing the Effects of the Experimenter's Expectations and Theoretical Biases on the Data

Your expectations and biases can influence your answers to questions and the interpretations you make of them without your being aware of it happening (Rosenthal & Rosnow, 1969; Whitaker, Dill, & Whitaker Jr., 1990). While these effects cannot be completely eliminated from therapy outcome research, there may be ways to reduce their impact, including the following:

1. Have someone *other than the clinician* interpret the data used to document therapy outcome. Hopefully, the expectations of the person, or persons, performing this task will be relatively neutral with regard to the effectiveness of the therapy being evaluated.
2. If possible, the person who analyzes the data should not know whether it was collected prior to, during, or following the termination of therapy.
3. If both experimental and control group subjects were used, the person who analyzes the data should not know to which of the groups each subject belongs.
4. In studies of the relative effectiveness of several therapies, it would be best if the same clinician did not administer them. The outcome—and consequently the data—could be biased by the clinician expecting one to be more effective than the other.

Identifying Relevant Organismic Variables

Organismic variables are properties or attributes of the individual. Examples are sex, chronological age, socioeconomic status, intellectual level, and educational level. The effectiveness of a therapy can be influenced by such variables. An approach to teaching the American Sign Language, for example, may be more effective with adults than with children.

There are at least two reasons in therapy outcome research for identifying relevant organismic variables. First, organismic variables may help to define the subpopulation(s) for which a particular intervention strategy is likely to be effective. If there are no relevant organismic variables, a strategy that is likely to be effective with some persons who have a particular communicative disorder should be likely to be effective with most, if not all, of those who have it (assuming that the disorder has only one cause). On the other hand, if the effectiveness of a strategy is influenced by one or more organismic variables, the strategy *may* only be usable with a subset of the population. The word *may* was italicized because even though a strategy may not be as effective with some persons as it is with others, it still may be the most effective one to use with all of them.

A second reason for identifying relevant organismic variables is concerned with the meaningfulness of combining subjects into groups. Data on the effects of an intervention strategy can be biased and/or transformed into "mathematical artifact" by combining data from subjects who differ with respect to relevant organismic variables. If an intervention strategy were effective with children and not with adults, for example, combining data from children and adults could make it appear to have been ineffective (particularly if there were more adults than children in the sample).

Identifying Relevant Therapist Variables

An intervention strategy administered by one therapist may not have the same effect as the same strategy administered by a second therapist. Certain attitudes and attributes of therapists can enhance or reduce the effectiveness of a therapy. One such attribute is amount of clinical experience. A therapy administered by a clinician who has had considerable experience may be more effective than the same one administered by a beginning clinician. Also, a clinician who expects a therapy to be effective may get a different result than one who expects it to be ineffective. Other therapist variables that could influence the effectiveness of an intervention strategy are sex, chronological age, socioeconomic status, degree of confidence in self, ability to communicate, and professional title (Dr. versus Mr., Ms., Miss, or Mrs.).

The effectiveness of an intervention strategy being at least partially a function of therapist variables has several implications. First, it limits the generality of research findings on the effectiveness of that strategy. Perhaps an intervention strategy would not be recommended for beginning clinicians and/or for those who lack confidence in its effectiveness. Second, it may not be possible to combine, or "lump," data from different clinicians. If such data are combined, an intervention strategy that is only effective for some clinicians may appear to be ineffective, particularly if it is ineffective for the majority of them.

Controlling Positive and Negative Placebo Effect Contamination

A placebo is

> . . . *any therapeutic procedure (or that component of any therapeutic procedure) which is given deliberately to have an effect, or unknowingly has an effect on a patient, symptom, syndrome, or disease, but which is objectively without specific activity for the condition being treated. The therapeutic procedure may be given with or without conscious knowledge that the procedure is a placebo, may be an active (non-inert) or nonactive (inert) procedure, and include, therefore, all medical procedures no matter how specific—oral and parenteral medication, topical preparations, inhalants, and mechanical, surgical, and psychotherapeutic procedures. The placebo must be differentiated from the placebo effect which may or may not occur and which may be favorable or unfavorable. The placebo effect is defined as the changes produced by placebos. (Shapiro, 1964, p. 75)*

Consequently, the placebo effect can either enhance or reduce the effectiveness of an intervention strategy. That is, the placebo effect can make it appear more effective or less effective than it really is. In therapy outcome research, therefore, one should recognize the possibility of, and control for, the placebo effect whenever possible.

What factors may be responsible for the placebo effect? According to Shapiro (1964), any of the following can result in a placebo effect:

1. The client's faith in the ability of the clinician, the therapy, or both, to help him or her. This can result in either a positive or negative placebo effect.

2. The clinician's attitude toward the intervention strategy—his or her faith or confidence in its effectiveness. This also can result in either a positive or a negative placebo effect.
3. The clinician's relationship to the client. The interested clinician "who imparts confidence, who performs a thorough examination, and who is not anxious, conflicted, or guilty about the patient or his treatment is more likely to elicit positive placebo reactions. Negative placebo reactions are more likely when the doctor [or clinician] is angry, rejecting, and contemptuous toward patients or seriously preoccupied with his own problems" (Shapiro, 1964, p. 77).

How can a placebo effect be distinguished from an effect of intervention? One approach would be to do the therapy again using a client and clinician who are relatively neutral in their expectations about its effectiveness. If the therapy was ineffective, this would suggest (not prove) that the previous positive results were a function of something other than it. On the other hand, the same results would provide additional support for the hypothesis that the therapy is effective.

What Are the Impacts of the Intervention Strategy on Other Attributes of a Client's Communicative Behavior at Given Points in Space-Time?

What Are the Impacts of the Intervention Strategy on a Client Other Than Those Directly Related to Communicative Behavior at Given Points in Space-Time?

The methodological considerations for answering these questions are the same as for the previous one.

What Are the Client's Attitudes toward the Intervention Strategy and Its Impacts on His or Her Communicative and Other Behaviors at Given Points in Space-Time?

Many of the methodological considerations discussed previously are relevant for designing research to answer this question. One that has not been mentioned in this chapter is the selection of a methodology for documenting attitudes. Several that have been used for this purpose—including the *semantic differential* technique (Osgood, Suci, & Tannenbaum, 1957)—are described in Chapter 8.

What Are the Attitudes of a Client's Clinician, Family, Friends, and Others toward the Intervention Strategy and toward Its Impacts on the Client's Communicative Behavior at Given Points in Space-Time?

The methodological considerations are the same as for the previous question. The semantic differential in Figure 8-10 was developed to partially answer this question for a stuttering intervention strategy (Silverman & Trotter, 1973).

What Investments Are Required of Client and Clinician at Given Points in Space-Time?

Time, financial, and emotional investments must be assessed. Both the client and clinician will have to keep track of their time and financial investments. The client's emotional investments can be inferred from comments he or she makes to the clinician during the course of therapy and/or from interviews conducted by the clinician (or someone else) following its termination.

What Is the Probability of Relapse Following Termination of Therapy?

You should assess the long-term effects of an intervention in addition to its immediate effects. It would be naive to assume that a client's status following termination of therapy is certain to remain unchanged over a relatively long period of time.

If you want to incorporate some type of follow-up into your assessment, you will have to make three decisions: (1) the behaviors to describe and how to describe them, (2) the intervals at which to describe them, and (3) the length of time to continue to do so.

You should decide whether your assessment will include follow-up before you select behaviors to describe and decide how to describe them. Some observational procedures would not be practical following termination of therapy, particularly for clients who do not live or are unlikely to continue to live close to your facility. It may be necessary, therefore, to select procedures that would enable you to gather the data you need by telephone or by mail.

How frequently should assessments be made following termination of therapy? This is a decision for which it is difficult to provide guidelines. However, if you made periodic assessments during therapy (e.g., once a month), it may be both desirable and possible to continue doing so at the same interval following termination—particularly for the first year.

The final decision—the length of time to follow up—is also a difficult one for which to provide guidelines. There is insufficient data on the long-term effects of at least some interventions for communicative disorders to provide a sound basis for making this decision. Perhaps until adequate data are available, it would be advisable to be conservative and adopt a five-year follow-up period, as have many investigators in medicine and psychotherapy as well as speech-language pathology (e.g., Van Riper, 1958).

Evaluation Checklist for Assessing the Adequacy of Therapy Outcome Research

Seven questions are discussed in this chapter that you should attempt to answer when assessing the adequacy of an intervention program for a communicative disorder. You can use the checklist in Figure 14-2 to structure you assessment of the adequacy of the data available for answering them. The word *adequacy* here refers to the levels of validity, reliability, and generality (see Chapter 12) of the data for the purposes for which they are used. For further information about this checklist, see Silverman (1977b).

Indicate beside each finding whether its validity, reliability, and generality appear adequate for the answering the question. If the validity, reliability or generality of a finding is uncertain, place a question mark in the appropriate space. Room is provided on the form for evaluating two findings that are relevant to each question.

1. WHAT ARE THE EFFECTS OF THE INTERVENTION PROGRAM UPON SPECIFIC BEHAVIORS THAT CONTRIBUTE TO A CLIENT'S COMMUNICATIVE DISORDER AT GIVEN POINTS IN SPACE-TIME?

   FINDING #1:

   VALIDITY _____   RELIABILITY _____   GENERALITY _____

   FINDING #2:

   VALIDITY _____   RELIABILITY _____   GENERALITY _____

2. WHAT ARE THE EFFECTS OF THE INTERVENTION PROGRAM UPON OTHER ATTRIBUTES OF A CLIENT'S COMMUNICATIVE BEHAVIOR AT GIVEN POINTS IN SPACE-TIME?

   FINDING #1:

   VALIDITY _____   RELIABILITY _____   GENERALITY _____

   FINDING #2:

   VALIDITY _____   RELIABILITY _____   GENERALITY _____

3. WHAT ARE THE EFFECTS OF THE INTERVENTION PROGRAM ON A CLIENT OTHER THAN THOSE DIRECTLY RELATED TO HIS OR HER COMMUNICATIVE DISORDER AT GIVEN POINTS IN SPACE-TIME?

   FINDING #1:

   VALIDITY _____   RELIABILITY _____   GENERALITY _____

   FINDING #2:

   VALIDITY _____   RELIABILITY _____   GENERALITY _____

4. WHAT ARE THE CLIENT'S ATTITUDES TOWARD THE INTERVENTION PROGRAM AND ITS EFFECTS ON HIS OR HER COMMUNICATIVE AND OTHER BEHAVIORS AT GIVEN POINTS IN SPACE-TIME?

   FINDING #1:

   VALIDITY _____   RELIABILITY _____   GENERALITY _____

   FINDING #2:

   VALIDITY _____   RELIABILITY _____   GENERALITY _____

FIGURE 14-2   Evaluation checklist for adequacy of therapy outcome research.

5. WHAT ARE THE ATTITUDES OF A CLIENT'S CLINICIAN, FAMILY, FRIENDS, AND OTHERS WITH WHOM HE OR SHE COMMUNICATES TOWARD THE INTERVENTION PROGRAM AND ITS EFFECTS ON HIS OR HER COMMUNICATIVE BEHAVIOR AND OTHER BEHAVIOR AT GIVEN POINTS IN SPACE-TIME?

FINDING #1:

VALIDITY _____   RELIABILITY _____   GENERALITY _____

FINDING #2:

VALIDITY _____   RELIABILITY _____   GENERALITY _____

6. WHAT INVESTMENTS ARE REQUIRED BY A CLIENT AND HIS OR HER CLINICIAN AT GIVEN POINTS IN SPACE-TIME?

FINDING #1:

VALIDITY _____   RELIABILITY _____   GENERALITY _____

FINDING #2:

VALIDITY _____   RELIABILITY _____   GENERALITY _____

7. WHAT IS THE PROBABILITY OF "RELAPSE" FOLLOWING TERMINATION OF THE INTERVENTION PROGRAM?

FINDING #1:

VALIDITY _____   RELIABILITY _____   GENERALITY _____

FINDING #2:

VALIDITY _____   RELIABILITY _____   GENERALITY _____

FIGURE 14-2   *Continued*

Exercises and Discussion Topics

1. Use the checklist in this chapter for evaluating some of the outcome research on an intervention program (therapy method) of your choice.

2. What items on the checklist included in this chapter are usable *clinically* for evaluating therapy outcome?

3. Use the semantic differential reproduced in Chapter 8 for evaluating the attitudes of three persons toward one of your clients. Have them listen to an audiotape or videotape (preferably the latter) of your client speaking.

Chapter 15

Legal and Ethical Considerations in Clinical Research

Almost all of the research conducted by speech-language pathologists and audiologists involves the use of human subjects. Persons who have participated in such research have been harmed by the failure of investigators to foresee possible undesirable effects of their experimental procedures on them (e.g., Silverman, 1988). There has been considerable interest since the Nuremberg trials (which were conducted after World War II) in the mental and physical welfare of persons who serve as subjects in research studies. This interest has resulted in the creation of regulations on both national and international levels (see Appendix D) that are intended to protect the rights of such persons. It also has stimulated considerable discussion about ethical aspects of how human subjects are used in clinical research (see Gostin, 1991; Grodin & Glantz, 1994; National Institutes of Health, 1993a; Penslar, 1993; Rosnow, 1990; Strohmetz & Skleder, 1992).

A number of legal and ethical considerations in clinical research are discussed in this chapter. Much of this discussion is also applicable to other kinds of research in which human subjects are used.

Need for Protecting Research Subjects

Persons who volunteer to serve as subjects are likely to assume that they will be *protected by the experimenter* from being harmed in any way (Lawson, 1995). They would be particularly likely to make this assumption if they are volunteering to participate in an experiment from which they could not expect to benefit personally. (Subjects can benefit personally by participating in an experiment in several ways, such as gaining knowledge, improving physical and/or mental health, or being paid.) They also would be particularly likely to assume that they will be protected if the research was being conducted under the auspices of a respected institution (such as a university or hospital).

While subjects may assume that there is no possibility of their being harmed by participating in an experiment, such an assumption would not be valid. It is impossible to design an experiment that is entirely risk-free. One of the most difficult components of the ethical review of research proposals by institutional review boards (IRBs) is assessing potential risks of harm to research participants (Meslin, 1990; Rosnow, Rotheram-Borus, Ceci, & Blanck, 1993; Thompson, 1990).

Although it would be unrealistic for subjects to assume that their participation in an experiment is entirely risk free, it would not be unreasonable for them to assume that their risk of being harmed is almost nonexistent if they are not informed to the contrary. Consequently, an experimenter who exposed subjects to more than extremely minimal risks of harm *without first informing them* about these risks would probably be viewed as behaving irresponsibly. The subjects, if they were harmed, could sue both the experimenter and the institution under whose auspices the research was conducted for negligence and/or some other tort (possibly battery) with a reasonable expectation of winning (Silverman, 1992). This is one of the reasons why institutions have committees to evaluate research proposals.

It is important that the actual risk of harm to a subject be consistent with the subject's assumption regarding the nature of this risk. How can one ensure that this will be the case? Several approaches can be used to ensure that a subject's *consent* to participate in an experiment is *informed* (Applebaum, Lidz, & Meisel, 1987; White, 1994). One would be to rely on the *experimenter* both to minimize risks to subjects and to inform them voluntarily about the risks remaining. While this would be the simplest (and probably the most common) approach, it has several limitations. Perhaps its main limitation is that the goals of collecting desired data and of protecting the persons from whom these data are being collected may not be compatible. Ordinarily an experimenter's primary objective is to gather the data needed to answer specific questions or to test specific hypotheses. While few experimenters would knowingly expose their subjects to highly dangerous experimental conditions without informing them about the risks, they might be tempted to be less forthright when there are potential risks associated with them that have not been demonstrated unequivocally to exist. Experimenters may hesitate to inform potential subjects about such risks because it could discourage enough of them from volunteering to make it impossible for the study to be undertaken or completed.

A second approach that can be used for ensuring that a subject's consent to participate is informed and that potential risks have been minimized and are within acceptable limits is to require the designs of all research studies that wish to use institutional clients as subjects to be scrutinized by an *institutional review board* (IRB). The mission of this committee would be to identify potential risks and to determine both whether they are within acceptable limits and whether subjects will be fully informed about them (Metz & Folkins, 1985; Rosnow, Rotheram-Borus, Ceci, & Blanck, 1993). This approach has been adopted by many institutions, including school systems, universities, and hospitals. Requiring such a board to approve the design for a study can protect subjects in several ways. First, it would probably motivate the experimenter to design the study so as to minimize the risks to subjects and thus maximize the odds of the proposal's being approved by the committee. Also, the experimenter would hesitate to propose a study that would expose subjects to unacceptably high risks of harm because doing so could damage his or her professional reputation. Second, such a board provides a mechanism for monitoring the degree to which subjects are informed about potential hazards and hence the degree to which their consent constitutes *informed consent* (see Applebaum, Lidz, & Meisel, 1987; White, 1994). Institutional review boards may require experimenters to submit to them copies of the consent forms that subjects will be asked to sign. The committee would then decide whether the presentation of possible hazards on them is sufficiently complete and accurate for a subject's consent to constitute fully informed consent. If a subject is not fully informed about potential hazards before signing a consent form, his or her consent probably would not be recognized by a court (Applebaum, Lidz, & Meisel, 1987; White, 1994). The concept of informed consent is dealt with in depth elsewhere in this chapter.

While the second approach (using institutional review boards) tends to be superior to the first (relying solely on the experimenter) for protecting the rights of subjects, it is not perfect. One of its limitations is that board members may not be familiar with the methodology an investigator proposes to use and consequently, they may fail to recognize potential hazards to subjects. It is even conceivable that no board members will be familiar with the methodology outlined in a proposal.

Informed Consent as a Vehicle for Protecting Investigators and Institutions

Clinical research in the previous section was viewed from the perspective of the need for protecting the rights of research subjects. In this section it will be viewed from a different perspective—that of the need for protecting the rights of investigators and the institutions under whose auspices they are doing their research. If our legal system did not protect these rights, little (if any) clinical research would be undertaken, which would have an obvious detrimental impact on the health of persons in our society.

Securing subjects' *informed consent* to participate in a study can provide both the investigator(s) and the institution under whose auspices the research is being conducted with some protection against litigation arising from allegations that they were physically or mentally harmed by doing so. If they were aware of a particular risk before consenting to participate in the study and if they were harmed in a manner predictable from this risk, they would be unlikely to be successful if they sued either the investigator or the institution.

One of the main types of litigation against which a subject's informed consent to participate in a study can provide some protection is *battery*. According to Fried:

> The central concept of battery is the offense to personal dignity that occurs when another impinges on one's bodily integrity without full and valid consent. A punch in the stomach or being doused with a pail of water are classic examples. It is not necessary to show that one has been physically injured, much less that one has suffered financial loss. The injury is to dignity. That being the case, law suits have been brought and won against doctors who performed needed and successful operations, but without consent of their patients. (Fried, 1974, p. 15)

Consequently, experimenting on people without their "full and valid consent" can result in litigation for battery even if they were not physically injured and even if they did not suffer financial loss. Such litigation also can result from subjecting clients to *therapy programs* without their "full and valid consent." For further information about battery and other torts for which an investigator can be sued, see Chapter 6 in Silverman (1992).

The requirement that must be satisfied to justify intentionally invading another's bodily integrity is securing his or her *free and informed* consent to do so. According to Fried:

> To be effective the consent must be to the particular contact with the person in question, and if procured by "fraud or mistake as to the essential character" of the conduct it is invalid. . . . And it is not just active fraud or concealment which destroys consent. The doctor [or experimenter] who obtains consent has the duty to give the facts the patient [or subject] needs to make an informed choice. . . . He must tell the patient [or subject] about the benefits and risks of the treatment [or experimental condition(s)], and how likely they are. And some courts have said that the patient must also be told about the hazards and advantages of alternative forms of treatment. (Fried, 1974, pp. 19–20)

Consequently, for consent to participate in an experiment to be regarded by a court as having been *free and informed,* the experimenter would have to be able to prove that subjects were not coerced into giving their consent and that they had been fully informed about the risks involved before they gave it.

Under some circumstances a subject's free and informed consent to participate in a study *may* not be sufficient. One such circumstance would be when the subject is a *child,* particularly a very young child who would be unable to understand the study and consequently would be incapable of giving informed consent. Consent in such a circumstance would have to be obtained from the child's legal guardian, who in most instances would be a parent (Grodin & Glantz, 1994). However, a guardian's ability to consent to a child's serving as a research subject is limited: "The tendency of the law has been to limit what may be done to children and incompetents just because they are unable to give effective consent. And those who act for them are strictly charged to act only in the manifest interests of these persons. They may not, for instance, volunteer them for experimentation which will *not directly* [italics mine] benefit them" (Fried, 1974, p. 23). The message here appears to be that securing a guardian's consent for his or her child to serve as a subject may not be adequate to protect against litigation against either the experimenter or the institution under whose auspices the research is being conducted.

A subject's free and informed consent also may not be sufficient if he or she is an adult whom the court would classify as *incompetent.* Adults are likely to be classified as incompetent if they are thought to be unable to make rational decisions regarding their own welfare. Persons diagnosed as psychotic or severely mentally retarded are likely to be classified as incompetent. Persons who are *severely communicatively handicapped* (e.g., global aphasics) also may be classified as incompetent. A court-appointed guardian could consent to such a person's serving as a subject. The restrictions on the guardian's ability to do so are the same as were given for guardians of children.

A subject can *withdraw* consent to participate in a study at any time, even if the subject promised when giving consent not to withdraw it (Fried, 1974). The National Institutes of Health policy statement on the protection of human subjects, in fact, not only mandates that subjects be allowed to withdraw consent at any time but requires that subjects *be informed* that they have this right.

For further information about informed consent as it applies to clinical research, see Applebaum, Lidz, and Meisel (1987), Lawson (1995), and White (1994).

Legal-Ethical Implications of the Therapeutic-Nontherapeutic Continuum in Clinical Research

The legal doctrines that apply to a particular clinical study are determined in part by whether the experimental conditions administered to subjects are intended to be therapeutic to them. Some studies are *entirely therapeutic* in their intent. An example would be a study of the impacts of a particular intervention program that the clinician would have used even if the research was not being done.

At the other end of the continuum would be studies in which the investigator had *no therapeutic intent.* The subjects in such studies would be unlikely to benefit personally from participating in them. They may, however, be providing data that could contribute to improving therapy programs for others with similar communicative disorders at some future date. An example would be an investigation by an audiologist of the responses of persons having a particular type of lesion in the auditory system to a particular type of auditory test. The audiologist's intent is to use their responses to the test stimuli to refine the test rather than to benefit them directly.

There are clinical studies that fall on the continuum between these extremes. In these studies some of the experimental conditions have a therapeutic intent and others do not. Or the experimental conditions are intended to be therapeutic for some subjects but not for others. An example of the first would be a study in which clients are given one or more diagnostic tests in addition to those they would ordinarily be given for clinical purposes. Those that ordinarily would be administered for clinical purposes constitute experimental conditions having a therapeutic intent; the others constitute experimental conditions that are not intended to be therapeutic.

An example of a clinical study in which the experimental conditions are intended to be therapeutic for some subjects but not for others would be a study in which subjects are *randomly assigned* to one of two treatment groups. The subjects assigned to the first group (the experimental group) would be administered a treatment (experimental condition) that was intended to be therapeutic and consequently could directly benefit them. Those assigned to the second group (the control group) either would be administered no treatment or would be administered a treatment that the experimenter did not expect to be as successful as the one administered to subjects in the first group. Thus, the subjects in the first group would be expected to benefit directly, and those in the second group either would not be expected to benefit directly or would not be expected to benefit to the same extent as those in the first group.

Nontherapeutic Clinical Research

While the persons who function as subjects in nontherapeutic clinical research may receive a small sum of money and/or personal satisfaction for doing so, they are unlikely to benefit directly in any substantial way from the experience. And by participating in the research they are risking their mental and/or physical health. In some types of research the risks to their health would be almost nonexistent; in others the risks would be substantial.

It has been argued (Fried, 1974) that there are no special legal doctrines that apply to nontherapeutic clinical research and that those that do apply (particularly with regard to the need for disclosing potential hazards) are the same as those that apply to the selling of products:

> *In general, the law imposes a strict duty of disclosure, wherever an individual with a great deal to lose is exposed to a risk or is asked to relinquish rights by some-one with considerably greater knowledge* [italics mine]. And this is true, whether the relation is one of buyer and seller or involves some public interest. Persons selling cosmetics, automobiles, or pharmaceuticals are required to make full disclosure of all the hazards involved in the products they sell. . . . There is no reason why the case should be any different where a researcher asks an experimental subject to risk his health. (Fried, 1974, p. 27)

Since experimenters would ordinarily have considerably greater knowledge of the potential risks associated with the methodology being used than would their subjects and since their subjects are risking their health by participating in the experiment, experimenters are obliged to make a full disclosure of potential hazards to subjects when seeking their consent to participate. It could be argued that the failure of the experimenter to do so would be more damaging with this type of research if a subject sued for battery than it would be with research having a therapeutic intent.

While it is almost always desirable to be able to document a subject's informed consent to participate in research, there are some types of nontherapeutic studies for which failure to do so ordinarily would result in minimal risks to either investigators or the institutions under whose auspices their research is being conducted. These are studies that involve only slight or remote risks of harm to subjects. The U.S. Department of Health and Human Services, for example, in its "Final Regulations Amending Basic HHS Policy for the Protection of Human Research Subjects" (*Federal Register*, January 26, 1981) classified the following types of research as having no, slight, or only remote risks of harm to subjects:

1. Research conducted in established or commonly accepted educational settings, involving normal educational practices, such as (i) research on regular and special education instructional strategies, or (ii) research on the effectiveness of or the comparison among instructional techniques, curricula, or classroom management methods.

2. Research involving the use of educational tests (cognitive, diagnostic, aptitude, achievement), if information taken from these sources are recorded in such a manner that subjects cannot be identified, directly or through identifiers linked to the subjects.

3. Research involving survey or interview procedures, except where all of the following conditions exist: (i) responses are recorded in such a manner that the

human subjects can be identified, directly or through identifiers linked to the subjects, (ii) the subject's responses, if they became known outside the research, could reasonably place the subject at risk of criminal or civil liability or be damaging to the subject's financial standing or employability, and (iii) the research deals with sensitive aspects of the subject's own behavior, such as illegal conduct, drug use, sexual behavior, or the use of alcohol.

Research involving the observation (including the observation by participants) of public behavior, except where all of the following conditions exist: (i) observations are recorded in such a manner that the human subjects can be identified, directly or through identifiers linked to the subjects, (ii) the observations recorded about the individual, if they become known outside the research, could reasonably place the subject at risk of criminal or civil liability or be damaging to the subject's financial standing or employability, and (iii) the research deals with sensitive aspects of the subject's own behavior such as illegal conduct, drug use, sexual behavior, or use of alcohol.

4. Research involving the collection or study of existing data, documents, pathological specimens, or diagnostic specimens, if these sources are publicly available or if the information is recorded by the investigator in such a manner that subjects cannot be identified, directly or through identifiers linked to the subjects. (*Federal Register,* January 26, 1981, pp. 8371–8372)

How would a person be compensated for harm resulting from his or her participation (as a subject) in a nontherapeutic research study? Such a person probably would have to initiate some type of litigation against the investigator and/or the institution under whose auspices the research was being conducted. A number of authorities on legal-ethical implications of using human subjects in research (e.g., Fried, 1974; Ladimer, 1970) have stated that investigators and their institutions have a moral obligation to voluntarily compensate subjects harmed in nontherapeutic research. Perhaps a special liability insurance could be carried by investigators or their institutions for this purpose.

For further information about legal-ethical aspects of nontherapeutic research, see Freund (1970), Fried (1974), Gostin (1991), Greenwald, Ryan, and Mulvihill (1982), Grodin and Glantz (1994), Lawson (1995), Metz and Folkins (1985), National Institutes of Health (1993a), Penslar (1993), and the publications of the Office for Protection from Research Risks, National Institutes of Health, Bethesda, Maryland 20205.

Therapeutic Clinical Research

Speech-language pathologists, audiologists, and other clinicians legally are justified only in using accepted therapies unless their clients specifically consent to the use of an experimental therapy. An *accepted therapy,* in this context, is a treatment program that at least some of one's professional peers would regard as appropriate for the particular condition being treated. If a speech-language pathologist treated a stutterer with a therapy program that at least some authorities on stuttering would regard as appropriate, this program would be likely to be classified as *accepted* therapy by the courts. It would not be necessary that all authorities on stuttering regard it as appropriate. The courts recognize that there are often different schools of thought on the appropriate therapy for a condition, and consequently, they will classify as accepted almost any therapy advocated by a recognized authority.

So long as the therapy program being used in the research is one that would be classified by the courts as accepted, the legal-ethical considerations (e.g., informed consent) would be essentially the same as for *clinical treatment.*

The further away an experimental therapy program lies from the standard and the accepted, the more acute the need for subjects to be fully informed about risks and *alternative treatment programs,* and the greater the need for the investigator to be able to document the subjects' free and informed consent to participate in research. The investigator's obligation to inform subjects about alternative treatment programs ordinarily does not extend to other alternative programs (Fried, 1974). The information presented about the experimental program should include a statement summarizing research findings and professional opinion relevant to its efficacy.

A situation that may pose a legal-ethical dilemma for an investigator is one in which there are alternative treatment programs that are regarded by other professionals as *effective* for treating the condition the experimental program is intended to treat. Full disclosure requires that the subjects be informed about these alternatives. However, informing potential subjects about such alternatives may cause them to refuse to participate in the experimental program. An investigator may be tempted, therefore, to make a less than full disclosure about alternative treatment programs in order to insure having an adequate number of subjects for the research. While doing so may increase the probability of having an adequate number of subjects for the research, it also could invalidate the subjects' consent to participate in the research, leaving the investigator vulnerable to several types of litigation, including battery. An investigator, when confronted with this situation, would be wise to make a full disclosure, including a statement summarizing research and professional opinion relevant to why the experimental therapy *may* be superior to existing accepted alternative treatment programs. An investigator should be able to develop such a statement—otherwise, one could reasonably question whether it would be *ethical* to expose subjects to an experimental treatment program that there is no reason to believe is superior to existing accepted ones. Institutional review boards have a responsibility to determine whether proposed experimental treatment programs have a reasonable chance of satisfying a *real need.*

Mixed Therapeutic and Nontherapeutic Clinical Research

The type of clinical research that tends to have the greatest legal-ethical perplexities associated with it is that which has both therapeutic and nontherapeutic aspects. A speech-language pathologist or audiologist, for example, who was engaged in therapy outcome research would indeed be attempting to ameliorate the client's communicative disorder (which would be the *therapeutic aspect*). The intervention strategy chosen, however, would not be selected *solely* from the perspective of the client's needs. Therapy would be administered in the context of a research program that was intended either to test new procedures or to compare the efficacy of various established procedures (which would be the *nontherapeutic aspect.*) Consequently, the treatment that a client received would be dictated, at least partially, by the requirements of the research design. In a study of the relative efficacy of two established procedures, the one the client is administered is likely to be determined by a table of random numbers. And in a study of the efficacy of a new procedure (experimental therapy), the decision whether a particular subject would be given it would be partially a function of the investigator's need for subjects with particular *demographic characteristics* (e.g., age and sex) to meet the requirements of the research design.

If the treatment dictated by a research design is the one that a client would have received anyway, then the presence of a research design ordinarily would not create any special legal-ethical problems. However, if the treatment dictated by a research design is *not* the one that a client ordinarily would have received, then the presence of a research design could indicate legal-ethical problems.

In clinical research having both therapeutic and nontherapeutic aspects there obviously is a legal obligation to make a full disclosure of *possible benefits and hazards*. This would be necessary even if the therapy that the clients were receiving was not part of a research project. Would it also be necessary to disclose (1) that at least some of the therapy they will be receiving *is part of a research project* and (2) the *nature* of the research project and the experimental design? A speech-language pathologist who was planning to describe the therapy program used with a client in an individual case study in an article published in a professional journal would have to answer that question. Would the client's consent be needed to publish the case study? If it were *impossible* for anyone to recognize the client from the information included in the case study, the answer to this question probably would be *no*. A client may be recognizable not only from a name or initials but also from specific information about his or her life history, such as the names of schools attended. An investigator would be wise, therefore, to carefully examine the life history data on subjects of case studies and to delete any nonessential information that would make them recognizable. Of course, the client (or the client's guardian) in some instances would be very willing to have a description of the therapy received published, particularly if (1) the client felt treatment was successful and/or (2) the client was convinced that the information presented could help in the treatment of others with similar conditions.

While clinicians who do not disclose to a client that the therapy is part of a research project or do not describe the *impact* that being part of a research project will have on the therapy the client will be receiving may be relatively safe legally, clinicians may find themselves vulnerable from a *public relations* perspective. Most clients, for example, probably would feel that they had been deceived if they discovered they received the therapy program they did because they were randomly assigned to a particular treatment group. Such a discovery would be likely to adversely affect their relationship with their clinician if they are still in therapy. And the disclosure of such a discovery in the media could severely damage the reputation of both the investigator and the institution under whose auspices the research was conducted. The general public would tend to regard the random assignment of subjects to treatment groups without their knowledge as irresponsible, even if the therapy subjects received had been successful.

Documenting a Person's Informed Consent to Serve as a Research Subject

An outline of a form for documenting a person's informed consent to serve as a subject in a research project is presented in Figure 15-1. This outline includes the information that ordinarily is necessary for explaining to potential subjects (1) the purpose and value of the study, (2) what they will be asked to do and what will be done to them, and (3) the possible benefits and risks to them. It also provides a means for documenting that subjects were informed that they may withdraw their consent at any time and that they have consented to having information about them published (if they cannot be recognized). In addition, it provides documentation that their consent was given freely (that it was not coerced or forced). Paragraph *g* in Figure 15-1 would be included only if provision had been made for com-

---

RESPONSIBLE INVESTIGATOR:

TITLE OF PROTOCOL:

TITLE OF CONSENT FORM *(if different from protocol)*:

I have been asked to participate in a research study that is investigating *(describe purpose of the study)*. In participating in this study I agree to *(describe briefly and in lay terms procedures to which subject is consenting)*.

I understand that

(a) The possible risks of the procedure include *(list known risks or side effects; if none, so state)*. Alternative treatments include *(list alternative treatments and briefly describe advantages and disadvantages of each; if none, so state)*.

(b) The possible benefits of the study to me are *(enumerate; if none, so state)*.

(c) Any questions I have concerning my participation in the study will be answered by *(list names and degrees of people who will be available to answer questions)*.

(d) I may withdraw from the study at any time without prejudice.

(e) The results of this study may be published, but my name or identify will not be revealed and my records will remain confidential unless disclosure of my identity is required by law.

(f) My consent is given voluntarily without being coerced or forced.

(g) In the event of injury resulting from the study, medical care and treatment will be available at *(state name of institution)*.

Compensation (damages) would be limited to situations where negligence occurred and would be controlled by provisions of the Federal Tort Claims Act.

DATE   PATIENT OR RESPONSIBLE PARTY

PATIENT'S SOCIAL SECURITY NUMBER

AUDITOR/WITNESS

INVESTIGATOR/CLINICIAN REPRESENTATIVE

FIGURE 15-1 Outline for a consent form for documenting a person's informed consent to serve as a subject in a research project. *(From Purtilo, R.D., and Cassel, C.K., Ethical Dimensions in the Health Professions. Philadelphia: W.B. Saunders, 1981.)*

pensating subjects for injuries that they receive (e.g., if the investigator or the institution had liability insurance that covered such injuries). Note that subjects' signatures should be witnessed. Obviously, if the information presented in the form was inaccurate or incomplete, a subject's signature on it might not constitute *informed* consent. Whether it would constitute informed consent would depend on how essential the inaccurate or incomplete information was for alerting subjects to potential risks.

Utilization of Data from Research in Which Subjects Were Abused

Is it ethical to utilize data from research in which subjects were abused, particularly from that in which they were knowingly abused? Perhaps the most extreme, contemporary example of such data would be that gathered in Nazi Germany during World War II that motivated the development of the Nuremberg Code (see Appendix D). Each of us must answer this question for ourself. The following comment by Dr. Tomas Radil-Weiss, a psychiatrist and head of the Section on Neurophysiology of the Czechoslovak Academy of Sciences, who was imprisoned at Auschwitz Concentration Camp when he was 14 years old may be helpful when doing so:

> The second world war ended many years ago. Most of those who survived the stay at the German concentration camp at Auschwitz have already died of the consequences of their imprisonment; those still alive are already in the last third of their life. Is there any point to returning to the experiences of those days? Consideration of the mental hygiene of former prisoners cautions us that perhaps we should not do it. *But consideration of the general interest holds that we are not entitled to ignore any knowledge that can contribute to social development—including medicine and psychology—even if acquired under unspeakably awful conditions* [italics mine]. (Radil-Weiss, 1983, p. 259)

The utilization of such data may allow a little good to come from the suffering of those research subjects who have been abused physically or psychologically, purposefully or through negligence.

Exercises and Discussion Topics

1. Read the "monster" study (Silverman, 1988). What would be the ethical arguments, both pro and con, for utilizing these data?

2. Is it ethical to do research in which the methodology includes response-contingent punishment (e.g., "time out")? Why?

3. Is it ethical in therapy outcome research either to deprive a client of therapy for a period of time or to use one with him or her that you don't expect to be effective in order to have a baseline or "control" condition? Why?

4. Should a client's informed consent by sought and documented if a therapy being used is "experimental"—that is, if its efficacy has not been established empirically? Why?

Conducting and Funding Research in a Clinical Setting

This book hopefully has acquainted you with some of the benefits a clinician can derive from doing clinical research (i.e., functioning as clinician-investigators) and has provided the information you need to begin doing it. If you are employed as a clinician in a school or medical setting and want to function as a clinician-investigator, how would you go about securing the necessary administrative and financial support? The information presented in this chapter will provide a partial answer to this question.

Securing Administrative Support

It would be difficult (though certainly not impossible) for you to do clinical research without at least some administrative support. Doing such research obviously necessitates an investment of time. Since most master's-level speech-language pathologists and audiologists are hired to provide clinical services, they probably will have to convince their supervisor and/or other administrators that it would be advantageous to the institution (including its administrators) if they were given time for clinical research. The time investment required is likely to be relatively small if your questions can be answered by observations you can make while providing clinical services, particularly if they are ones that you make routinely to document therapy outcome for IEPs and insurance companies.

Some reasons for your doing clinical research that administrators at your institution may find compelling include the following:

- Your research can provide useful documentation for the impacts of intervention on your clients that can be used for marketing services for persons who are communicatively impaired and for satisfying the documentation requirements of third party payers, including governmental agencies and insurance companies.

- Carefully documenting therapy outcome provides the information you need to maximize your effectiveness. If you do not systematically document the impacts of intervention on your clients, how can you tell how well you are achieving your objectives?
- The presence of an ongoing clinical research program is likely to bring local and possibly even state, national, and international recognition to the institution. This should be helpful in attracting grants and gifts from individuals, private foundations, and governmental sources.
- The research you want to do will not be expensive (either in time or money) because you will be gathering the data you need to answer your questions while providing clinical services.

Of course, your administrator is unlikely to regard all of these reasons as being equally compelling. You must decide, based on your previous experience with him or her, which ones are likely to be most effective. Furthermore, you may be able to use some of the reasons mentioned in Chapter 2 for why it would be desirable for you to function as a clinician-investigator for this purpose.

Preparing a Research Proposal

We have considered several arguments that you may be able to use to secure administrative support for your doing a clinical research project. You can present them to the administrator or administrators whose support you are seeking in a written proposal (prospectus) that is structured like a memorandum. The kinds of information you should include are the following:

- The question(s) you want to answer
- Possible practical implications of the answer(s) for your clients and those of other clinicians
- Why it would be advantageous to your institution for you to undertake the project
- Why you believe you are qualified to undertake the project
- The time and financial investment that is necessary and the source or sources from which you would seek funding (assuming that the level of funding necessary exceeded that which could be provided by your operating budget)
- Where you would plan to report the results of the project
- Coinvestigators and consultants who would be involved in the project and a statement describing their roles and qualifications for performing them
- A description of the methodology that would be used to answer each question, including a statement concerning possible dangers to subjects and how you plan to document their informed consent to participate (see Chapter 15)
- A description of how the data would be analyzed for answering each question

Some suggestions for communicating each of these in a proposal are presented in the following paragraphs.

Your statement about the question(s) you wish to answer should communicate the topic of the project to someone who is not familiar with the technical jargon used by speech-language pathologists and audiologists. Technical terms should be used only when absolutely necessary; those that are used should be clearly defined. If data have been reported that are relevant to your question(s), they should be summarized and you should indicate why additional data are needed.

Next, you should indicate why it would be advantageous to do the project in your clinical setting. You should indicate as cogently as you can why doing it is likely to be helpful to both your clients and employer. You may be able to use here some of the arguments for doing clinical research that are mentioned in Chapter 2.

Your next task is to demonstrate that you are qualified to do the project. It is particularly important that you document the specific training and experience that qualifies you to administer any diagnostic tests or intervention strategies that you are planning to use.

The time and funding necessary to complete the proposed project and the source or sources from which the funding might be obtained should be indicated. You should provide an estimate of the total number of hours or the average number of hours per week it probably would be necessary to spend on the project. And you should include a detailed budget, with justification for each item.

Some information should be included about how you plan to disseminate your questions, answers, and interpretations. If this information is going to be disseminated in a written report or a convention presentation, specify the journal(s) or convention(s) through which you hope to disseminate it (unless, of course, it is to be disseminated solely to persons at your institution).

Others (e.g., coinvestigators and consultants) who would be involved in the project should be mentioned. The role of each should be indicated, and there should be a statement about his or her qualifications to perform it.

You should include a detailed description of the methodology you would use to answer each question—that is, who you would observe and how you would observe them. You should describe the scenarios by which subjects could be harmed by participating (if there are any) and indicate the likelihood of each occurring. An investigator has both an ethical and a legal responsibility to not expose subjects to experimental procedures that could cause them harm without their informed consent (see Chapter 15).

The manner in which the data will be analyzed for answering each question should be indicated. See Chapters 9, 10, and 11 for descriptions of statistical and other methods that can be used for doing so.

The types of information mentioned here may not be the only ones that it is necessary to include in a research proposal. Before beginning to prepare a proposal, you should inquire whether your institution has a form for this purpose. Some of the larger public school systems and medical institutions that employ speech-language pathologists and audiologists have them.

Research Funding

All research projects require some funding. The amount that you need to do a project may be so little that you can get it from your operating budget. This is often the case for therapy outcome research.

If the funding needed for a project exceeds that available from your operating budget, you will probably have to apply for some sort of grant. Speech-language pathologists and audiologists have received funding for their research activities from a variety of sources, some of which were internal (institutional) and some external (extramural).

Internal grants are awarded by the institution (school system, hospital, rehabilitation center, and so on) with which the person applying is affiliated. Their maximum size tends to be relatively small. They usually are intended either to support research that only requires a relatively low level of funding (which would include almost all therapy outcome research in speech-language pathology and audiology) or to provide "seed" money for the preliminary ("pilot") research of investigators who plan to apply for extramural funding. These grants are usually easier for beginning investigators to obtain than extramural ones. They also tend to require a less complex application procedure than the latter.

If the funding needed to answer your question(s) exceeds several thousand dollars, you will probably have to apply for an extramural grant. An extramural grant is one from any source other than the institution by which you are employed. Such a source could be a corporation (e.g., IBM), an organization (e.g., the Heart Association or United Cerebral Palsy), a private foundation (e.g., the Ford Foundation), or a governmental agency (e.g., the National Institutes of Health, the Office of Education, or the National Science Foundation). Funds for research in speech-language pathology and audiology have been obtained from all four sources. The federal government, through such agencies as the National Institutes of Health (NIH), the Office of Education (OE), and the National Science Foundation (NSF), has provided more funds for this purpose than any other source. These agencies offer a variety of research support programs, including some for which beginning investigators are eligible.

How do you identify the agencies, corporations, foundations, and organizations that are most likely to fund a particular project? The decision about where to submit a grant proposal is one of the most important in the grantsmanship/grant-seeking process (Gelatt, 1989; Hall, 1988; Ogden & Goldberg, 1995; Sparks, 1989). An excellent proposal is unlikely to get funded if it is submitted to an agency, corporation, foundation, or organization that does not have as a part of its mission supporting the type of research that is being proposed. Also, if there are several appropriate places to which a proposal could be submitted, the odds of being funded may not be the same for all of them—that is, some may be more competitive than others (Gelatt, 1989).

Information about programs that support research on communication disorders can be acquired from a number of sources, including the following:

- The *Catalog of Federal Domestic Assistance (CFDA)*, a catalog that is published annually by the Government Printing Office, is one of the most valuable reference sources for finding out about federal programs. It contains a number of indexes to help users locate specific programs of interest, determine eligibility, and obtain information about application deadlines. The *Federal Automated Program Retrieval Information System (FAPRIS)* is a computer database version of this catalog.
- The *Foundation Center* is a national clearinghouse for information on foundation and corporate giving. One way that it disseminates such information is through a national

network of more than 150 library reference collections. The Center offered its services to the public free of charge when this chapter was written.

- The *Annual Register of Grant Support* is a directory of fellowship and grant support programs of government agencies, foundations, business, professional, and other organizations.
- The *Directory of Biomedical and Health Care Grants* covers funding programs supported by government agencies, private foundations, corporations, and professional organizations.
- The *Federal Grants and Contracts Weekly* lists selected grant and contract programs. A contract program is one in which an agency describes what it wants to have done and invites interested persons to submit proposals for doing it.
- The *Taft Corporate Giving Directory* is a guide to over 500 corporate foundations or direct giving programs.
- The *Sponsored Programs Information Network (SPIN)* is a computer database that contained information about more than 3000 funding opportunities (federal, nonfederal, and corporate) when this chapter was written.
- The *Computer Retrieval of Information on Scientific Projects (CRISP)* database contains information on research programs supported by the U.S. Public Health Service.

After you have identified one or more places to apply for funding, your next task is to prepare a grant proposal. There are several sources from which you may be able to obtain assistance when doing so. One is from persons who have applied for research grants, particularly from those who have been successful. Help from a person whose research has been supported by an organization to which you plan to apply can be particularly valuable.

A second source from which you should be able to get some help is the office of research support at your institution. Many educational and medical facilities that employ speech-language pathologists and audiologists have such an office.

A third source from which help can be sought is publications on grantsmanship. Several very informative ones were published in the February 1989 issue of *Asha* (Catlett, 1989; Gelatt, 1989; "How to Be Sure You Don't Get Funded," 1989; Sparks, 1989). Others that can be helpful include Bauer (1995), Carlson (1995), Decker (1993), Gitlin (1996), Locke (1993), Lucas (1992), National Institutes of Health (1993b), Reif-Lehrer (1995), Ries (1995), Schumacher (1992), and Schwartz (1992).

Almost all extramural funding programs are highly competitive, and their proposal processing procedures tend to be quite complex and time-consuming (see Lore & Gutter, 1968, and Summers, 1987, for descriptions of such procedures at NIH). More proposals usually are submitted than can be funded. Furthermore, most granting organizations look for evidence of "demonstrated research competence"—that is, the ability to successfully complete research projects as evidenced by publication. This, of course, would tend to put a beginning investigator at a disadvantage. Such an investigator probably would be wise, therefore, to select as his or her first research projects ones that could be funded internally.

Use of Consultants

This book can acquaint you much of the information you need to function as a clinician-investigator. However, the information provided is not sufficient to bring you to the point where it is unnecessary to have your methodology checked by someone. Many institutions with speech and hearing facilities (including colleges, hospitals, and school systems) employ persons knowledgeable about statistics and research methodology who consult with members of their staff. If your institution has no such consultant, there may be faculty at local colleges and universities who are competent in statistics and research methodology who would be willing to consult with you.

It is important to contact a research design consultant before you begin collecting data. If something is wrong with your design, the data you collect may be worthless. That is, they may not possess an adequate level of validity, reliability, and generality for accurately answering your question(s).

A consultant's recommendations can be inappropriate. They may not result in a design that will yield the data necessary to answer your questions. Or they may not result in the most efficient or practical design for doing so.

Why might a consultant's recommendations be inappropriate? There can be several possible reasons. First, he or she may commit what Kimball (1957) has referred to as an "error of the third kind"—that is, giving the right answer to the wrong question. Here, the consultant does not understand the question or questions the investigator is attempting to answer. Consequently, his or her recommendations are appropriate not for answering these questions but for those he or she thinks the investigator is trying to answer. A consultant is most likely to make this type of error when he or she is completely unfamiliar with the content area in which the research is being done.

A consultant's recommendations may also be inappropriate because they are not sufficiently practical or efficient. For assessing the impact of a particular therapy, a consultant may recommend using a design in which forty persons who have a particular communicative disorder are randomly assigned to one of two groups: the members of one group receive the experimental therapy and the members of the other do not. Such a design may not be practical because forty persons with that communicative disorder may not be available to serve as subjects, and it would not be ethical (or possible) to deprive half of them of the therapy for the duration of the program (see Chapter 15). Even if it were practical to use such a design, it might not be efficient because of the time needed to administer therapy to twenty clients and evaluate its impact on a group of this size. A single subject design using ten persons, in which each served as his or her own "control," could well be both more efficient and more practical for collecting the necessary data.

A third reason a consultant's recommendations may be inappropriate is that he or she has made a mistake. Consultants, like all humans, are fallible. A certain percentage of the time their recommendations will be wrong.

What should you do if you are uncertain about the appropriateness of a consultant's recommendation? Get a "second opinion" and then make the best decision you can. This, of course, is similar to the situation you find yourself in when you are forced to make clinical decisions from equivocal or incomplete data.

Our focus in this discussion has been on research design consultants. Most of the comments are relevant to other types as well.

Exercises and Discussion Topics

1. Based upon your clinical experience, formulate an answerable question you probably could answer while employed as a speech-language pathologist or audiologist in a clinical setting that probably would not require an unrealistic time investment or external funding.

2. Write a short proposal you could submit to your employer that should motivate him or her to support your attempting to answer the question you formulated (see Exercise 1).

3. Describe how you would make the observations needed to answer this question (i.e., formulate a research design for answering it). The material in Chapters 6 through 11 should be helpful.

Chapter *17*

Cultural Considerations in the Design and Interpretation of Clinical Research

As a profession we are becoming increasingly aware of the ways that cultural diversity impacts on our functioning as clinicians (Anderson, 1991, 1992; Battle, 1993; Bebout & Arthur, 1992; Cheng, 1989; Erickson & Iglesias, 1986; Hammer, 1994; Lee, 1989; Maestas & Erickson, 1992; Matsuda, 1989; Nellum-Davis, 1993; Scott, 1995; Screen & Anderson, 1994; Taylor, 1986, 1992; Terrell & Hale, 1992; Van Kleeck, 1994). We now realize that it isn't safe to assume that our diagnostic procedures (particularly tests) are insensitive to cultural differences. Furthermore, we are becoming increasingly aware of the impacts that such differences can have on learning styles and consequently, on approaches to management.

Before we begin our discussion of cultural considerations in designing and interpreting clinical research, let's briefly consider what there is about culture that makes such considerations necessary. The following definition of culture by Porter and Samovar (1976, p. 7) provides some insight into this. They define culture as:

> *the cumulative deposit of knowledge, experience, meanings, beliefs, values, attitudes, religions, concepts of self, the universe, and self-universe relationships, hierarchies of status, role expectations, spatial relations, and time concepts acquired by a large group of people in the course of generations through individual and group striving. Culture manifests itself both in patterns of language and thought and in forms of activity and behavior. These patterns become models for common adaptive acts and styles of expressive behavior, which enable people to*

> *live in a society within a given geographical environment at a given state of technical development. (1976, p. 7)*

We will focus in this chapter on implications of these manifestations of culture and ethnicity for suggesting questions that are relevant clinically and/or for making the observations needed to answer such questions.

While there has been considerable interest in the role that culture and ethnicity play in clinical practice, this does not appear to be the case for clinical research judging by the paucity of references to them in the literature. Obviously, if they affects one, it would have to affect the other. Some ways will be suggested in this chapter that manifestations of culture and ethnicity could impact on the design and interpretation of clinical research based, in large part, on how they are thought to impact on the assessment and management of communicative disorders.

Implications for Questions to Ask

Research throughout this book has been equated to the asking and answering of questions. Manifestations of culture and ethnicity can affect both the questions that are asked and the strategies used to answer them. With regard to the former, it could result in questions being asked that seek to identify cultural factors that could affect clinical practice and/or clinical research methodology. The following are examples of such questions that were suggested by comments in the papers and books cited in the first paragraph:

- In what ways is it necessary for clinicians and researchers to change how they usually interview and communicate verbally and nonverbally to accommodate an informant's or subject's cultural background?
- Do the stimuli utilized in a diagnostic test elicit the same behaviors (responses) from persons in a certain culture as they do from persons in the culture in which the test was standardized?
- Are the norms for a diagnostic test appropriate for persons having a particular cultural background? See Lahey (1992) and Seymour (1992) for discussions of several relevant issues.
- Are persons having a particular cultural background as familiar with the tasks a test requires them to do as are those in the culture in which the test was standardized?
- Do persons having a particular cultural background tend to be as motivated to do well on a test as those in the culture in which the test was standardized?
- Do language acquisition milestones tend to occur at the same ages in children in a particular culture as they do in the cultural groups on which existing norms are based?
- At what ages do children in a culture tend to acquire each of the phonological, morphological, syntactic, and semantic "rules" that do not occur in English?
- What questions should be added to and deleted from case history forms to make them appropriate for families in the culture?
- What habits, customs, values, and beliefs do persons having a particular cultural/ ethnological background tend to hold or practice that could affect the client-clinician

relationship? Also, what attitudes toward expression of emotion and feelings, privacy, courtesy, respect for elders, behaviors related to family roles and sex roles, and the work ethic are they likely to have that could affect this relationship?

- How important do families in the culture tend to believe it is that children speak well? Is the importance given to speaking well different for girls than for boys?
- What speech/language differences call adverse attention to speakers in a culture?
- What beliefs appear to be widely accepted by families in a culture about the etiology of communicative disorders? According to Anderson and Fenichel (1989), cultures differ markedly with regard to their beliefs about the etiology of disorders.
- From whom are the families in a culture likely to seek help for a person who has a communicative disorder—for example, a speech-language pathologist or audiologist, a physician, a chiropractor, a priest, a medicine man, an herbalist, an acupuncturist, a voodoo practitioner, a faith healer, a spiritualist, a minister? Service providers other than speech-language pathologists and audiologists would tend to be consulted in some cultures (Cole, 1989).
- What role (if any) do religious beliefs, sacred practices, or talismans tend to play in a culture in the treatment of communicative disorders? Supernatural sources such as fate, evil spirits, or the punitive or retributive actions of a deity are regarded in some cultures as likely causes of disorders—including communicative disorders (Anderson & Fenichel, 1989; Fain, 1990; Maestas & Erickson, 1992; Wayman, Lynch, & Hanson, 1990).
- What beliefs appear to be widely accepted by families in a culture about the management of communicative disorders? In some cultures, for example, there is a belief that "a [communicative] disorder represents an act of God or demons and should not be tampered with" (Fain, 1990, p. 45).
- What beliefs appear to be widely accepted by families in a culture about factors that determine the efficacy of therapy. Bebout and Arthur (1992), for example, reported data that suggest that many Asians believe a willingness to "try hard" is the most important one.
- What stereotypes are there in a culture for persons who have various communicative disorders?
- How does having a communicative disorder tend to affect the self-concept of persons who have a particular cultural background?
- What communicative behaviors would tend to be considered abnormal in the clinician's culture that would not tend to be regarded as being so in the client's?
- What modes of service delivery for clients having a particular cultural background are likely to come closest to being both efficient and effective?
- What stereotypes are clinicians who have one cultural background likely to have about clients who have another that could adversely affect their clinical relationship?
- What alternative strategy can be devised for reducing the severity of a particular communicative disorder in a culture in which the strategy of choice in the clinician's culture is not economically feasible?
- How might volunteers from a client's culture (under the clinician's supervision) be helpful in facilitating the management of his or her communicative disorder?

- In what ways might the families of clients in a particular culture (under a clinician's supervision) be helpful in facilitating the management of their communicative disorders?
- What are the attitudes of persons in a cultural group toward seeking help? Doing so is widely regarded as "shameful" in some of them (Wayman, Lynch, & Hanson, 1990).
- What child-rearing practices in a cultural group are likely to impact either positively or negatively on the relationship between the family of a child and his or her clinician?
- For a cultural minority group in the United States, what deviations from the phonological, morphological, syntactic, and semantic "rules" of standard American English are "language differences rather than language disorders?"
- For a cultural minority group in the United States, what pragmatic deviations in the choice of verbal and nonverbal code while communicating are differences rather than disorders?

Implications for Answering Questions

Cultural factors can also influence the choice of tasks for making the observations needed to answer questions. Ones that would tend to yield valid data when administered to persons who share your cultural background may not tend to do so when administered to persons having another. There are a number of ways that performance on tasks could be influenced by cultural factors sufficiently to significantly reduce the validity of data yielded by them. The following are examples that were suggested by comments in the papers and books cited in the first paragraph of this chapter:

- The questions asked on "generic" case history and background information forms may not allow for the collection of information that is appropriate for answering clinicians' and researchers' questions about persons who have a particular cultural background. Some of the questions that appear on such forms may not be relevant and others that are relevant do not appear. *Bloch's Ethnic/Cultural Assessment Guide* (in Orque, Block, & Monroy, 1983) may be helpful to you when modifying such forms to make them culturally/ethnologically appropriate.
- Certain case history information obtained from informants (e.g., parents) may not be as accurate, complete, and/or appropriate for answering your questions as it would tend to be if obtained from persons in your culture. People differ in what they abstract and remember from what they observe—what they hear, see, smell, taste, and/or touch that they regard as significant and worth remembering. Their "filters" are affected by manifestations of their culture and ethnicity, including their language (see Whorf, 1956). People tend to abstract things for which they have words and there are cultural differences in vocabulary, even among persons who speak the same language. There are also cultural differences in the meanings that particular words have for people. Consequently, your questions may not be interpreted as you expect them to be by informants whose culture and ethnicity differs from your own. And as a result of such breakdowns in communication, the information you obtain may be inaccurate or not as complete as you probably would assume it to be if it was provided by an informant who shared your

culture and ethnicity. For information about structuring a case history interview to maximize the probability of getting accurate, relevant information from persons whose cultural background differs from yours, see Patton (1990, Chapter 7), Spradley (1979), Stewart and Cash (1988), and Taylor (1992).

- Persons having a client's cultural background and ethnicity may not be as familiar with a diagnostic or research task (particularly the stimuli used) as are the persons on whom its validity was established. If they are not as familiar with a task as its developer assumed, then poor performance on it could result (at least in part) from such a lack of familiarity rather than from the deficit that the task was designed to detect. Some of the picture stimuli used in language tests, for example, may not be as familiar to clients having some cultural backgrounds as to those having others; consequently, inappropriate responses to such stimuli would not necessarily indicate that a client has a deficit.

- If a task is a test, the published norms may not be appropriate for persons having a client's (subject's) cultural background and ethnicity. The reason for a client's (subject's) poor performance could be (at least in part) a lack of familiarity with the test stimuli and/or situations about which he or she is required to make judgments rather than a deficit in what the test was designed to measure.

- A client's (subject's) motivation to do a particular task well may be influenced by his or her cultural background and ethnicity. We all have priorities that determine how well we have to do a task for us to be satisfied with our performance. While we have to do some tasks very well to satisfy ourselves, for others this is not the case. Our priorities are determined, in part, by the expected performance levels in our culture for the various tasks we are required to do. While earning high grades in school is a priority in some cultures, it is not so in others; consequently, children in the former are more likely to be motivated to achieve high grades than those in the latter. They are also more likely to be motivated to do well on diagnostic and research tasks than those in the latter.

- The language in which instructions and stimuli are communicated to a client or subject can affect his or her performance. If a client or subject is multilingual and the language used is not his or her first one, he or she may not perform as well as expected on a task because of a breakdown in communication. Also, if the instructions and/or stimuli for a task are translated from one language into another, performance may be affected by the translation not being equivalent to the original: It often is difficult to find words in two languages that convey exactly the same meaning.

- The sex and age of the clinician (researcher) and the manner in which he or she interacts with the client (subject) may affect the person's performance. In some cultures, for example, males and females are not permitted to work together and consequently task performance may be affected by a person being uncomfortable working with someone of the opposite sex (Nellum-Davis, 1993).

It is crucial that when a cultural difference is observed in the performance on a task that *it not be interpreted as a deficit* (Cole, 1986; Martinez, Bedore, & Ludwig, 1994; Sue, 1983). This is likely to occur if a clinician or researcher uses his or her culture as the "yard stick" against which other cultures are measured. If persons from another culture tend to perform differently on a task than they do in yours, this does not necessarily mean that their performance is less mature or inferior. The same, of course, is true for differences in attitude between persons from another culture and yours.

Exercises and Discussion Topics

1. Locate an article in one of the ASHA journals in which the failure to consider cultural differences may have resulted in a question being answered incorrectly. How might the methodology used to answer the question be modified to make it culturally appropriate and consequently, more likely to yield a correct answer?

2. Formulate an "answerable" question pertaining to cultural differences that would be likely to have clinical implications. How would you make the observations needed to answer it?

Appendixes

Selected Descriptive and Inferential Statistics: Computational Formulas with Worked Examples, Minitab Commands, and Exercises

Introduction

This appendix provides the information you need to compute most of the statistics that are described in Chapters 9 and 10. Consequently, the material presented here is really an extension of that presented in these two chapters. The *interpretation* of these statistics is described in the chapters (descriptive statistics in Chapter 9 and inferential ones in Chapter 10), but not their *computation*. Computational procedures for statistics were not described in the chapters because some research design courses offered in speech-language pathology and audiology training programs do not include a unit on computing statistics. The reason usually is that the students who take them have already had a statistics course. However, regardless of whether you have had a statistics course, if you want to review the computational procedures for certain descriptive or inferential statistics, you can do so using the exercises in this appendix because the approximate values (answers) you should get for them are given.

The computations required for these statistics can be made with either a calculator or a computer. Computational formulas and worked examples are provided for doing so with a calculator. While it is practical to make most of them in this way, it is almost always less time-consuming to work the examples with a computer.

Programs that will compute the statistics in this appendix (as well as others) are available for all computers. It is only necessary with these programs to issue a few commands to compute a statistic after the data have been inputted. Unfortunately, the commands you would use to compute a particular statistic are not the same for all of these programs.

The commands that are included in this appendix are those for computing statistics with the Minitab Statistical Software. There are detailed instructions for using these commands in the manual that comes with the Minitab program. This program can compute all of the statistics mentioned in Chapters 9 and 10, as well as many others. Versions of this program— which are available for most computers, including IBM-compatible and Macintosh ones—all utilize the same command set. Consequently, someone who has learned to use Minitab on one type of computer can easily learn to use it on another. This program was developed at Pennsylvania State University to help teach introductory courses in statistics and is relatively easy to learn to use. While it was originally developed to be a teaching tool and is being used for this purpose at more than 2000 colleges and universities, it is now being utilized by researchers and other professionals at more than 3000 facilities because of its power and ease of use. For further information about the program, contact Minitab, Inc., 3081 Enterprise Drive, State College, PA 16801-3008 (Telephone: 814-238-3280).

A single set of data is used for all statistical analyses in this appendix (see Table A-1). The data are frequencies per 100 words of four disfluency types in samples of the spontaneous speech of 56 elementary-school-age children who do not stutter. The children made up "once upon a time" stories about each of the ten *Children's Apperception Test* (CAT) cards. The stories were recorded and transcribed and the frequency of interjection, part-word repetition, word repetition, and revision-incomplete phrase per 100 words spoken was determined for the sample from each child. The labels *C1* to *C8* in Table A-1 stand for Column 1 to Column 8; these labels are used both when inputting these data and analyzing them with the Minitab program.

TABLE A-1   Frequencies per 100 words of interjection of sounds, syllables, words, and phrases (I), part-word repetition (PW), word repetition (W), and revision-incomplete phrase (R-IP) produced by 56 second-through sixth-grade nonstutterers during the performance of a spontaneous speech task.

Subject	GRADE (C1)	I (C2)	PW (C3)	W (C4)	R-IP (C5)
1	2	0.50	1.16	0.50	2.16
2	2	2.13	1.42	0.35	5.67
3	2	1.40	0.00	0.00	5.14
4	2	0.40	1.21	0.40	1.62
5	2	0.31	0.94	0.63	2.52
6	2	0.00	0.35	0.35	1.74
7	2	0.00	0.00	1.28	3.21
8	2	0.47	2.37	0.95	1.90
9	2	0.30	1.80	1.50	4.49
10	2	0.50	1.00	1.33	6.16
11	2	8.53	0.34	2.39	2.73
12	2	1.04	1.04	1.04	1.56
13	2	1.46	0.29	0.44	4.54
14	2	0.36	0.36	0.72	1.08
15	2	1.87	0.00	0.75	2.24
16	3	0.46	1.14	1.60	3.65
17	3	3.78	1.13	2.64	3.02

TABLE A-1   *Continued*

Subject	GRADE (C1)	I (C2)	PW (C3)	W (C4)	R-IP (C5)
18	3	2.23	1.49	2.97	4.83
19	3	0.33	0.99	0.99	1.64
20	3	0.49	0.00	0.49	0.49
21	3	1.07	1.43	1.07	6.79
22	3	0.55	4.42	3.31	6.08
23	3	0.84	0.28	0.28	1.68
24	3	0.28	0.41	0.28	3.72
25	3	3.40	1.51	1.89	1.89
26	3	1.80	0.90	0.60	2.40
27	4	0.44	1.54	0.00	3.30
28	4	0.94	1.57	0.78	2.83
29	4	0.00	2.41	2.78	3.33
30	4	0.33	0.65	0.49	3.41
31	4	0.56	1.29	0.88	5.31
32	4	0.00	0.12	0.12	0.97
33	4	0.43	0.22	0.65	4.13
34	4	0.00	1.21	2.02	4.48
35	4	3.67	0.83	0.83	3.33
36	5	0.84	0.84	0.42	3.38
37	5	0.16	0.82	0.82	8.20
38	5	1.61	0.00	0.36	1.97
39	5	1.76	1.58	3.25	4.55
40	5	0.28	0.14	1.14	1.99
41	5	2.92	0.93	0.80	4.77
42	5	1.72	0.81	1.26	2.80
43	5	0.72	0.21	0.21	1.65
44	5	0.00	0.54	0.27	2.41
45	5	1.82	0.61	1.70	3.64
46	5	0.52	0.34	2.41	4.83
47	6	0.00	0.28	0.28	0.86
48	6	0.00	0.19	0.77	0.96
49	6	1.99	0.00	0.85	3.42
50	6	0.00	0.47	0.47	1.10
51	6	0.00	0.93	0.00	1.39
52	6	0.69	0.00	0.00	1.72
53	6	0.00	0.66	0.99	1.32
54	6	0.73	0.91	0.18	3.09
55	6	0.78	0.26	0.26	1.03
56	6	0.30	0.41	0.51	2.03

The format that is used for each statistic is as follows. A question is asked about the data in Table A-1 that the statistic can help to answer. The question is followed by the computational formula for the statistic and the calculations required to compute it. Following this, the answer to the question is given based on the value computed for the statistic. Next, the Minitab command for computing the statistic is presented. Finally, there is an exercise in which you are asked to use different data from Table A-1 to compute the statistic. The approximate value you should get for the statistic is given. Your value (answer) may differ a little from mine because of "rounding" error. That is, you may not have carried intermediate computations to the same number of decimal places that I did before rounding them.

Entering Data in a Minitab Worksheet

Before you can compute statistics on a set of data using the Minitab Statistical Software, you must first enter the data into a worksheet. The worksheet (which is a spreadsheet) consists of a matrix of rows and columns (see Figure A-1). All of the criterion measures (data) from a subject are recorded in the same row; consequently, the number of rows in a worksheet equals the number of subjects. The number of columns in a worksheet is equal to the number of criterion measures recorded for each subject on which statistics are to be computed.

You can enter data in a worksheet in several ways. If the version of Minitab you are using has a *data window,* you can issue the command to display it and then enter your criterion measures (data) in the appropriate rows and columns. You can do this by using the arrow keys to place the cursor in each cell in which you want to enter a criterion measure and then enter it with the keyboard. If the version of Minitab you are using does not have a data window, you can enter criterion measures by issuing commands. The first command

	C1	C2	C3	C4	C5	C6	C7
→	PW	R-IP					
1	1.16	2.16					
2	1.42	5.67					
3	0.00	5.14					
4	1.21	1.62					
5	0.04	2.52					
6	0.35	1.74					
7	0.00	3.21					
8	2.37	1.90					
9	1.80	4.49					
10	1.00	6.16					
11	0.34	2.73					
12	1.04	1.56					
13							

File   Edit   Calc   Stat   Window   Graph   Editor

Disfluency Data.MTW

FIGURE A-1   A Minitab worksheet.

READ C1 C2 C3 C4

tells the computer to take the criterion measures from the line that follows the READ command and put them into columns C1, C2, C3, and C4 of the next row of the worksheet. The number of columns can be in the hundreds. A READ command is issued for each row. After all of the criterion measures have been entered, the command

END

is issued. The display on the monitor screen will look something like that in Figure A-2. There may, of course, be more rows and columns in the worksheet than your screen can display at one time. If you wanted to print the data in a four-column worksheet, the appropriate command would be

PRINT C1 C2 C3 C4

Such a printout could be useful when checking for data entry errors. After the data are entered in the worksheet, various statistical analyses can be performed on them.

```
MTB   >   READ   C1    C2    C3
DATA  >   0.50   1.16  0.50
DATA  >   2.13   1.42  0.35
DATA  >   1.40   0.00  0,00
DATA  >   0.40   1.21  0.40
DATA  >   0.13   0.94  0.63
DATA  >   0.00   0.35  0.35
DATA  >   0.00   0.00  1.28
DATA  >   0.47   2.37  0.95
DATA  >   0.30   1.80  1.50
DATA  >   0.50   1.00  1.33
DATA  >   8,53   0.34  2.39
DATA  >   1.04   1.04  1.04
DATA  >   1.46   0.29  0.44
DATA  >   0.36   0.36  0.72
DATA  >   1.87   0.00  0.75
DATA  >   0.46   1.14  1.60
DATA  >   3.78   1.13  2.64
DATA  >   2.23   1.49  2.97
DATA  >   0.33   0.99  0.99
DATA  >   0.49   0.00  0.49
DATA  >   1.07   1.43  1.07
DATA  >   0.55   4.42  3.31
DATA  >   0.84   0.28  0.28
DATA  >   0.28   0.41  0.28
DATA  >   3.40   1.51  1.89
DATA  >   1.80   0.90  0.60
DATA  >   END
MTB   >
```

FIGURE A-2   A monitor screen for a Minitab worksheet in which data were entered by issuing READ commands.

Some Notation Used in This Appendix

Symbol	Meaning
ΣX	Sum [or add] scores on variable labeled X.
ΣX^2	Square scores on variable labeled X and then sum [or add] them.
$(\Sigma X)^2$	Sum (or add) scores on variable labeled X and then square this sum.
$\overline{X}$	Sum (or add) scores on the variable X and then divide total by the number of scores summed.
$\overline{X}^2$	Compute mean of variable labeled X (as indicated above) and square it.
ΣY	Sum (or add) scores on variable labeled Y.
ΣY^2	Square scores on variable labeled Y and then sum (or add) them.
$(\Sigma Y)^2$	Sum (or add) scores on variable labeled Y and then square this sum.
$\overline{Y}$	Sum (or add) scores on variable labeled Y and then divide total by number of scores summed.
$\overline{Y}^2$	Compute mean of variable labeled Y (as indicated above) and square it.
ΣXY	Multiply each person's X-score by his or her Y-score and then sum (or add) the results of these multiplications.
N	The number of persons in the sample.
$\sqrt{}$	Compute square root.
$\vert\ \vert$	Compute absolute value.

Other notation is defined when used.

Descriptive Statistics: Measures of Central Tendency

1. Mean

QUESTION: How many instances of interjection per 100 words did the *average* child produce during his or her performance of the spontaneous speech task?

$$\overline{X} = \frac{\Sigma X}{N} = \frac{57.71}{56} = 1.03$$

MINITAB: DESCRIBE C2

ANSWER: The average child produced 1.03 instances of interjection per 100 words during the performance of the spontaneous speech task.

EXERCISE: Determine the mean number of word repetitions per 100 words that were produced by the 56 children. (Your answer should be approximately 0.97.)

2. Median

QUESTION: How many instances of interjection per 100 words did the *typical* child produce during his or her performance of the spontaneous speech task? The first step in computing the median to answer the question is to order the 56 interjection frequencies from lowest to highest.

0.00	0.30	0.52	1.61
0.00	0.30	0.55	1.72
0.00	0.31	0.56	1.76
0.00	0.33	0.69	1.80
0.00	0.33	0.72	1.82
0.00	0.36	0.73	1.87
0.00	0.40	0.78	1.99
0.00	0.43	0.84	2.13
0.00	0.44	0.84	2.23
0.00	0.46	0.94	2.92
0.00	0.47	1.04	3.40
0.16	0.49	1.07	3.67
0.28	0.50	1.40	3.78
0.28	0.50	1.46	8.53

Since there are an *even* number of scores, the median score would be midway between the $N/2$ (0.50) and $N/2$ +1 score (0.52). The median interjection frequency, therefore, would be 0.51. (If there had been an *odd* number of scores, the median score would have been the middle one.)

MINITAB: DESCRIBE C2

ANSWER: The typical child produced 0.51 instances of interjection per 100 words during his or her performance of the spontaneous speech task.

REMARK: Note that the mean interjection frequency (1.03) is approximately twice as high as the median interjection frequency (0.51). This discrepancy is primarily due to five children who had relatively high interjection frequencies—that is, greater than 2.5 per 100 words. A few persons who have relatively high (or relatively low) scores on a task can substantially influence the mean score on that task.

EXERCISE: Determine the median number of word repetitions per 100 words that were produced by 56 children. (Your answer should be approximately 0.76.)

3. Mode

QUESTION: What frequency of interjection per 100 words was most typical (i.e., occurred most often) during the children's performance of the spontaneous speech task?

   The type of data table that we used for computing the median (see p. 297) can also be used for computing the mode. Since the mode is the most frequently occurring score, the modal interjection frequency per 100 words would be 0.00. Note that 0.00 occurred 11 times. No other frequency occurred this often.

MINITAB: SORT C2

PRINT C2

(**Note**: The SORT command orders the 56 interjection frequencies from lowest to highest. The PRINT command prints these frequencies after they are ordered. The mode is determined by examining the printout.)

ANSWER: The frequency of interjection per 100 words that was most typical during the children's performance of the spontaneous speech task was 0.00.

EXERCISE: Determine the modal numbers of word repetitions per 100 words that were produced by these 56 children. (Your answer should be 0.00.)

Descriptive Statistics: Measures of Variability

1. Range

QUESTION: What was the range of interjection frequencies produced by these children during their performance of the spontaneous speech task?

The range in a set of measures is defined by two scores: the lowest score and the highest score. To identify these scores, the measures are ordered from lowest to highest. The lowest score and the highest score in the set would define the range. The interjection frequencies for the 56 children range from 0.00 to 8.53 (see p. 297).

MINITAB: DESCRIBE C2

ANSWER: The interjection frequencies produced by these children during their performance of the spontaneous speech task ranged from 0.00 to 8.53.

EXERCISE: Determine the range of word repetition frequencies for these 56 children. (Your answer should be 0.00 and 3.31.)

2. Interquartile Range

QUESTION: Within what range of interjection frequencies did the middle 50 percent of the 56 children fall during the performance of their spontaneous speech task?

The interquartile range is defined by two scores: the third quartile (Q_3)—that is, the score below which 75 percent of the scores fall—and the first quartile (Q_1)—that is, the score below which 25 percent of the scores fall. These scores can be converted into an index (Q) by calculating the difference between them.

$$Q = Q_3 - Q_1 = 1.535 - 0.29 = 1.245$$

Q_1 and Q_3 were determined from the frequency distribution on p. 297.

MINITAB: DESCRIBE C2

ANSWER: The interjection frequencies for the middle 50 percent of the children ranged from 0.29 to 1.535. The magnitude of the interquartile range (i.e., the maximum amount that the middle 50 percent of children differed from each other) was 1.245 instances per 100 words.

EXERCISE: Determine the interquartile range for word repetition frequencies (Q) for these 56 children. (Your answer should be approximately 0.92.)

3. Standard Deviation

QUESTION: How different were the children's interjection frequencies from each other during their performance of the spontaneous speech task?

The standard deviation is a measure of how different various scores are from each other. The larger the standard deviation, the more different they would be. The standard deviation for the children's interjection frequencies (S) is:

$$S = \sqrt{\frac{\Sigma X^2}{N} - \bar{X}^2} = \sqrt{\frac{166.92}{56} - (1.03)^2} = \sqrt{1.92} = 1.39$$

MINITAB: DESCRIBE C2

ANSWER: The children's interjection frequencies were quite different from each other judging by the fact that the standard deviation (1.39) was larger than the mean.

EXERCISE: Determine the standard deviation for the children's word repetition frequencies. (Your answer should be approximately 0.85.)

Descriptive Statistics: Measures of Association

1. Contingency Coefficient

QUESTION: Were the children who produced the highest frequency of interjection per 100 words on the spontaneous speech task the same ones who produced the highest frequencies of part-word repetition per 100 words on this task and vice versa?

The first step in computing the contingency coefficient is to assign each of the 56 children to one of the four cells of a 2×2 table.

INTERJECTION

	Below Median	Above Median
Above Median	13 a	15 b
Below Median	15 c	13 d

PART-WORD REPETITION

A

If a child's interjection frequency was below the median (i.e., less than 0.51) and the part-word repetition frequency was above the median (i.e., greater than 0.815), the child was assigned to cell *a*. If the child's interjection frequency was above the median and the part-word repetition frequency was above the median, the child was assigned to cell *b*. If both the interjection and part-word repetition frequencies were below their respective medians, the child was assigned to cell *c*. And if the interjection frequency was above the median and the part-word repetition frequency was below the median, the child was assigned to cell *d*.

The next step is to compute the value of chi square (χ^2) for the frequencies in the table. The value of chi square that was computed for this table (see p. 304) is 0.07. (Note that χ^2 has a different meaning here than it had previously.) The contingency coefficient for this table would be:

$$C = \sqrt{\frac{\chi^2}{N + \chi^2}} = \sqrt{\frac{0.07}{56 + 0.07}} = \sqrt{0.0012} = .035$$

Since the possible values of the contingency coefficient vary between 0.00 and a number less than 1.00, and the closer the value is to 0.00 the weaker the association between the two variables, the degree of association for these children between level of interjection production and level of part-word repetition production would appear to be quite weak.

MINITAB: Enter the two interjection frequencies for below the median in C1 and the two interjection frequencies for above the median in C2. Issue the command CHISQUARE C1-C2. To compute C from the resulting chi-square statistic, enter the statistic in C3, N in C4, and then issue the following command:

```
LET C5 = SQRT (C3 / (C4 + C3))
```

The contingency coefficient will be in C5.

ANSWER: There was little, if any, tendency for children who produced the highest frequencies of interjection on the spontaneous speech task to be the same children who produced the highest frequencies of part-word repetition on this task, and vice versa.

EXERCISE: Determine whether the children who produced the highest frequencies of word repetition per 100 words on the spontaneous speech task were the same ones who produced the highest frequencies of revision-incomplete phrase per 100 words on this task, and vice versa, through the use of a contingency coefficient. (The value of the contingency coefficient you compute should be approximately 0.31.)

2. Phi Coefficient

QUESTION: Were the children who produced the highest frequencies of interjection per 100 words on the spontaneous speech task the same ones that produced the highest frequencies of part-word repetition per 100 words on this task, and vice versa?

The first step in computing the phi coefficient is to assign each of the 56 children to one of the four cells of a 2 × 2 table in the same manner as for the contingency coefficient (see p. 299). The next step is to compute the value of phi for the frequencies in the table through the use of the following formula:

$$\Phi = \frac{(bc - ad)}{\sqrt{(a + b)(c + d)(a + c)(b + d)}}$$

$$= \frac{(15)(15) - (13)(13)}{\sqrt{(13 + 15)(15 + 13)(13 + 15)(15 + 13)}} = \frac{56}{\sqrt{614656}}$$

$$= \frac{56}{784} = 0.071$$

Since the possible values of the phi coefficient range from -1.00 to $+1.00$, and the closer the value is to 0.00 the weaker the association between the two variables, the degree of association for these children between level of interjection production and level of part-word repetition production would appear to be quite weak.

MINITAB: Insert the frequency from cell a in C1, cell b in C2, cell c in C3, and cell d in C4 and issue the following command:

```
LET C5 = ((C2*C3) - (C1*C4)) / SQRT ((C1 + C2)*(C3 + C4)*
(C1 + C3)*(C2 + C4))
```

The phi coefficient will be in C5.

ANSWER: There was little, if any, tendency for the children who produced the highest frequencies of interjection on the spontaneous speech task to be the same children who produced the highest frequencies of part-word repetition on this task, and vice versa.

EXERCISE: Determine whether the children who produced the highest frequencies of word repetition per 100 words on the spontaneous speech task were the same ones who produced the highest frequencies of revision-incomplete phrase per 100 words on this task, and vice versa, through the use of a phi coefficient. (The value of the phi coefficient you compute should be approximately 0.36.)

3. Spearman Rank-Order Coefficient

QUESTION: How similar was the ordering of the second graders with regard to their interjection frequencies and part-word repetition frequencies during their performance of the spontaneous speech task?

   The first step in computing a Spearman rank-order correlation coefficient between the interjection frequencies and part-word repetition frequencies of the fifteen second graders (see Table A-1) is to determine each child's rank for interjection frequency and each child's rank for part-word repetition frequency. The child who had the lowest frequency of part-word repetition would be assigned the rank 1; the one who had the next lowest, the rank 2; the one who had the third lowest the rank 3; and so on. If more than one child had the same frequency, each would be assigned the mean of the tied ranks. The ranks assigned to the fifteen children for their interjection frequencies and part-word repetition frequencies are indicated in the table that follows. Also included in the table is the difference between each child's two ranks (d_j) and this difference squared (d_j^2). The sum of the squared differences between ranks for the fifteen children is used for computing the Spearman rank-order coefficient.

Subject Number	Rank		d_i	d_i^2
	I	*PW*		
1	8.5	11.0	− 2.5	6.25
2	14.0	13.0	1.0	1.00
3	11.0	2.0	9.0	81.0
4	6.0	12.0	− 6.0	36.0
5	4.0	8.0	4.0	16.00
6	1.5	6.0	− 4.5	20.25
7	1.5	2.0	− 0.5	0.25
8	7.0	15.0	− 8.0	64.00
9	3.0	14.0	−11.0	121.00
10	8.5	9.0	− 0.5	0.25
11	15.0	5.0	10.0	100.00
12	10.0	10.0	0.0	0.00
13	12.0	4.0	8.0	64.00
14	5.0	7.0	− 2.0	4.00
15	13.0	2.0	11.0	121.00
				$\Sigma d_i^2 = 635.00$

The value of the Spearman rank-order coefficient for these data would be:

$$r_s = 1 - \frac{6\Sigma\, d_i^2}{N^3 - N} = 1 - \frac{(6)(635)}{(15)^3 - 15}$$

$$= 1 - \frac{3810}{3375 - 15} = 1 - 1.13 = -0.13$$

Since the possible values range from −1.00 to +1.00, and the closer the value is to 0.00 the weaker the association between the two variables, the degree of association for these children between level of interjection production and level of part-word repetition production would appear to be quite weak.

MINITAB: Enter the two sets of data to be correlated in C1 and C2 and issue the following three commands:

```
RANK C1 C3
RANK C2 C4
CORRELATION C3 C4
```

If the data are ranks, only the third is necessary.

ANSWER: There was little, if any, similarity in the ordering of the second graders with regard to their interjection frequencies and part-word repetition frequencies during their performance of the spontaneous speech task.

EXERCISE: Determine the degree of similarity of the ordering of the third graders with regard to their interjection frequencies and part-word repetition frequencies during their performance of the spontaneous speech task, using the Spearman rank-order coefficient. (The value for the correlation you compute should be approximately 0.40.)

4. Pearson Product-Moment Correlation Coefficient

QUESTION: Were the levels of the children's interjection frequencies related to those of their part-word repetition frequencies during their performance of the spontaneous speech task?

The first step in computing a Pearson product-moment correlation coefficient between interjection frequencies and part-word repetition frequencies for the 56 children (see Table A-1) is to compute the following sums:

$$\Sigma X = \text{sum of the 56 interjection frequencies} = 57.71$$

$$\Sigma Y = \text{sum of the 56 part-word repetition frequencies} = 46.75$$

$$\Sigma X^2 = \text{sum of the squares of the 56 interjection frequencies} = 166.92$$

$$\Sigma Y^2 = \text{sum of the squares of the 56 part-word repetition frequencies} = 71.68$$

$$\Sigma XY = \text{sum of the products of the 56 pairs of frequencies} = 47.00$$

The Pearson product-moment correlation coefficient for these data would be:

$$r = \frac{N\Sigma XY - (\Sigma X)(\Sigma Y)}{\sqrt{\left[N\Sigma X^2 - (\Sigma X)^2\right]\left[N\Sigma Y^2 - (\Sigma Y)^2\right]}}$$

$$= \frac{(56)(47.00) - (57.71)(46.75)}{\sqrt{\left[(56)(166.92) - (57.71)^2\right]\left[(56)(71.68) - (46.75)^2\right]}}$$

$$= \frac{2632.00 - 2697.94}{\sqrt{\left[9347.52 - 3330.44\right]\left[4014.08 - 2185.56\right]}}$$

$$= \frac{-65.94}{\sqrt{11,002,351}} = \frac{-65.94}{3316.98}$$

$$= -0.02$$

Since the possible values of this correlation coefficient *(r)* range from –1.00 to +1.00, and the closer the value is to 0.00, the weaker the association between the two variables, there doesn't appear to be any relationship between these children's interjection and part-word repetition frequencies.

MINITAB: Enter the 56 interjection frequencies in C1 and the 56 part-word repetition frequencies in C2 and issue the following command:

```
CORRELATION C1 C2
```

The value of *r* would be shown on the screen. If you also wanted a scattergram to be plotted on the screen, you would issue the following command:

PLOT C1 VERSUS C2

ANSWER: There doesn't appear to be any relationship between these children's interjection frequency levels and part-word repetition frequency levels.

EXERCISE: Determine the degree of relationship between the children's word repetition frequencies and revision-incomplete phrase frequencies. (The value of *r* you compute should be approximately 0.37).

Inferential Statistical Tests: Nominal Data

1. Chi Square Test

QUESTION: Was there a tendency for children who had interjection frequencies above the median for the group also to have part-word repetition frequencies above the median for the group, or vice versa?

The first step in performing a chi square test is selecting a *level of confidence* (alpha level)—the maximum acceptable probability for a *Type I error* (see Chapter 10). We will use the 0.05 level of confidence. The region of rejection will be *two-tailed* (see Chapter 10) because to answer the question it is necessary to be able to detect both positive and negative relationships between the two disfluency types.

The next step is to compute the value of chi square. Each of the 56 children is assigned to one of the four cells in a 2×2 table in the same manner as for the contingency coefficient (see p. 299). The value of chi square would be computed from this table as follows:

$$\chi^2 = \frac{N\left(|ad - bc| - \frac{N}{2}\right)^2}{(a + b)(c + d)(a + c)(b + d)}$$

$$= \frac{56\left(|(13)(13) - (15)(15)| - \frac{56}{2}\right)^2}{(13 + 15)(15 + 13)(13 + 15)(15 + 13)}$$

$$= \frac{56(|169 - 225| - 28)^2}{(28)(28)(28)(28)} = \frac{56(28)^2}{614,656}$$

$$= \frac{43,904}{614.656} = 0.07$$

To determine whether the value of chi square computed is large enough for the null hypothesis to be rejected, the chi square value required for rejection is located in Table A-2. The degrees of freedom *(df)* here would be 1 (i.e., the number of rows minus one times the number of columns minus one). The value of chi square required for rejection at the 0.05 alpha level when *df* = 1 is 3.84. Since the value computed is smaller than this (i.e., 0.07), the null hypothesis would not be rejected.

TABLE A-2   Table of Critical Values of Chi Square.*

					Probability under H_0 that $\chi^2 \geq$ chi square								
df	.99	.98	.95	.90	.80	.70	.50	.30	.20	.10	.05	.02	.01	.001
1	.00016	.00063	.0039	.016	.064	.15	.46	1.07	1.64	2.71	3.84	5.41	6.64	10.83
2	.02	.04	.10	.21	.45	.71	1.39	2.41	3.22	4.60	5.99	7.82	9.21	13.82
3	.12	.18	.35	.58	1.00	1.42	2.37	3.66	4.64	6.25	7.82	9.84	11.34	16.27
4	.30	.43	.71	1.06	1.65	2.20	3.36	4.88	5.99	7.78	9.49	11.67	13.28	18.46
5	.55	.75	1.14	1.61	2.34	3.00	4.35	6.06	7.29	9.24	11.07	13.39	15.09	20.52
6	.87	1.13	1.64	2.20	3.07	3.83	5.35	7.23	8.56	10.64	12.59	15.03	16.81	22.46
7	1.24	1.56	2.17	2.83	3.82	4.67	6.35	8.38	9.80	12.02	14.07	16.62	18.48	24.32
8	1.65	2.03	2.73	3.49	4.59	5.53	7.34	9.52	11.03	13.36	15.51	18.17	20.09	26.12
9	2.09	2.53	3.32	4.17	5.38	6.39	8.34	10.66	12.24	14.68	16.92	19.68	21.67	27.88
10	2.56	3.06	3.94	4.86	6.18	7.27	9.34	11.78	13.44	15.99	18.31	21.16	23.21	29.59
11	3.05	3.61	4.58	5.58	6.99	8.15	10.34	12.90	14.63	17.28	19.68	22.62	24.72	31.26
12	3.57	4.18	5.23	6.30	7.81	9.03	11.34	14.01	15.81	18.55	21.03	24.05	26.22	32.91
13	4.11	4.76	5.89	7.04	8.63	9.93	12.34	15.12	16.98	19.81	22.36	25.47	27.69	34.53
14	4.66	5.37	6.57	7.79	9.47	10.82	13.34	16.22	18.15	21.06	23.68	26.87	29.14	36.12
15	5.23	5.98	7.26	8.55	10.31	11.72	14.34	17.32	19.31	22.31	25.00	28.26	30.58	37.70
16	5.81	6.61	7.96	9.31	11.15	12.62	15.34	18.42	20.46	23.54	26.30	29.63	32.00	39.29
17	6.41	7.26	8.67	10.08	12.00	13.53	16.34	19.51	21.62	24.77	27.59	31.00	33.41	40.75
18	7.02	7.91	9.39	10.86	12.86	14.44	17.34	20.60	22.76	25.99	28.87	32.35	34.80	42.31
19	7.63	8.57	10.12	11.65	13.72	15.35	18.34	21.69	23.90	27.20	30.14	33.69	36.19	43.82
20	8.26	9.24	10.85	12.44	14.58	16.27	19.34	22.78	25.04	28.41	31.41	35.02	37.57	45.32
21	8.90	9.92	11.59	13.24	15.44	17.18	20.34	23.86	26.17	29.62	32.67	36.34	38.93	46.80
22	9.54	10.60	12.34	14.04	16.31	18.10	21.24	24.94	27.30	30.81	33.92	37.66	40.29	48.27
23	10.20	11.29	13.09	14.85	17.19	19.02	22.34	26.02	28.43	32.01	35.17	38.97	41.64	49.73
24	10.86	11.99	13.85	15.66	18.06	19.94	23.34	27.10	29.55	33.20	36.42	40.27	42.98	51.18
25	11.52	12.70	14.61	16.47	18.94	20.87	24.34	28.17	30.68	34.38	37.65	41.57	44.31	52.62
26	12.20	13.41	15.38	17.29	19.82	21.79	25.34	29.25	31.80	35.56	38.88	42.86	45.64	54.05
27	12.88	14.12	16.15	18.11	20.70	22.72	26.34	30.32	32.91	36.74	40.11	44.14	46.96	55.48
28	13.56	14.85	16.93	18.94	21.59	23.65	27.34	31.39	34.03	37.92	41.34	45.42	48.28	56.89
29	14.26	15.57	17.71	19.77	22.48	24.58	28.34	32.46	35.14	39.09	42.56	46.69	49.59	58.30
30	14.95	16.31	18.49	20.60	23.36	25.51	29.34	33.53	36.25	40.26	43.77	47.96	50.89	59.70

Adapted from Table IV of Fisher and Yates: Statistical Tables for Biological, Agricultural, and Medical Research (6th edition). Copyright 1974 by Longman Group, Ltd. With permission of Longman Group, Ltd.

MINITAB: Enter the two interjections frequencies for below the median in C1 and the two interjection frequencies for above the median in C2 and then issue the following command:

CHISQUARE C1-C2

The value for chi-square displayed on the screen would be compared to the one in Table A-2 required for rejection of the null hypothesis.

ANSWER: There was no tendency for the children who had interjection frequencies above the median for the group to also have part-word repetition frequencies above the median for the group, or vice versa (chi square test; alpha = 0.05).

EXERCISE: Determine whether there was a tendency for the children who had word repetition frequencies above the median for the group also to have revision-incomplete phrase frequencies above the median for the group and vice versa. (The value of chi square you compute should be approximately 5.78.)

Inferential Statistical Tests: Ordinal Data

1. Sign Test

QUESTION: Did the second graders tend to produce higher frequencies of interjection than of part-word repetition?

The first step in performing a sign test is selecting a *level of confidence,* or the maximum acceptable probability for a *Type I error* (i.e., concluding there was a tendency for the second graders to produce higher frequencies of interjection than of part-word repetition when there was no such tendency). We will use the 0.05 level of confidence. The region of rejection for the test will be *one-tailed* because it is only necessary to detect a difference in one direction to answer the question.

The next step is to compute the value for the sign test. Each of the second graders is assigned a + or a – , depending on whether his or her interjection frequency or part-word repetition frequency is higher. If the child's interjection frequency is higher than his or her part-word repetition frequency, the child is assigned a +; if the child's part-word repetition frequency is higher than his or her interjection frequency, the child is assigned a –. If the child's part-word repetition frequencies and interjection frequencies are the same, he or she is assigned a 0. The sign assignments for the fifteen children are as follows:

Subject	Sign	Subject	Sign
1	–	9	–
2	+	10	–
3	+	11	+
4	–	12	0
5	–	13	+
6	–	14	0
7	0	15	+
8	–		

The number of subjects for whom the two frequencies are not the same (N), and the number of times the sign occurs that occurs *least* often (x) are determined for this distribution. The values of N and x are 12 and 5, respectively. Based on the binomial distribution (see Table A-3), when $N = 12$, the probability of five pluses (x) occurring by chance is 0.387. Since this value is larger than 0.05, the null hypothesis would not be rejected.

MINITAB: Enter minuses in C1 as –1s and pluses as +1s. Then issue the following command:

```
STEST C1
```

The probability associated with the number of pluses (or minuses) in the data set will be displayed on the screen.

ANSWER: The second graders did not exhibit a tendency to produce higher frequencies of interjection than of part-word repetition (sign test; alpha = 0.05).

REMARK: This procedure can be used to compute the probability value for the sign test when the number of subjects for whom the two frequencies are not the same (N) is 25 or fewer. When the value of N exceeds 25, the procedure used to answer the next question is appropriate.

QUESTION: Did the second, third, and fourth graders tend to produce higher frequencies of interjection than of part-word repetition?

We will use the 0.05 level of confidence here. The region of rejection will be *one-tailed*.

Next, each of the 35 second, third, and fourth graders is assigned a sign in the same manner as for the previous question. The sign assignments for these children are as follows:

Subject	Sign	Subject	Sign
1	−	19	−
2	+	20	+
3	+	21	−
4	−	22	−
5	−	23	+
6	−	24	−
7	0	25	+
8	−	26	+
9	−	27	−
10	−	28	−
11	+	29	−
12	0	30	−
13	+	31	−
14	0	32	−
15	+	33	+
16	−	34	−
17	+	35	+
18	+		

The values of N and x for this distribution (which were determined in the same manner as for the previous question) are 32 and 13 respectively. The probability of 13 pluses (x) occurring by chance when $N = 32$ can be determined by means of the following formula (which is based on the "normal curve"):

$$Z = \frac{(x \pm 0.5) - \frac{1}{2} N}{\frac{1}{2} \sqrt{N}} \quad \text{where } x + 0.5 \text{ is used when } x < \tfrac{1}{2} N,$$
$$\text{and } x - 0.5 \text{ is used when } x > \tfrac{1}{2} N.$$

$$= \frac{(13 + 0.5) - \frac{1}{2}(32)}{\frac{1}{2}\sqrt{32}}$$

$$= \frac{13.5 - 16.0}{\frac{1}{2}(5.66)} = \frac{-2.5}{2.83} = -0.88$$

Based on the normal distribution (see Table A-4) the probability of this outcome occurring by chance is 0.189. Since this value is larger than 0.05, the null hypothesis would not be rejected.

TABLE A-3   Table of probabilities associated with values as small as observed values of x in the sign test.*

Given in the body of this table are one-tailed probabilities under H_0 for the binomial test when $P = Q = \frac{1}{2}$. To save space, decimal points are omitted in the p's.

N \ x	0	1	2	3	4	5	6	7	8	9	10	11	12	13	14	15
5	031	188	500	812	969	†										
6	016	109	344	656	891	984	†									
7	008	062	227	500	773	938	992	†								
8	004	035	145	363	637	855	965	996	†							
9	002	020	090	254	500	746	910	980	998	†						
10	001	011	055	172	377	623	828	945	989	999	†					
11		006	033	113	274	500	726	887	967	994	†	†				
12		003	019	073	194	387	613	806	927	981	997	†	†			
13		002	011	046	133	291	500	709	867	954	989	998	†	†		
14		001	006	029	090	212	395	605	788	910	971	994	999	†	†	
15			004	018	059	151	304	500	696	849	941	982	996	†	†	†
16			002	011	038	105	227	402	598	773	895	962	989	998	†	†
17			001	006	025	072	166	315	500	685	834	928	975	994	999	†
18			001	004	015	048	119	240	407	593	760	881	952	985	996	999
19				002	010	032	084	180	324	500	676	820	916	968	990	998
20				001	006	021	058	132	252	412	588	748	868	942	979	994
21				001	004	013	039	095	192	332	500	668	808	905	961	987
22					002	008	026	067	143	262	416	584	738	857	933	974
23					001	005	017	047	105	202	339	500	661	798	895	953
24					001	003	011	032	076	154	271	419	581	729	846	924
25						002	007	022	054	115	212	345	500	655	788	885

†1.0 or approximately 1.0

*Adapted from Table IV, B, of Walker and Lev. 1953. Statistical Inference. New York: Holt, p. 458.

MINITAB: The procedure is the same as for the small N example. It computes probabilities directly, rather than estimating them with the normal curve.

ANSWER: The second, third, and fourth graders did not exhibit a tendency to produce higher frequencies of interjection than of part-word repetition (sign test; alpha = 0.05).

EXERCISE: Determine whether the second and third graders exhibited a tendency to produce higher frequencies of revision-incomplete phrase than of word repetition. (The probability value that you compute should be approximately 0.001.)

2. Mann-Whitney U Test

QUESTION: Did the typical (i.e., median) second or third grader have a higher frequency of interjection than did the typical fourth, fifth or sixth grader?

The first step in performing a Mann-Whitney U test is selecting an *alpha* level, or a

TABLE A-4   Table of probabilities associated with values as extreme as observed values of z in the normal distribution.*

z	.00	.01	.02	.03	.04	.05	.06	.07	.08	.09
.0	.5000	.4960	.4920	.4880	.4840	.4801	.4761	.4721	.4681	4641
.1	.4602	.4562	.4522	.4483	.4443	.4404	.4364	.4325	.4286	.4247
.2	.4207	.4168	.4129	.4090	.4052	.4013	.3974	.3936	.3897	.3859
.3	.3821	.3783	.3745	.3707	.3669	.3632	.3594	.3557	.3520	.3483
.4	.3446	.3409	.3372	.3336	.3300	.3264	.3228	.3192	.3156	.3121
.5	.3085	.3050	.3015	.2981	.2946	.2912	.2877	.2843	.2810	.2776
.6	.2743	.2709	.2676	.2643	.2611	.2578	.2546	.2514	.2483	.2451
.7	.2420	.2389	.2358	.2327	.2296	.2266	.2236	.2206	.2177	.2148
.8	.2119	.2090	.2061	.2033	.2005	.1977	.1949	.1922	.1894	.1867
.9	.1841	.1814	.1788	.1762	.1736	.1711	.1685	.1660	.1635	.1611
1.0	.1587	.1562	.1539	.1515	.1492	.1469	.1446	.1423	.1401	.1379
1.1	.1357	.1335	.1314	.1292	.1271	.1251	.1230	.1210	.1190	.1170
1.2	.1151	.1131	.1112	.1093	.1075	.1056	.1038	.1020	.1003	.0985
1.3	.0968	.0951	.0934	.0918	.0901	.0885	.0869	.0853	.0838	.0823
1.4	.0808	.0793	.0778	.0764	.0749	.0735	.0721	.0708	.0694	.0681
1.5	.0668	.0655	.0643	.0630	.0618	.0606	.0594	.0582	.0571	.0559
1.6	.0548	.0537	.0526	.0516	.0505	.0495	.0485	.0475	.0465	.0455
1.7	.0446	.0436	.0427	.0418	.0409	.0401	.0392	.0384	.0375	.0367
1.8	.0359	.0351	.0344	.0336	.0329	.0322	.0314	.0307	.0301	.0294
1.9	.0287	.0281	.0274	.0268	.0262	.0256	.0250	.0244	.0239	.0233
2.0	.0228	.0222	.0217	.0212	.0207	.0202	.0197	.0192	.0188	.0183
2.1	.0179	.0174	.0170	.0166	.0162	.0158	.0154	.0150	.0146	.0143
2.2	.0139	.0136	.0132	.0129	.0125	.0122	.0119	.0116	.0113	.0110
2.3	.0107	.0104	.0102	.0099	.0096	.0094	.0091	.0089	.0087	.0084
2.4	.0082	.0080	.0078	.0075	.0073	.0071	.0069	.0068	.0066	.0064
2.5	.0062	.0060	.0059	.0057	.0055	.0054	.0052	.0051	.0049	.0048
2.6	.0047	.0045	.0044	.0043	.0041	.0040	.0039	.0038	.0037	.0036
2.7	.0035	.0034	.0033	.0032	.0031	.0030	.0029	.0028	.0027	.0026
2.8	.0026	.0025	.0024	.0023	.0023	.0022	.0021	.0021	.0020	.0019
2.9	.0019	.0018	.0018	.0017	.0016	.0016	.0015	.0015	.0014	.0014
3.0	.0013	.0013	.0013	.0012	.0012	.0011	.0011	.0011	.0010	.0010
3.1	.0010	.0009	.0009	.0009	.0008	.0008	.0008	.0008	.0007	.0007
3.2	.0007									
3.3	.0005									
3.4	.0003									
3.5	.00023									
3.6	.00016									
3.7	.00011									
3.8	.00007									
3.9	.00005									
4.0	.00003									

Adapted from Table A of Siegel. Nonparametric Statistics for the Behavioral Sciences. Copyright 1956 by McGraw-Hill Inc. With permission of McGraw-Hill Book Company.

maximum acceptable probability for a *Type I* error (i.e., concluding the median second or third grader had a higher frequency of interjection than did the median fourth, fifth, or sixth grader when there was no such difference). The 0.05 alpha level will be used for this test. Since to answer the question it only would be necessary to detect a difference between the two groups in one direction, the region of rejection for the test will be one-tailed.

The next step is to compute the value for the Mann-Whitney *U* Test. The 56 children are ordered on the basis of their interjection frequencies, and the rank is assigned to each child that designates his or her place in the ordering. The child who had the lowest interjection frequency would be assigned the rank 1; the one who had the second lowest, the rank 2; the one who had the third lowest, the rank 3; and so on. If more than one child had the same frequency, each would be assigned the mean of the tied ranks. The ranks assigned to the children are indicated as follows:

Second & Third Graders		Fourth, Fifth, & Sixth Graders	
Frequency	Rank	Frequency	Rank
0.00	6.0	0.00	6.0
0.00	6.0	0.00	6.0
0.28	13.5	0.00	6.0
0.30	15.5	0.00	6.0
0.31	17.0	0.00	6.0
0.33	18.5	0.00	6.0
0.36	20.0	0.00	6.0
0.40	21.0	0.00	6.0
0.46	24.0	0.00	6.0
0.47	25.0	0.16	12.0
0.49	26.0	0.28	13.5
0.50	27.5	0.30	15.5
0.50	27.5	0.33	18.5
0.55	30.0	0.43	22.0
0.84	36.5	0.44	23.0
1.04	39.0	0.52	29.0
1.07	40.0	0.56	31.0
1.40	41.0	0.69	32.0
1.46	42.0	0.72	33.0
1.80	46.0	0.73	34.0
1.87	48.0	0.78	35.0
2.13	50.0	0.84	36.5
2.23	51.0	0.94	38.0
3.40	53.0	1.61	43.0
3.78	55.0	1.72	44.0
8.53	56.0	1.76	45.0
		1.82	47.0
		1.99	49.0
		2.92	52.0
		3.67	54.0
$R_1 = 835.0$		$R_2 = 761.0$	
$n_1 = 26$		$n_2 = 30$	

Next, two estimates of U are computed from the sums of the ranks of the second and third graders (R_1) and the fourth, fifth, and sixth graders (R_2). In these formulas, n_1 refers to the number of second and third graders and n_2 refers to the number of fourth, fifth, and sixth graders.

$$U = n_1 n_2 + \frac{n_1(n_1 + 1)}{2} - R_1$$

$$= (26)(30) + \frac{26(26 + 1)}{2} - 835.0$$

$$= 780.0 + 351.0 - 835.0 = 296.0$$

$$U = n_1 n_2 + \frac{n_2(n_2 + 1)}{2} - R_2$$

$$= (26)(30) + \frac{30(30 + 1)}{2} - 761.0$$

$$= 780.0 + 465.0 - 761.0 = 484.0$$

The lowest estimate of U then is used to compute the value of Z, the test statistic.

$$Z = \frac{U - \frac{n_1 n_2}{2}}{\sqrt{\frac{(n_1)(n_2)(n_1 + n_2 + 1)}{12}}}$$

$$= \frac{296 - \frac{(26)(30)}{2}}{\sqrt{\frac{(26)(30)(26 + 30 + 1)}{12}}}$$

$$= \frac{296 - 390}{\sqrt{3705}} = \frac{-94}{60.87} = -1.54$$

Based on the normal distribution (see Table A-4), the probability of this outcome occurring by chance is 0.062. Since this value is larger than 0.05, the null hypothesis would not be rejected.

MINITAB: After the data for the two groups (the second and third graders and the fourth, fifth, and sixth graders) are in columns C1 and C2, issue the following command:

MANN-WHITNEY C1 C2

Minitab assigns ranks, computes the statistic (which it labels W rather than U), and indicates the level of confidence at which the statistic is significant.

ANSWER: The typical second or third grader did not have a higher frequency of interjection than the typical fourth, fifth, or sixth grader (Mann-Whitney U Test; alpha = 0.05).

REMARK: This computational procedure is appropriate when the number of subjects in the larger groups is more than twenty. For appropriate computational procedures when this number is twenty or smaller, see Siegel (1956, 1988).

EXERCISE: Determine whether the typical (i.e., median) second or third grader had a higher frequency of part-word repetition than did the typical fourth, fifth, or sixth grader through the use of the Mann-Whitney U Test. (The value you compute for Z should be approximately -1.40.)

3. Friedman Two-Way Analysis of Variance (χ_r^2)

QUESTION: Did the second graders tend to produce higher frequencies of some of the four disfluency types (i.e., interjection, part-word repetition, word repetition, and revision-incomplete phrase) than of others?

The first step in performing a Friedman Two-Way Analysis of Variance is selecting an *alpha* level, or a maximum acceptable probability for a *Type I* error (i.e., concluding that there was a tendency for the second graders to produce higher frequencies of some of the disfluency types than of others when there was no such tendency). A 0.05 alpha level will be used for this test.

The next step is to compute the value of χ_r^2. Each second grader's disfluency frequencies for interjection, part-word repetition, word repetition, and revision-incomplete phrase are ordered from lowest to highest. The rank is then assigned to each that designates its position in the ordering (1 is assigned to the lowest frequency, 2 to the second lowest frequency, and so on). If more than one disfluency type has the same frequency, each is assigned the mean of the tied ranks. The ranks assigned to the fifteen second graders, based on the frequencies of the four disfluency types they produced (see p. 292), are as follows:

Subject Number	I	PW	W	R-IP
1	1.5	3.0	1.5	4.0
2	3.0	2.0	1.0	4.0
3	3.0	1.5	1.5	4.0
4	1.5	3.0	1.5	4.0
5	1.0	3.0	2.0	4.0
6	1.0	2.5	2.5	4.0
7	1.5	1.5	3.0	4.0
8	1.0	4.0	2.0	3.0
9	1.0	3.0	2.0	4.0
10	1.0	2.0	3.0	4.0
11	4.0	1.0	2.0	3.0
12	2.0	2.0	2.0	4.0
13	3.0	1.0	2.0	4.0
14	1.5	1.5	3.0	4.0
15	3.0	1.0	2.0	4.0
R_j	29.0	32.0	31.0	58.0

The formula for computing the value of χ_r^2 is:

$$\chi_r^2 = \frac{12}{Nk(k+1)} \sum_{j=1}^{k} \left(R_j\right)^2 - 3N(k+1)$$

where

$R_j =$ a column sum (i.e., total)
$N =$ number of rows
$k =$ number of columns

The value of χ_r^2 for these data is:

$$\chi_r^2 = \frac{12}{(15)(4)(4+1)} \left[(29)^2 + (32)^2 + (31)^2 + (58)^2\right] - (3)(15)(4+1)$$

$$= \frac{12}{300}(6190) - 225$$

$$= 247.6 - 225.0 = 22.6$$

To determine whether this value of χ_r^2 is large enough for the null hypothesis to be rejected, the value of chi square required for rejection is located in Table A-2. The degrees of freedom *(df)* here would be 3 (i.e., the number of columns minus one). The value of chi square required for rejection at the 0.05 alpha level when *(df)* = 3 is 7.82. Since the value computed is larger than this (i.e., 22.6), the null hypothesis would be rejected.

MINITAB: Data are entered into the first three columns and the first 60 rows of the Data Window spreadsheet. The number 1 should be entered into first 15 rows of the first column (C1), the number 2 into rows 16 through 30, the number 3 into rows 31 through 45, and the number 4 into rows 46 through 60. The numbers 1 through 15 should be entered into the first 15 rows of the second column (C2), as well as the second 15, third 15, and final 15. Consequently, the sequence 1 through 15 is repeated four times in C2. The 60 disfluency frequencies should be entered in the third column (C3). The interjection frequencies should be in rows 1 through 15 of C3 , the part-word repetition frequencies in rows 16 through 30, the word repetition frequencies in rows 31 through 45, and the revision-incomplete phrase frequencies in rows 46 through 60. Next, the following command should be issued:

FRIEDMAN C3 C1 C2

The probability that the differences in the frequencies of the four disfluency types are due to chance is displayed on the screen.

ANSWER: The second graders tended to produce higher frequencies of some of the disfluency types than of others (Friedman Two-Way Analysis of Variance; alpha = 0.05).

EXERCISE: Determine whether the third graders tended to produce higher frequencies of some of the four disfluency types than of the others through the use of the Friedman Two-Way Analysis of Variance. (The value you compute should be approximately 12.74.)

4. Kruskal-Wallis One-Way Analysis of Variance

QUESTION: Was there a tendency for the amount of part-word repetition produced by the children to vary as a function of grade level?

The first step in performing a Kruskal-Wallis One-Way Analysis of Variance is selecting an *alpha* level, or a maximum acceptable probability for a *Type I* error (i.e., concluding that there was a tendency for the amount of part-word repetition produced by the children to vary as a function of grade level when there was not such tendency). A 0.05 alpha level will be used for this test.

The next step is to compute the value of H. First, the 56 children are ordered on the basis of their part-word repetition frequency. The rank is then assigned to each that represents his or her position in the ordering (1 is assigned to the child with the lowest frequency, 2 to the child with the second lowest frequency, and so on). If more than one child has the same frequency, each is assigned the mean of the tied ranks. The ranks assigned to the children in each grade are as follows:

Second	Third	Fourth	Fifth	Sixth
4.0	4.0	8.0	4.0	4.0
4.0	14.5	12.0	9.0	4.0
4.0	21.5	26.0	11.0	10.0
16.0	32.0	30.0	17.5	13.0
17.5	37.0	43.5	24.0	14.5
19.0	40.0	45.0	25.0	21.5
20.0	41.0	50.0	28.0	23.0
36.0	47.0	51.0	29.0	27.0
38.0	48.0	55.0	31.0	33.0
39.0	49.0		34.5	34.5
42.0	56.0		52.0	
43.5				
46.0				
53.0				
54.0				
$R_j = 436.0$	390.0	320.5	265.0	184.5

The formula for computing the value of H is:

$$H = \frac{12}{N(N + 1)} \sum_{j=1}^{k} \frac{R_j^2}{n_j} - 3(N + 1)$$

where

R_j = a column sum (i.e., total)
N = the total number of subjects
n_j = the number of subjects in a column

The value of *H* for these data is:

$$H = 12/56(56 + 1)[(436)^2/15 + (390)^2/11 + (320.5)^2/9 + (265)^2/11 +$$
$$(184.5)^2/10] - 3(56 + 1)$$

$$= 0.003759[47,701.81] - 171$$

$$= 8.31$$

To determine whether the value of H is large enough for the null hypothesis to be rejected, the value of H required for rejection is located in Table A-2. (H is distributed as chi square, provided that the number of groups is greater than 3 and there are more than 5 subjects in each of the groups.) The degrees of freedom *(df)* here would be 4 (i.e., the number of columns minus one). The value of chi square required for rejection at the 0.05 alpha level when *df* = 4 is 9.49. Since the value of H computed is smaller than this (i.e., 8.31), the null hypothesis would not be rejected.

MINITAB: Data are entered into the first two columns and the first 56 rows of the Data Window spreadsheet. The 56 part-word repetition frequencies should be entered in the first column (C1). The number designating the grade of the child contributing each frequency should be inserted beside it in column two (C2):1 should be entered for second graders, the number 2 for third graders, the number 3 for fourth graders, and the number 4 for fifth graders. Next, the following command should be issued:

KRUSKAL-WALLIS C1 C2

The probability that the differences in the frequencies of part-word repetition are due to chance is displayed on the screen.

ANSWER: There wasn't a tendency for the amount of part-word repetition produced by the children to vary as a function of grade level (Kruskal-Wallis One-Way Analysis of Variance; alpha = 0.05).

EXERCISE: Determine whether there was a tendency for the amount of word repetition produced by the children to vary as a function of grade level through the use of the Kruskal-Wallis One-Way Analysis of Variance.

Inferential Statistical Tests: Interval and Ratio Data

1. t-Test for Related Measures

QUESTION: Did the children on the average tend to produce higher frequencies of interjection than of part-word repetition?

The first step in performing a t-test for related measures is selecting an *alpha* level, or a maximum acceptable probability for a *Type I* error (i.e., concluding that the children on the average tended to produce higher frequencies of interjection than of part-word repetition when there was no such tendency). A 0.05 alpha level will be used for this test. Since to answer the question it only would be necessary to detect a difference between interjection frequency and part-word repetition frequency in one direction, the region of rejection for the test will be *one tailed*.

The next step is to compute the value of *t*. Each child's part-word repetition frequency is subtracted from his or her interjection frequency (see Table A-1). If the part-word repetition frequency is smaller than the interjection frequency, this difference is assigned a + sign. If the part-word repetition frequency is larger than the interjection frequency, this difference is assigned a − sign. The difference frequencies for the 56 children are as follows:

Subject	Difference (D)	Subject	Difference (D)
1	−0.66	29	−2.41
2	+0.71	30	−0.32
3	+1.40	31	−0.73
4	−0.81	32	−0.12
5	−0.63	33	+0.21
6	−0.35	34	−1.21
7	0.00	35	+2.84
8	−1.90	36	0.00
9	−1.50	37	−0.66
10	−1.50	38	+1.61
11	+8.19	39	+0.18
12	0.00	40	+0.14
13	+1.17	41	+1.99
14	0.00	42	+0.91
15	+1.87	43	+0.51
16	−0.68	44	−0.54
17	+2.65	45	+1.21
18	+0.74	46	+0.18
19	−0.66	47	−0.28
20	+0.49	48	−0.19
21	−0.36	49	+1.99
22	−3.87	50	−0.47
23	+0.56	51	−0.93
24	−0.13	52	+0.69
25	+1.89	53	−0.66
26	+0.90	54	−0.18
27	−1.10	55	+0.52
28	−0.63	56	−0.11

The following are computed from these difference frequencies:

ΣD = the algebraic difference between the sum of the differences that have plus signs and the sum of the differences that have minus signs = 33.55 (i.e., plus sum) − 22.59 (i.e., minus sum) = 10.96

$\overline{D}$ = The mean of the algebraic sum of the differences = 10.96/56 = 0.196

ΣD^2 = The sum of the squared difference frequencies = 144.596

The value of t here is:

$$t = \frac{\overline{D}\sqrt{N-1}}{\sqrt{\dfrac{\Sigma D^2}{N} - \overline{D}^2}}$$

$$= \frac{0.196\sqrt{56-1}}{\sqrt{\dfrac{144.596}{56} - (0.196)^2}}$$

$$= \frac{0.196(7.416)}{\sqrt{2.582 - 0.038}} = \frac{1.454}{1.579}$$

$$= 0.92$$

To determine whether this value of t is large enough for the null hypothesis to be rejected, the value of t required for rejection is located in Table A-5. The degrees of freedom *(df)* here would be 55 (i.e., the number of subjects minus one). The value of t required for rejection at 0.05 alpha level when $df = 55$ is 1.67. Since the value computed—0.92—is smaller than this, the null hypothesis would not be rejected.

MINITAB: Data are entered into the first two columns and the first 56 rows of the Data Window spreadsheet. The 56 part-word repetition frequencies should be entered in the first column (C1)and the 56 interjection frequencies in the second column (C2) . Next, the following commands should be issued:

```
LET C3 = C1 - C2
TTEST C3
ALTERNATIVE = -1
```

The value used for the alternative subcommand was –1 because it was desired to determine if the children's interjection frequencies tended to be larger than their part-word repetition frequencies: If it had been desired to determine whether their part-word repetition frequencies tended to be higher than their interjection frequencies, the value used for the alternative subcommand would have been +1.

The probability that the differences in the frequencies of part-word repetition and interjection frequencies are due to chance is displayed on the screen.

ANSWER: The children on the average did not tend to produce higher frequencies of interjection than of part-word repetition (*t*-test for related measures; alpha = 0.05).

EXERCISE: Determine whether the children on the average exhibited a tendency to produce higher frequencies of revision-incomplete phrase than of word repetition through the use of the *t*-test for related measures. (The value of t you compute should be approximately 9.88.)

2. t-Test for Independent Measures

QUESTION: Did the second and third graders tend to produce higher frequencies of interjection on the average than the fourth, fifth, and sixth graders?

TABLE A-5   Table of critical values of *t*.*

df	Level of significance for one-tailed test					
	.10	.05	.025	.01	.005	.0005
	Level of significance for two-tailed test					
	.20	.10	.05	.02	.01	.001
1	3.078	6.314	12.706	31.821	63.657	636.619
2	1.886	2.920	4.303	6.965	9.925	31.598
3	1.638	2.353	3.182	4.541	5.841	12.941
4	1.533	2.132	2.776	3.747	4.604	8.610
5	1.476	2.015	2.571	3.365	4.032	6.859
6	1.440	1.943	2.447	3.143	3.707	5.959
7	1.415	1.895	2.365	2.998	3.499	5.405
8	1.397	1.860	2.306	2.896	3.355	5.041
9	1.383	1.833	2.262	2.821	3.250	4.781
10	1.372	1.812	2.228	2.764	3.169	4.587
11	1.363	1.796	2.201	2.718	3.106	4.437
12	1.356	1.782	2.179	2.681	3.055	4.318
13	1.350	1.771	2.160	2.650	3.012	4.221
14	1.345	1.761	2.145	2.624	2.977	4.140
15	1.341	1.753	2.131	2.602	2.947	4.073
16	1.337	1.746	2.120	2.583	2.921	4.015
17	1.333	1.740	2.110	2.567	2.898	3.965
18	1.330	1.734	2.101	2.552	2.878	3.922
19	1.328	1.729	2.093	2.539	2.861	3.883
20	1.325	1.725	2.086	2.528	2.845	3.850
21	1.323	1.721	2.080	2.518	2.831	3.819
22	1.321	1.717	2.074	2.508	2.819	3.792
23	1.319	1.714	2.069	2.500	2.807	3.767
24	1.318	1.711	2.064	2.492	2.797	3.745
25	1.316	1.708	2.060	2.485	2.787	3.725
26	1.315	1.706	2.056	2.479	2.779	3.707
27	1.314	1.703	2.052	2.473	2.771	3.690
28	1.313	1.701	2.048	2.467	2.763	3.674
29	1.311	1.699	2.045	2.462	2.756	3.659
30	1.310	1.697	2.042	2.457	2.750	3.646
40	1.303	1.684	2.021	2.423	2.704	3.551
60	1.296	1.671	2.000	2.390	2.660	3.460
120	1.289	1.658	1.980	2.358	2.617	3.373
∞	1.282	1.645	1.960	2.326	2.576	3.291

*Adapted from Table III of Fisher and Yates. Statistical Tables for Biological, Agricultural, and Medical Research (6th edition). Copyright 1974 by Longman Group, Ltd. With permission of Longman Group, Ltd.

The first step in performing a *t*-test for independent measures is selecting an *alpha* level, or maximum acceptable probability for a *Type I* error (i.e., concluding that the second and third graders tended to produce higher frequencies of interjection on the average than the fourth, fifth, and sixth graders when there was no such tendency). A 0.05 alpha level will be used for this test. Since to answer the question it only would be necessary to detect a difference between second and third graders and fourth, fifth, and sixth graders in one direction, the region of rejection for the test will be *one-tailed*.

The next step is to compute the value for *t*. The following values are computed from the interjection frequencies in Table A-1 for each group of children:

<table>
<tr><td>2nd and 3rd Grade</td><td>4th, 5th, and 6th Grade</td></tr>
<tr><td>$n_1 = 26$</td><td>$n_2 = 30$</td></tr>
<tr><td>$\Sigma X_1 = 34.50$</td><td>$\Sigma X_2 = 23.21$</td></tr>
<tr><td>$\overline{X}_1 = 1.33$</td><td>$\overline{X}_2 = 0.77$</td></tr>
<tr><td>$\Sigma X_1^2 = 124.02$</td><td>$\Sigma X_2^2 = 42.91$</td></tr>
</table>

$$S_1^2 = \frac{\Sigma X_1^2}{N_1} - \overline{X}_1^2 \qquad\qquad S_2^2 = \frac{\Sigma X_2^2}{N_2} - \overline{X}_2^2$$

$$= \frac{124.02}{26} - (1.33)^2 \qquad\qquad = \frac{42.91}{30} - (0.77)^2$$

$$= 4.77 - 1.77 = 3.00 \qquad\qquad = 1.43 = 0.59 = 0.84$$

The value of *t* here would be:

$$t = \frac{\overline{X}_1 - \overline{X}_2}{\sqrt{\frac{n_1 S_1^2 + n_2 S_2^2}{n_1 + n_2 - 2}\left(\frac{1}{n_1} + \frac{1}{n_2}\right)}}$$

$$= \frac{1.33 - 0.77}{\sqrt{\frac{(26)(3.00) + (30)(0.84)}{26 + 30 - 2}\left(\frac{1}{26} + \frac{1}{30}\right)}}$$

$$= \frac{0.56}{\sqrt{\frac{103.2}{54}(0.07)}}$$

$$= \frac{0.56}{\sqrt{0.1337777}} = \frac{0.56}{0.37}$$

$$= 1.51$$

To determine whether the value of *t* is large enough for the null hypothesis to be rejected, the value of *t* required for rejection is located in Table A-5. The degrees of freedom *(df)* here would be 54 (i.e., the number of subjects minus two). The value of *t* required for rejection at the 0.05 alpha level when *df* = 54 is 1.67. Since the value computed—i.e., 1.51—is smaller than this, the null hypothesis would not be rejected.

MINITAB: Data are entered into the first two columns of the Data Window spreadsheet. The second and third graders' interjection frequencies should be entered in the first column (C1)and the fourth, fifth, and sixth graders' interjection frequencies in the second column (C2). Next, the following command and subcommand should be issued:

```
TWOSAMPLE C1 C2
ALTERNATIVE = +1
```

The value used for the alternative subcommand was +1 because it was desired to determine if the second and third graders tended to be higher interjection frequencies than the fourth, fifth, and sixth graders: If it had been desired to determine whether their interjection frequencies tended to be lower, the value used for the alternative subcommand would have been –1.

The probability that the differences in the frequencies of part-word repetition and interjection frequencies are due to chance is displayed on the screen.

ANSWER: The second and third graders did not tend to produce higher frequencies of interjection on the average than the fourth, fifth, and sixth graders (*t*-test for independent measures; alpha = 0.05).

EXERCISE: Determine whether the second and third graders tended to produce higher frequencies of part-word repetition on the average than the fourth, fifth, and sixth graders through the use of the *t*-test for independent measures. (The value of *t* you compute should be approximately 1.52.)

3. *t-Test for the Significance of Pearson Product-Moment Correlation Coefficients*

QUESTION: Was there any relationship between the children's interjection frequencies and part-word repetition frequencies during their performances of the spontaneous speech task?

The first step in performing a *t*-test for the significance of the Pearson product-moment correlation coefficient *(r)* is selecting an *alpha* level, or a maximum acceptable probability for a *Type I* error (i.e., concluding that there was a relationship between the children's interjection frequencies and part-word repetition frequencies when there was no such relationship). A 0.05 alpha level will be used for this test. Since to answer this question it would be necessary to detect both positive and negative relationships between interjection frequency and part-word repetition frequency, the region of rejection for the test will be *two-tailed*.

The next step is to compute the value of *t*. The Pearson product-moment correlation coefficient for the relationship between interjection frequency and part-word repetition frequency is –0.02 (see p. 303). The value of *t* here would be:

$$t = \frac{r}{\sqrt{1 - r^2}} \sqrt{N - 2}$$

$$= \frac{-0.02}{\sqrt{1 - (-0.02)^2}} \sqrt{56 - 2}$$

$$= \frac{-0.2}{\sqrt{1 - 0.0004}} \sqrt{54}$$

$$= \frac{-0.02}{0.9998} \, 7.3485 = (-0.0200)(7.3485)$$

$$= -0.1470$$

To determine whether this value of t is large enough for the null hypothesis to be rejected, the value of t required for rejection is located in Table A-5. The degrees of freedom *(df)* here would be 54 (i.e., the number of subjects minus two). The value of t required for rejection at the 0.05 alpha level, when $df = 54$ and the region of rejection is two-tailed, is 2.00. Since the value computed, –0.147, is smaller than this, the null hypothesis would not be rejected.

MINITAB: Enter the correlation coefficient *(r)* in the top row of the first column (C1) and the number of subjects *(N)* in the top row of the second column (C2) of the Data Window spreadsheet. Next, the following command should be issued:

```
LET C3 = (C1 / SQRT (1 - C1**2)) (SQRT (C2 - 2))
```

The value for t is displayed on the screen. To determine whether it is large enough for the null hypothesis to be rejected, the value of t required for rejection is located in Table A-5.

ANSWER: There was no relationship between the children's interjection frequencies and part-word repetition frequencies during their performance of the spontaneous speech task (t-test for a Pearson product-moment correlation coefficient; alpha = 0.05).

EXERCISE: Determine whether there was any relationship between the children's word repetition frequencies and revision-incomplete phrase frequencies during their performance of the spontaneous speech task through the use of the t-test for the significance of Pearson product-moment correlation coefficients. (The value of t you compute should be approximately 3.02.)

3. Analysis of Variance (F-Test) for Dependent Measures

QUESTION: Did the second graders on the average tend to produce higher frequencies of some of the four disfluency types (i.e., interjection, part-word repetition, word repetition, and revision-incomplete phrase) than of the others?

The first step in performing an analysis of variance for dependent measures *(F)* is selecting an *alpha* level, or a maximum acceptable probability for a *Type I* error (i.e., concluding that there was a tendency for the second graders on the average to produce higher frequencies of some of the four disfluency types than of others when there was no such tendency). A 0.05 alpha level will be used for this test.

The next step is to compute the value of F. The sums of the second grader's four disfluency frequencies (T) and the square of the sum of their four disfluency frequencies divided by the number of disfluency frequencies summed $(T^2/4)$ based on Table A-1 are as follows:

Subject	T_r	$T_r^2/4$
1	4.32	4.666
2	9.57	22.896
3	6.54	10.693
4	3.63	3.294
5	4.40	4.840
6	2.44	1.488
7	4.49	5.040
8	5.69	8.094
9	8.09	16.362
10	8.99	20.205
11	13.99	48.930
12	4.68	5.476
13	6.73	11.323
14	2.52	1.588
15	4.86	5.905
	$T_r = 90.94$	$\Sigma T_r^2/4 = 170.800$

The following computations are them made from the frequencies in each column—that is, the disfluency frequencies of each of the four types produced by the fifteen second graders.

Measure	I	PW	W	R-IP	
T_c	19.27	12.28	12.63	46.76	$T = 90.34$
$\overline{X}_c$	1.285	0.819	0.842	3.117	
$T_c^2/15$	24.756	10.053	10.634	145.766	$\Sigma T_c^2/15 = 191.209$
ΣX^2	87.164	17.100	15.680	183.938	$\Sigma\Sigma X^2 = 303.782$

Next, four sum of square (SS) are computed from these row and column data analyses. The first is the sum of squares (SS) for columns (c), or disfluency types.

$$SS_c = \frac{\Sigma T_c^2}{r} - \frac{T^2}{cr}$$

$$= 191.209 - \frac{(90.94)^2}{(4)(15)}$$

$$= 191.209 - 137.835 = 53.374$$

The second is the sum of squares *(SS)* for rows *(r)*, or subjects.

$$SS_r = \frac{\Sigma T_r^2}{c} - \frac{T^2}{cr}$$

$$= 170.800 - \frac{(90.94)^2}{(4)(15)}$$

$$= 170.800 - 137.835 = 32.965$$

The third is the total *(T)* sum of squares.

$$SS_T = \Sigma\Sigma X^2 - \frac{T^2}{cr} = 303.782 - \frac{(90.94)^2}{(4)(15)}$$

$$= 303.782 - 137.835 = 165.947$$

The fourth is the residual sum of squares (labeled SS_{cr}), which is assumed to represent random measurement error.

$$SS_{cr} = SS_T - SS_c - SS_r = 165.947 - 53.374 - 32.965$$

$$= 79.608$$

The value of *F* can be computed by means of the following formula:

$$F = \frac{SS_c/c - 1}{SS_{cr}/(c - 1)(r - 1)}$$

where $c - 1$ is the degrees of freedom for SS_c and $(c - 1)(r - 1)$ is the degrees of freedom for SS_{cr}. The first is df_1 and the second df_2 (see Table A-6).

The value of *F* here is:

$$F = \frac{53.374/3}{79.608 / 42} = \frac{17.791}{1.895} = 9.39$$

To determine whether the value of *F* is large enough for the null hypothesis to be rejected, the value of *F* required for rejection is located in Table A-6. There are two degrees of freedom: df_1 would be 3 (i.e., the number of columns minus one) and df_2 would be 42 (i.e., the number of columns minus one times the number of rows minus one). The value of *F* required for rejection at the 0.05 alpha level when $df_1 = 3$ and $df_2 = 42$ is 2.84. Since the value computed—that is, 9.39—exceeds this value, the null hypothesis would be rejected.

MINITAB: Data are entered into the first three columns and the first 60 rows of the Data Window spreadsheet. The 60 disfluency frequencies should be entered in the first column (C1). A number for designating the type of disfluency should be inserted beside each in column two (C2): 1 should be entered for interjections, 2 for part-word repetitions, 3 for word repetitions, and 4 for revisions-incomplete phrases. A number from 1 to 15 designating the sub-

TABLE A-6   Percent points in the distribution of F.*

df₂ \ df₁		1	2	3	4	5	6	8	12	24	∞
1	0.1%	405284	500000	540379	562500	576405	585937	598144	610667	623497	636619
	0.5%	16211	20000	21615	22500	23056	23437	23925	24426	24940	25465
	1 %	4052	4999	5403	5625	5764	5859	5981	6106	6234	6366
	2.5%	647.79	799.50	864.16	899.58	921.85	937.11	956.66	976.71	997.25	1018.30
	5 %	161.45	199.50	215.71	224.58	230.16	233.99	238.88	243.91	249.05	254.32
	10 %	39.86	49.50	53.59	55.83	57.24	58.20	59.44	60.70	62.00	63.33
	20 %	9.47	12.00	13.06	13.73	14.01	14.26	14.59	14.90	15.24	15.58
2	0.1	998.5	999.0	999.2	999.2	999.3	999.3	999.4	999.4	999.5	999.5
	0.5	198.50	199.00	199.17	199.25	199.30	199.33	199.37	199.42	199.46	199.51
	1	98.49	99.00	99.17	99.25	99.30	99.33	99.36	99.42	99.46	99.50
	2.5	38.51	39.00	39.17	39.25	39.30	39.33	39.37	39.42	39.46	39.50
	5	18.51	19.00	19.16	19.25	19.30	19.33	19.37	19.41	19.45	19.50
	10	8.53	9.00	9.16	9.24	9.29	9.33	9.37	9.41	9.45	9.49
	20	3.56	4.00	4.16	4.24	4.28	4.32	4.36	4.40	4.44	4.48
3	0.1	167.5	148.5	141.1	137.1	134.6	132.8	130.6	128.3	125.9	123.5
	0.5	55.55	49.80	47.47	46.20	45.39	44.84	44.13	43.39	42.62	41.83
	1	34.12	30.81	29.46	28.71	28.24	27.91	27.49	27.05	26.60	26.12
	2.5	17.44	16.04	15.44	15.10	14.89	14.74	14.54	14.34	14.12	13.90
	5	10.13	9.55	9.28	9.12	9.01	8.94	8.84	8.74	8.64	8.53
	10	5.54	5.46	5.39	5.34	5.31	5.28	5.25	5.22	5.18	5.13
	20	2.68	2.89	2.94	2.96	2.97	2.97	2.98	2.98	2.98	2.98
4	0.1	74.14	61.25	56.18	53.44	51.71	50.53	49.00	47.41	45.77	44.05
	0.5	31.33	26.28	24.26	23.16	22.46	21.98	21.35	20.71	20.03	19.33
	1	21.20	18.00	16.69	15.98	15.52	15.21	14.80	14.37	13.93	13.46
	2.5	12.22	10.65	9.98	9.60	9.36	9.20	8.98	8.75	8.51	8.26
	5	7.71	6.94	6.59	6.39	6.26	6.16	6.04	5.91	5.77	5.63
	10	4.54	4.32	4.19	4.11	4.05	4.01	3.95	3.90	3.83	3.76
	20	2.35	2.47	2.48	2.48	2.48	2.47	2.47	2.46	2.44	2.43
5	0.1	47.04	36.61	33.20	31.09	29.75	28.84	27.64	26.42	25.14	23.78
	0.5	22.79	18.31	16.53	15.56	14.94	14.51	13.96	13.38	12.78	12.14
	1	16.26	13.27	12.06	11.39	10.97	10.67	10.29	9.89	9.47	9.02
	2.5	10.01	8.43	7.76	7.39	7.15	6.98	6.76	6.52	6.28	6.02
	5	6.61	5.79	5.41	5.19	5.05	4.95	4.82	4.68	4.53	4.36
	10	4.06	3.78	3.62	3.52	3.45	3.40	3.34	3.27	3.19	3.10
	20	2.18	2.26	2.25	2.24	2.23	2.22	2.20	2.18	2.16	2.13
6	0.1	35.51	27.00	23.70	21.90	20.81	20.03	19.03	17.99	16.89	15.75
	0.5	18.64	14.54	12.92	12.03	11.46	11.07	10.57	10.03	9.47	8.88
	1	13.74	10.92	9.78	9.15	8.75	8.47	8.10	7.72	7.31	6.88
	2.5	8.81	7.26	6.60	6.23	5.99	5.82	5.60	5.37	5.12	4.85
	5	5.99	5.14	4.76	4.53	4.39	4.28	4.15	4.00	3.84	3.67
	10	3.78	3.46	3.29	3.18	3.11	3.05	2.98	2.90	2.82	2.72
	20	2.07	2.13	2.11	2.09	2.08	2.06	2.04	2.02	1.99	1.95
7	0.1	29.22	21.69	18.77	17.19	16.21	15.52	14.63	13.71	12.73	11.69
	0.5	16.24	12.40	10.88	10.05	9.52	9.16	8.68	8.18	7.65	7.08
	1	12.25	9.55	8.45	7.85	7.46	7.19	6.84	6.47	6.07	5.65
	2.5	8.07	6.54	5.89	5.52	5.29	5.12	4.90	4.67	4.42	4.14
	5	5.59	4.74	4.35	4.12	3.97	3.87	3.73	3.57	3.41	3.23
	10	3.59	3.26	3.07	2.96	2.88	2.83	2.75	2.67	2.58	2.47
	20	2.00	2.04	2.02	1.99	1.97	1.96	1.93	1.91	1.87	1.83
8	0.1	25.42	18.49	15.83	14.39	13.49	12.86	12.04	11.19	10.30	9.34
	0.5	14.69	11.04	9.60	8.81	8.30	7.95	7.50	7.01	6.50	5.95
	1	11.26	8.65	7.59	7.01	6.63	6.37	6.03	5.67	5.28	4.86
	2.5	7.57	6.06	5.42	5.05	4.82	4.65	4.43	4.20	3.95	3.67
	5	5.32	4.46	4.07	3.84	3.69	3.58	3.44	3.28	3.12	2.93
	10	3.46	3.11	2.92	2.81	2.73	2.67	2.59	2.50	2.40	2.29
	20	1.95	1.98	1.95	1.92	1.90	1.88	1.86	1.83	1.79	1.74
9	0.1	22.86	16.39	13.90	12.56	11.71	11.13	10.37	9.57	8.72	7.81
	0.5	13.61	10.11	8.72	7.96	7.47	7.13	6.69	6.23	5.73	5.19
	1	10.56	8.02	6.99	6.42	6.03	5.80	5.47	5.11	4.73	4.31
	2.5	7.21	5.71	5.08	4.72	4.48	4.32	4.10	3.87	3.61	3.33
	5	5.12	4.26	3.86	3.63	3.48	3.37	3.23	3.07	2.90	2.71
	10	3.36	3.01	2.81	2.69	2.61	2.55	2.47	2.38	2.28	2.16
	20	1.91	1.94	1.90	1.87	1.85	1.83	1.80	1.76	1.72	1.67

Adapted from Table V of Fisher and Yates: Statistical Tables for Biological, Agricultural, and Medical Research *(6th edition). Copyright 1974 by Longman Group, Ltd. With permission of Longman Group, Ltd. The 0.5% and 2.5% points are reprinted by permission of the Biometrika Trustees from* Biometrika, *volume 33 (April, 1943), pp. 73–78.*

TABLE A-6   *Continued*

df_2 \ df_1		1	2	3	4	5	6	8	12	24	∞
10	0.1%	21.04	14.91	12.55	11.28	10.48	9.92	9.20	8.45	7.64	6.76
	0.5%	12.83	9.43	8.08	7.34	6.87	6.54	6.12	5.66	5.17	4.64
	1%	10.04	7.56	6.55	5.99	5.64	5.39	5.06	4.71	4.33	3.91
	2.5%	6.94	5.46	4.83	4.47	4.24	4.07	3.85	3.62	3.37	3.08
	5%	4.96	4.10	3.71	3.48	3.33	3.22	3.07	2.91	2.74	2.54
	10%	3.28	2.92	2.73	2.61	2.52	2.46	2.38	2.28	2.18	2.06
	20%	1.88	1.90	1.86	1.83	1.80	1.78	1.75	1.72	1.67	1.62
11	0.1	19.69	13.81	11.56	10.35	9.58	9.05	8.35	7.63	6.85	6.00
	0.5	12.23	8.91	7.60	6.88	6.42	6.10	5.68	5.24	4.76	4.23
	1	9.65	7.20	6.22	5.67	5.32	5.07	4.74	4.40	4.02	3.60
	2.5	6.72	5.26	4.63	4.28	4.04	3.88	3.66	3.43	3.17	2.88
	5	4.84	3.98	3.59	3.36	3.20	3.09	2.95	2.79	2.61	2.40
	10	3.23	2.86	2.66	2.54	2.45	2.39	2.30	2.21	2.10	1.97
	20	1.86	1.87	1.83	1.80	1.77	1.75	1.72	1.68	1.63	1.57
12	0.1	18.64	12.97	10.80	9.63	8.89	8.38	7.71	7.00	6.25	5.42
	0.5	11.75	8.51	7.23	6.52	6.07	5.76	5.35	4.91	4.43	3.90
	1	9.33	6.93	5.95	5.41	5.06	4.82	4.50	4.16	3.78	3.36
	2.5	6.55	5.10	4.47	4.12	3.89	3.73	3.51	3.28	3.02	2.72
	5	4.75	3.88	3.49	3.26	3.11	3.00	2.85	2.69	2.50	2.30
	10	3.18	2.81	2.61	2.48	2.39	2.33	2.24	2.15	2.04	1.90
	20	1.84	1.85	1.80	1.77	1.74	1.72	1.69	1.65	1.60	1.54
13	0.1	17.81	12.31	10.21	9.07	8.35	7.86	7.21	6.52	5.78	4.97
	0.5	11.37	8.19	6.93	6.23	5.79	5.48	5.08	4.64	4.17	3.65
	1	9.07	6.70	5.74	5.20	4.86	4.62	4.30	3.96	3.59	3.16
	2.5	6.41	4.97	4.35	4.00	3.77	3.60	3.39	3.15	2.89	2.60
	5	4.67	3.80	3.41	3.18	3.02	2.92	2.77	2.60	2.42	2.21
	10	3.14	2.76	2.56	2.43	2.35	2.28	2.20	2.10	1.98	1.85
	20	1.82	1.83	1.78	1.75	1.72	1.69	1.66	1.62	1.57	1.51
14	0.1	17.14	11.78	9.73	8.62	7.92	7.43	6.80	6.13	5.41	4.60
	0.5	11.06	7.92	6.68	6.00	5.56	5.26	4.86	4.43	3.96	3.44
	1	8.86	6.51	5.56	5.03	4.69	4.46	4.14	3.80	3.43	3.00
	2.5	6.30	4.86	4.24	3.89	3.66	3.50	3.29	3.05	2.79	2.49
	5	4.60	3.74	3.34	3.11	2.96	2.85	2.70	2.53	2.35	2.13
	10	3.10	2.73	2.52	2.39	2.31	2.24	2.15	2.05	1.94	1.80
	20	1.81	1.81	1.76	1.73	1.70	1.67	1.64	1.60	1.55	1.48
15	0.1	16.59	11.34	9.34	8.25	7.57	7.09	6.47	5.81	5.10	4.31
	0.5	10.80	7.70	6.48	5.80	5.37	5.07	4.67	4.25	3.79	3.26
	1	8.68	6.36	5.42	4.89	4.56	4.32	4.00	3.67	3.29	2.87
	2.5	6.20	4.77	4.15	3.80	3.58	3.41	3.20	2.96	2.70	2.40
	5	4.54	3.68	3.29	3.06	2.90	2.79	2.64	2.48	2.29	2.07
	10	3.07	2.70	2.49	2.36	2.27	2.21	2.12	2.02	1.90	1.76
	20	1.80	1.79	1.75	1.71	1.68	1.66	1.62	1.58	1.53	1.46
16	0.1	16.12	10.97	9.00	7.94	7.27	6.81	6.19	5.55	4.85	4.06
	0.5	10.58	7.51	6.30	5.64	5.21	4.91	4.52	4.10	3.64	3.11
	1	8.53	6.23	5.29	4.77	4.44	4.20	3.89	3.55	3.18	2.75
	2.5	6.12	4.69	4.08	3.73	3.50	3.34	3.12	2.89	2.63	2.32
	5	4.49	3.63	3.24	3.01	2.85	2.74	2.59	2.42	2.24	2.01
	10	3.05	2.67	2.46	2.33	2.24	2.18	2.09	1.99	1.87	1.72
	20	1.79	1.78	1.74	1.70	1.67	1.64	1.61	1.56	1.51	1.43
17	0.1	15.72	10.66	8.73	7.68	7.02	6.56	5.96	5.32	4.63	3.85
	0.5	10.38	7.35	6.16	5.50	5.07	4.78	4.39	3.97	3.51	2.98
	1	8.40	6.11	5.18	4.67	4.34	4.10	3.79	3.45	3.08	2.65
	2.5	6.04	4.62	4.01	3.66	3.44	3.28	3.06	2.82	2.56	2.25
	5	4.45	3.59	3.20	2.96	2.81	2.70	2.55	2.38	2.19	1.96
	10	3.03	2.64	2.44	2.31	2.22	2.15	2.06	1.96	1.84	1.69
	20	1.78	1.77	1.72	1.68	1.65	1.63	1.59	1.55	1.49	1.42
18	0.1	15.38	10.39	8.49	7.46	6.81	6.35	5.76	5.13	4.45	3.67
	0.5	10.22	7.21	6.03	5.37	4.96	4.66	4.28	3.86	3.40	2.87
	1	8.28	6.01	5.09	4.58	4.25	4.01	3.71	3.37	3.00	2.57
	2.5	5.98	4.56	3.95	3.61	3.38	3.22	3.01	2.77	2.50	2.19
	5	4.41	3.55	3.16	2.93	2.77	2.66	2.51	2.34	2.15	1.92
	10	3.01	2.62	2.42	2.29	2.20	2.13	2.04	1.93	1.81	1.66
	20	1.77	1.76	1.71	1.67	1.64	1.62	1.58	1.53	1.48	1.40
19	0.1	15.08	10.16	8.28	7.26	6.61	6.18	5.59	4.97	4.29	3.52
	0.5	10.07	7.09	5.92	5.27	4.85	4.56	4.18	3.76	3.31	2.78
	1	8.18	5.93	5.01	4.50	4.17	3.94	3.63	3.30	2.92	2.49
	2.5	5.92	4.51	3.90	3.56	3.33	3.17	2.96	2.72	2.45	2.13
	5	4.38	3.52	3.13	2.90	2.74	2.63	2.48	2.31	2.11	1.88
	10	2.99	2.61	2.40	2.27	2.18	2.11	2.02	1.91	1.79	1.63
	20	1.76	1.75	1.70	1.66	1.63	1.61	1.57	1.52	1.46	1.39

(Continued)

TABLE A-6   *Continued*

df₂		1	2	3	4	5	6	8	12	24	∞
20	0.1%	14.82	9.95	8.10	7.10	6.46	6.02	5.44	4.82	4.15	3.38
	0.5%	9.94	6.99	5.82	5.17	4.76	4.47	4.09	3.68	3.22	2.69
	1 %	8.10	5.85	4.94	4.43	4.10	3.87	3.56	3.23	2.86	2.42
	2.5%	5.87	4.46	3.86	3.51	3.29	3.13	2.91	2.68	2.41	2.09
	5 %	4.35	3.49	3.10	2.87	2.71	2.60	2.45	2.28	2.08	1.84
	10 %	2.97	2.59	2.38	2.25	2.16	2.09	2.00	1.89	1.77	1.61
	20 %	1.76	1.75	1.70	1.65	1.62	1.60	1.56	1.51	1.45	1.37
21	0.1	14.59	9.77	7.94	6.95	6.32	5.88	5.31	4.70	4.03	3.26
	0.5	9.83	6.89	5.73	5.09	4.68	4.39	4.01	3.60	3.15	2.61
	1	8.02	5.78	4.87	4.37	4.04	3.81	3.51	3.17	2.80	2.36
	2.5	5.83	4.42	3.82	3.48	3.25	3.09	2.87	2.64	2.37	2.04
	5	4.32	3.47	3.07	2.84	2.68	2.57	2.42	2.25	2.05	1.81
	10	2.96	2.57	2.36	2.23	2.14	2.08	1.98	1.88	1.75	1.59
	20	1.75	1.74	1.69	1.65	1.61	1.59	1.55	1.50	1.44	1.36
22	0.1	14.38	9.61	7.80	6.81	6.19	5.76	5.19	4.58	3.92	3.15
	0.5	9.73	6.81	5.65	5.02	4.61	4.32	3.94	3.54	3.08	2.55
	1	7.94	5.72	4.82	4.31	3.99	3.76	3.45	3.12	2.75	2.31
	2.5	5.79	4.38	3.78	3.44	3.22	3.05	2.84	2.60	2.33	2.00
	5	4.30	3.44	3.05	2.82	2.66	2.55	2.40	2.23	2.03	1.78
	10	2.95	2.56	2.35	2.22	2.13	2.06	1.97	1.86	1.73	1.57
	20	1.75	1.73	1.68	1.64	1.61	1.58	1.54	1.49	1.43	1.35
23	0.1	14.19	9.47	7.67	6.69	6.08	5.65	5.09	4.48	3.82	3.05
	0.5	9.63	6.73	5.58	4.95	4.54	4.26	3.88	3.47	3.02	2.48
	1	7.88	5.66	4.76	4.26	3.94	3.71	3.41	3.07	2.70	2.26
	2.5	5.75	4.35	3.75	3.41	3.18	3.02	2.81	2.57	2.30	1.97
	5	4.28	3.42	3.03	2.80	2.64	2.53	2.38	2.20	2.00	1.76
	10	2.94	2.55	2.34	2.21	2.11	2.05	1.95	1.84	1.72	1.55
	20	1.74	1.73	1.68	1.63	1.60	1.57	1.53	1.49	1.42	1.34
24	0.1	14.03	9.34	7.55	6.59	5.98	5.55	4.99	4.39	3.74	2.97
	0.5	9.55	6.66	5.52	4.89	4.49	4.20	3.83	3.42	2.97	2.43
	1	7.82	5.61	4.72	4.22	3.90	3.67	3.36	3.03	2.66	2.21
	2.5	5.72	4.32	3.72	3.38	3.15	2.99	2.78	2.54	2.27	1.94
	5	4.26	3.40	3.01	2.78	2.62	2.51	2.36	2.18	1.98	1.73
	10	2.93	2.54	2.33	2.19	2.10	2.04	1.94	1.83	1.70	1.53
	20	1.74	1.72	1.67	1.63	1.59	1.57	1.53	1.48	1.42	1.33
25	0.1	13.88	9.22	7.45	6.49	5.88	5.46	4.91	4.31	3.66	2.89
	0.5	9.48	6.60	5.46	4.84	4.43	4.15	3.78	3.37	2.92	2.38
	1	7.77	5.57	4.68	4.18	3.86	3.63	3.32	2.99	2.62	2.17
	2.5	5.69	4.29	3.69	3.35	3.13	2.97	2.75	2.51	2.24	1.91
	5	4.24	3.38	2.99	2.76	2.60	2.49	2.34	2.16	1.96	1.71
	10	2.92	2.53	2.32	2.18	2.09	2.02	1.93	1.82	1.69	1.52
	20	1.73	1.72	1.66	1.62	1.59	1.56	1.52	1.47	1.41	1.32
26	0.1	13.74	9.12	7.36	6.41	5.80	5.38	4.83	4.24	3.59	2.82
	0.5	9.41	6.54	5.41	4.79	4.38	4.10	3.73	3.33	2.87	2.33
	1	7.72	5.53	4.64	4.14	3.82	3.59	3.29	2.96	2.58	2.13
	2.5	5.66	4.27	3.67	3.33	3.10	2.94	2.73	2.49	2.22	1.88
	5	4.22	3.37	2.98	2.74	2.59	2.47	2.32	2.15	1.95	1.69
	10	2.91	2.52	2.31	2.17	2.08	2.01	1.92	1.81	1.68	1.50
	20	1.73	1.71	1.66	1.62	1.58	1.56	1.52	1.47	1.40	1.31
27	0.1	13.61	9.02	7.27	6.33	5.73	5.31	4.76	4.17	3.52	2.75
	0.5	9.34	6.49	5.36	4.74	4.34	4.06	3.69	3.28	2.83	2.29
	1	7.68	5.49	4.60	4.11	3.78	3.56	3.26	2.93	2.55	2.10
	2.5	5.63	4.24	3.65	3.31	3.08	2.92	2.71	2.47	2.19	1.85
	5	4.21	3.35	2.96	2.73	2.57	2.46	2.30	2.13	1.93	1.67
	10	2.90	2.51	2.30	2.17	2.07	2.00	1.91	1.80	1.67	1.49
	20	1.73	1.71	1.66	1.61	1.58	1.55	1.51	1.46	1.40	1.30
28	0.1	13.50	8.93	7.19	6.25	5.66	5.24	4.69	4.11	3.46	2.70
	0.5	9.28	6.44	5.32	4.70	4.30	4.02	3.65	3.25	2.79	2.25
	1	7.64	5.45	4.57	4.07	3.75	3.53	3.23	2.90	2.52	2.06
	2.5	5.61	4.22	3.63	3.29	3.06	2.90	2.69	2.45	2.17	1.83
	5	4.20	3.34	2.95	2.71	2.56	2.44	2.29	2.12	1.91	1.65
	10	2.89	2.50	2.29	2.16	2.06	2.00	1.90	1.79	1.66	1.48
	20	1.72	1.71	1.65	1.61	1.57	1.55	1.51	1.46	1.39	1.30
29	0.1	13.39	8.85	7.12	6.19	5.59	5.18	4.64	4.05	3.41	2.64
	0.5	9.23	6.40	5.28	4.66	4.26	3.98	3.61	3.21	2.76	2.21
	1	7.60	5.42	4.54	4.04	3.73	3.50	3.20	2.87	2.49	2.03
	2.5	5.59	4.20	3.61	3.27	3.04	2.88	2.67	2.43	2.15	1.81
	5	4.18	3.33	2.93	2.70	2.54	2.43	2.28	2.10	1.90	1.64
	10	2.89	2.50	2.28	2.15	2.06	1.99	1.89	1.78	1.65	1.47
	20	1.72	1.70	1.65	1.60	1.57	1.54	1.50	1.45	1.39	1.29

TABLE A-6 *Continued*

df_2		df_1 1	2	3	4	5	6	8	12	24	∞
30	0.1%	13.29	8.77	7.05	6.12	5.53	5.12	4.58	4.00	3.36	2.59
	0.5%	9.18	6.35	5.24	4.62	4.23	3.95	3.58	3.18	2.73	2.18
	1%	7.56	5.39	4.51	4.02	3.70	3.47	3.17	2.84	2.47	2.01
	2.5%	5.57	4.18	3.59	3.25	3.03	2.87	2.65	2.41	2.14	1.79
	5%	4.17	3.32	2.92	2.69	2.53	2.42	2.27	2.09	1.89	1.62
	10%	2.88	2.49	2.28	2.14	2.05	1.98	1.88	1.77	1.64	1.46
	20%	1.72	1.70	1.64	1.60	1.57	1.54	1.50	1.45	1.38	1.28
40	0.1	12.61	8.25	6.60	5.70	5.13	4.73	4.21	3.64	3.01	2.23
	0.5	8.83	6.07	4.98	4.37	3.99	3.71	3.35	2.95	2.50	1.93
	1	7.31	5.18	4.31	3.83	3.51	3.29	2.99	2.66	2.29	1.80
	2.5	5.42	4.05	3.46	3.13	2.90	2.74	2.53	2.29	2.01	1.64
	5	4.08	3.23	2.84	2.61	2.45	2.34	2.18	2.00	1.79	1.51
	10	2.84	2.44	2.23	2.09	2.00	1.93	1.83	1.71	1.57	1.38
	20	1.70	1.68	1.62	1.57	1.54	1.51	1.47	1.41	1.34	1.24
60	0.1	11.97	7.76	6.17	5.31	4.76	4.37	3.87	3.31	2.69	1.90
	0.5	8.49	5.80	4.73	4.14	3.76	3.49	3.13	2.74	2.29	1.69
	1	7.08	4.98	4.13	3.65	3.34	3.12	2.82	2.50	2.12	1.60
	2.5	5.29	3.93	3.34	3.01	2.79	2.63	2.41	2.17	1.88	1.48
	5	4.00	3.15	2.76	2.52	2.37	2.25	2.10	1.92	1.70	1.39
	10	2.79	2.39	2.18	2.04	1.95	1.87	1.77	1.66	1.51	1.29
	20	1.68	1.65	1.59	1.55	1.51	1.48	1.44	1.38	1.31	1.18
120	0.1	11.38	7.31	5.79	4.95	4.42	4.04	3.55	3.02	2.40	1.56
	0.5	8.18	5.54	4.50	3.92	3.55	3.28	2.93	2.54	2.09	1.43
	1	6.85	4.79	3.95	3.48	3.17	2.96	2.66	2.34	1.95	1.38
	2.5	5.15	3.80	3.23	2.89	2.67	2.52	2.30	2.05	1.76	1.31
	5	3.92	3.07	2.68	2.45	2.29	2.17	2.02	1.83	1.61	1.25
	10	2.75	2.35	2.13	1.99	1.90	1.82	1.72	1.60	1.45	1.19
	20	1.66	1.63	1.57	1.52	1.48	1.45	1.41	1.35	1.27	1.12
∞	0.1	10.83	6.91	5.42	4.62	4.10	3.74	3.27	2.74	2.13	1.00
	0.5	7.88	5.30	4.28	3.72	3.35	3.09	2.74	2.36	1.90	1.00
	1	6.64	4.60	3.78	3.32	3.02	2.80	2.51	2.18	1.79	1.00
	2.5	5.02	3.69	3.12	2.79	2.57	2.41	2.19	1.94	1.64	1.00
	5	3.84	2.99	2.60	2.37	2.21	2.09	1.94	1.75	1.52	1.00
	10	2.71	2.30	2.08	1.94	1.85	1.77	1.67	1.55	1.38	1.00
	20	1.64	1.61	1.55	1.50	1.46	1.43	1.38	1.32	1.23	1.00

ject contributing the disfluency frequency should be inserted beside each in column three (C3). Next, the following command should be issued:

TWOWAY C1 C2 C3

The MS values for C2 and ERROR are displayed on the screen. Use the following formula to compute F:

$$F = MS_{C2}/MS_{ERROR}$$

To determine whether the value computed for F is large enough for the null hypothesis to be rejected, the value of F required for rejection is located in Table A-6.

ANSWER: The second graders on the average tended to produce higher frequencies of some of the disfluency types than of others (F-test; alpha = 0.05)

REMARK: This example and the one that follows illustrate the simplest possible applications of analysis of variance. More complex ones are described in Chapter 10 and in most intermediate and advanced statistical textbooks for psychologists. The Minitab Statistical Software is powerful enough to do almost any analysis of variance.

EXERCISE: Determine whether the third graders tended to produce higher frequencies of some of the four disfluency types than of others through the use of analysis of variance. (The value of *F* you compute should be approximately 7.77.)

3. Analysis of Variance (F-Test) for Independent Measures

QUESTION: Was there a tendency for the amount of part-word repetition produced by the children to vary as a function of grade level?

The first step in performing an analysis of variance for independent measures *(F)* is selecting an *alpha* level, or maximum acceptable probability for a *Type I* error (i.e., concluding that there was a tendency for the amount of part-word repetition produced by the children to vary as a function of grade level when there was no such tendency). A 0.05 alpha level will be used for this test.

The next step is to compute the value of *F.* The following computations are made from the part-word repetition frequencies of the children at each grade level (see Table A-1).

Measure	2nd Grade	3rd Grade	4th Grade	5th Grade	6th Grade	
n_c	15	11	9	11	10	$N = 56$
T_c	12.28	13.70	9.84	6.82	4.11	$T = 46.75$
$\overline{X}_c$	0.819	1.245	1.093	0.620	0.411	
T_c^2/n_c	10.053	17.063	10.758	4.228	1.689	$\Sigma T_c^2/n_c = 43.791$
ΣX_c^2	17.100	30.695	14.947	6.238	2.700	$\Sigma\Sigma X^2 = 71.680$

Next, three sum of square *(SS)* values are computed from these column data analyses. The first is the sum of squares *(SS)* for columns *(c)* or grade levels.

$$SS_c = \frac{\Sigma T_c^2}{n_c} - \frac{T^2}{N}$$

$$= 43.791 - \frac{(46.75)^2}{56}$$

$$= 43.791 - 39.028$$

$$= 4.763$$

The second is the total *(T)* sum of squares.

$$SS_T = \Sigma\Sigma X^2 - \frac{T^2}{N}$$

$$= 71.680 - \frac{(46.75)^2}{56}$$

$$= 71.680 - 39.028$$

$$= 32.652$$

The third is the within group *(w)*, or residual sum of squares, which is assumed to represent random measurement error.

$$SS_w = SS_T - SS_c = 32.652 - 4.763 = 27.889$$

The value of *F* can be computed by means of the following formula:

$$F = \frac{SS_c/c - 1}{SS_w/N - c}$$

where *c* − 1 is the degrees of freedom for SS_c and *N* − *c* is the degrees of freedom for SS_w. The first is df_1 and the second df_2 (see p. 190). The value of *F* here is:

$$F = \frac{4.763/5 - 1}{27.889/56 - 5} = \frac{1.191}{0.547} = 2.18$$

To determine whether the value of *F* is large enough for the null hypothesis to be rejected, the value of *F* required for rejection is located in Table A-6. There are two degrees of freedom: df_1 would be 4 (i.e., the number of columns minus one) and df_2 would be 51 (i.e., the number of subjects minus the number of columns). The value of *F* required for rejection at the 0.05 alpha level, when $df_1 = 4$ and $df_2 = 51$, is 2.56. Since the value computed—2.18—is smaller than this value, the null hypothesis would not be rejected.

MINITAB: Data should be entered in the first five columns of the Data Window spreadsheet: The part-word repetition frequencies for the second graders should be entered in the first column (C1); those for the third graders in the second column (C2); those for the fourth graders in the third column (C3); those for the fifth graders in the fourth column (C4); and those for the sixth graders in the fifth column (C5). Next, the following command should be issued:

```
AOVONEWAY C1-C5
```

The value for *F* will be displayed on the screen. To determine whether this value is large enough for the null hypothesis to be rejected, the value of *F* required for rejection is located in Table A-6.

ANSWER: There did not appear to be a tendency for the amount of part-word repetition produced by the children to vary as a function of grade level (*F*-test; alpha = 0.05).

EXERCISE: Determine whether there was a tendency for the amount of word repetition produced by the children to vary as a function of grade level through the use of analysis of variance. (The value of *F* you compute should be approximately 2.32.)

Confidence Interval Estimation

1. Mean

QUESTION: Within what range is the mean interjection frequency of the *population* from which the children were selected (i.e., second- through sixth-grade nonstutterers) most likely to fall?

To answer this question, a *95 percent confidence interval* will be computed. Theoretically, the limits of this interval define a range within which we can be 95 percent certain to find the mean interjection frequency for the population from which the sample was drawn. This 95 percent figure, however, should be regarded as only approximate, since certain assumptions underlying the computational procedures may not have been met (see Chapter 10).

The upper and lower limits of the confidence interval can be computed by means of the two formulas below. The first is for the upper limit and the second for the lower limit.

$$\overline{\mu} = \overline{X} + \frac{SD}{\sqrt{N-1}} (1.96)$$

$$\underline{\mu} = \overline{X} - \frac{SD}{\sqrt{N-1}} (1.96)$$

where

$\overline{X}$ = mean frequency for the sample = 1.03 (see p. 296)

SD = standard deviation for the sample = 1.39 (see p. 299)

N = number of subjects = 56

1.96 = a constant for 95 percent confidence intervals

The mean value that would represent the *upper* limit of the confidence interval would be:

$$\overline{\mu} = 1.03 + \frac{1.39}{\sqrt{56-1}} (1.96)$$

$$= 1.03 + (0.187)(1.96)$$

$$= 1.40$$

The mean value that would represent the *lower* limit of the confidence interval should be:

$$\underline{\mu} = 1.03 - \frac{1.39}{\sqrt{56-1}} (1.96)$$

$$= 1.03 - (0.187)(1.96)$$

$$= 0.66$$

MINITAB: Enter the mean in the first row of the first column (C1), the standard deviation in the first row of the second column (C2), and the number of subjects in the first row of the third column (C3) of the Data Window spreadsheet. Next, issue the following commands:

```
LET C1 = 1.03
LET C2 = 1.39
LET C3 = 56
C4 = C1 + (C2/(SQRT (C3 - 1))) * 1.96
C5 = C1 - (C2/(SQRT (C3 - 1))) * 1.96
```

The upper limit will be in the top row of C4 and the lower limit will be in the top row of C5.

ANSWER: The mean interjection frequency of the population from which the children were selected is *approximately* 95 percent certain to fall between 0.66 and 1.40.

REMARK: The width of the confidence interval can be changed by substituting a different constant for 1.96. For a 99 percent confidence interval, for example, 2.58 would be used as the constant.

EXERCISE: Compute a 95 percent confidence interval for the mean part-word repetition frequency of the population from which the children were selected. (The upper limit of the confidence interval you compute should be approximately 1.03, and the lower limit should be approximately 0.63.)

2. Median

QUESTION: Within what range is the median interjection frequency of the *population* from which the children were selected (i.e., second- through sixth-grade nonstutterers) most likely to fall?

To answer this question, a *95 percent confidence interval* will be computed. Theoretically, the limits of this interval define a range within which we can be 95 percent certain to find the median interjection frequency for the population from which the sample was drawn. This 95 percent figure, however, should be regarded as only approximate, since certain assumptions underlying the computational procedures may not have been met (see Chapter 10).

The upper and lower limits of the confidence interval can be computed by means of the two formulas below. The first is for the upper limit and the second for the lower limit.

$$\overline{\xi} = mdn + \frac{1.25SD}{\sqrt{N - 1}}(1.96)$$

$$\underline{\xi} = mdn - \frac{1.25SD}{\sqrt{N - 1}}(1.96)$$

where

mdn = median frequency for sample = 0.51 (see p. 297)

SD = standard deviation of sample = 1.39 (see p. 299)

N = number of subjects = 56

1.96 = a constant for 95 percent confidence intervals

1.25 = a constant

The median value that would represent the *upper boundary* of the confidence interval would be:

$$\overline{\xi} = 0.51 + \frac{(1.25)(1.39)}{\sqrt{56 - 1}}(1.96)$$

$$= 0.51 + (0.234)(1.96)$$

$$= 0.97$$

The median value that would represent the *lower boundary* of the confidence interval would be:

$$\underline{\xi} = 0.51 - \frac{(1.25)(1.39)}{\sqrt{56-1}}(1.96)$$

$$= 0.51 - (0.234)(1.96)$$

$$= 0.05$$

MINITAB: Enter the median in the first row of the first column (C1), the standard deviation in the first row of the second column (C2), and the number of subjects in the first row of the third column (C3) of the Data Window spreadsheet. Next, issue the following commands:

```
LET C1 = 0.51
LET C2 = 1.39
LET C3 = 56
C4 = C1 + ((1.25 * C2)/(SQRT (C3 - 1))) * 1.96
C5 = C1 - ((1.25 * C2)/(SQRT (C3 - 1))) * 1.96
```

The upper limit will be in the top row of C4 and the lower limit will be in the top row of C5.

ANSWER: The median interjection frequency of the population from which the children were selected is *approximately* 95 percent certain to fall between 0.05 and 0.97.

REMARK: The width of the confidence interval can be changed by substituting a different constant for 1.96. For a 99 percent confidence interval, for example, 2.58 would be used as the constant.

EXERCISE: Compute a 95 percent confidence interval for the median part-word repetition frequency of the population from which the children were selected. (The upper limit of the confidence interval you compute should be approximately 1.07, and the lower limit should be approximately 0.56.)

3. *Difference between Means*

QUESTION: Within what range is the *difference between mean* part-word repetition frequencies for third graders and sixth graders in the *populations* from which the children were selected (i.e., third grade nonstutterers and sixth grade nonstutterers) most likely to fall?

To answer this question, a *95 percent confidence interval* will be computed. Theoretically, the limits of this interval define a range within which we can be 95 percent certain to find the difference between mean part-word repetition frequencies for third graders and sixth graders in the populations from which the samples were drawn. This 95 percent figure, however, should be regarded as only approximate, since certain assumptions underlying the computational procedures may not have been met (see Chapter 10).

The upper and lower limits of the confidence interval can be computed by means of the two formulas below. The first is for the upper limit and the second for the lower limit.

$$\overline{\Delta} = \overline{D}_1 + (1.96)\sqrt{\frac{S_1^2}{n_1 - 1} + \frac{S_2^2}{n_2 - 1}}$$

$$\underline{\Delta} = \overline{D}_1 - (1.96)\sqrt{\frac{S_1^2}{n_1 - 1} + \frac{S_2^2}{n_2 - 1}}$$

where

$$\overline{D}_1 = \overline{X}_1 - \overline{X}_2 = 1.245 - 0.411 = 0.834$$

n_1 = number of third graders = 11

n_2 = number of sixth graders = 10

1.96 = a constant for 95 percent confidence intervals

S_1^2 = variance of third graders' part-word repetition frequencies

$$= \frac{\Sigma X_1^2}{n_1} - \overline{X}_1^2$$

$$= \frac{30.695}{11} - (1.245)^2$$

$$= 2.790 - 1.550 = 1.240$$

S_2^2 = variance of sixth graders' part-word repetition frequencies

$$= \frac{\Sigma X_2^2}{n_2} - \overline{X}_2^2$$

$$= \frac{2.700}{10} - (0.411)^2$$

$$= 0.270 - 0.169 = 0.101$$

The mean difference that would represent the *upper boundary* of the confidence interval would be:

$$\overline{\Delta} = 0.834 + (1.96)\sqrt{\frac{1.240}{11 - 1} + \frac{0.101}{10 - 1}}$$

$$= 0.834 + (1.96)(0.368) = 1.56$$

The mean difference that would represent the *lower boundary* of the confidence interval would be:

$$\underline{\Delta} = 0.834 - (1.96)\sqrt{\frac{1.240}{11 - 1} + \frac{0.101}{10 - 1}}$$

$$= 0.834 - (1.96)(0.368) = 0.11$$

MINITAB: Enter the difference between the means in the first row of the first column (C1), the variance of the third graders part-word repetition frequencies in the first row of the second column (C2), the variance of the sixth graders part-word repetition frequencies in the first row of the third column (C3), the number of third graders in the first row of the fourth column (C4), and the number of sixth graders in the first row of the fifth column (C5) of the Data Window spreadsheet. Next, issue the following commands:

```
LET C1 = 0.834
LET C2 = 1.240
LET C3 = 0.101
LET C4 = 11
LET C5 = 10
C6 = C1 + 1.96 * (SQRT (C2/C4 - 1 + C3/C5 - 1))
C7 = C1 - 1.96 * (SQRT (C2/C4 - 1 + C3/C5 - 1))
```

The upper limit will be in the top row of C6 and the lower limit will be in the top row of C7.

ANSWER: The difference between the means of the populations from which the children were selected is *approximately* 95 percent certain to fall between 0.11 and 1.56.

REMARK: The width of the confidence interval can be changed by substituting a different constant for 1.96. For a 99 percent confidence interval, for example, 2.58 would be used as the constant.

EXERCISE: Compute a 95 percent confidence interval for the difference between the mean part-word repetition frequencies for fourth graders and fifth graders in the populations from which the children were selected. (The upper limit of the confidence interval you compute should be approximately 1.01, and the lower limit should be approximately –0.07.)

3,500 Computer-Generated Random Digits

04433	80674	24520	18222	10610	05794	37515
60298	47829	72648	37414	75755	04717	29899
67884	59651	67533	68123	17730	95862	08034
89512	32155	51906	61662	64130	16688	37275
32653	01895	12506	88535	36553	23757	34209
95913	15405	13772	76638	48423	25018	99041
55864	21694	13122	44115	01601	50541	00147
35334	49810	91601	40617	72876	33967	73830
57729	32196	76487	11622	96297	24160	09903
86648	13697	63677	70119	94739	25875	38829
30574	47609	07967	32422	76791	39725	53711
81307	43694	83580	79974	45929	85113	72268
02410	54905	79007	54939	21410	86980	91772
18969	75274	52233	62319	08598	09066	95288
87863	82384	66860	62297	80198	19347	73234
68397	71708	15438	62311	72844	60203	46412
28529	54447	58729	10854	99058	18260	38765
44285	06372	15867	70418	57012	72122	36634
86299	83430	33571	23309	57040	29285	67870
84842	68668	90894	61658	15001	94055	36308
56970	83609	52098	04184	54967	72938	56834
83125	71257	60490	44369	66130	72936	69848
55503	52423	02464	26141	68779	66388	75242
47019	76273	33203	29608	54553	25971	69573
84828	32592	79526	29554	84580	37859	28504
68921	08141	79227	05748	51276	57143	31926
36458	96045	30424	98420	72925	40729	22337
95752	59445	36847	87729	81679	59126	59437
26768	47323	58454	56958	20575	76746	49878
42613	37056	43636	58085	06766	60227	96414
95457	30566	65482	25596	02678	54592	63607
95276	17894	63564	95958	39750	64379	46059
66954	52324	64776	92345	95110	59448	77249
17457	18481	14113	62462	02798	54977	48349
03704	36872	83214	59337	01695	60666	97410
21538	86497	33210	60337	27976	70661	08250
57178	67619	98310	70348	11317	71623	55510
31048	97558	94953	55866	96283	46620	52087
69799	55380	16498	80733	96422	58078	99643
90595	61867	59231	17772	67831	33317	00520
33570	04981	98939	78784	09977	29398	93896
15340	93460	57477	13898	48431	72936	78160
64079	42483	36512	56186	99098	48850	72527
63491	05546	67118	62063	74958	20946	28147
92003	63868	41034	28260	79708	00770	88643
52360	46658	66511	04172	73085	11795	52594
74622	12142	68355	65635	21828	39539	18988
04157	50079	61343	64315	70836	82857	35335
86003	60070	66241	32836	27573	11479	94114
41268	80187	20351	09636	84668	42486	71303

48611	62866	33963	14045	79451	04934	45576
78812	03509	78673	73181	29973	18664	04555
19472	63971	37271	31445	49019	49405	46925
51266	11569	08697	91120	64156	40365	74297
55806	96275	26130	47949	14877	69594	83041
77527	81360	18180	97421	55541	90275	18213
77680	58788	33016	61173	93049	04694	43534
15404	96554	88265	34537	38526	67924	40474
14045	22917	60718	66487	46346	30949	03173
68376	43918	77653	04127	69930	43283	35766
93385	13421	67957	20384	58731	53396	59723
09858	52104	32014	53115	03727	98624	84616
93307	34116	49516	42148	57740	31198	70336
04794	01534	92058	03157	91758	80611	45357
86265	49096	97021	92582	61422	75890	86442
65943	79232	45702	67055	39024	57383	44424
90038	94209	04055	27393	61517	23002	96560
97283	95943	78363	36498	40662	94188	18202
21913	72958	75637	99936	58715	07943	23748
41161	37341	81838	19389	80336	46346	91895
23777	98392	31417	98547	92058	02277	50315
59973	08144	61070	73094	27059	69181	55623
82690	74099	77885	23813	10054	11900	44653
83854	24715	48866	65745	31131	47636	45137
61980	34997	41825	11623	07320	15003	56774
99915	45821	97702	87125	44488	77613	56823
48293	86847	43186	42951	37804	85129	28993
33225	31280	41232	34750	91097	60752	69783
06846	32828	24425	30249	78801	26977	92074
32671	45587	79620	84831	38156	74211	82752
82096	21913	75544	55228	89796	05694	91552
51666	10433	10945	55306	78562	89630	41230
54044	67942	24145	42294	27427	84875	37022
66738	60184	75679	38120	17640	36242	99357
55064	17427	89180	74018	44865	53197	74810
69599	60264	84549	78007	88450	06488	72274
64756	87759	92354	78694	63638	80939	98644
80817	74533	68407	55862	32476	19326	95558
39847	96884	84657	33697	39578	90197	80532
90401	41700	95510	61166	33757	23279	85523
78227	90110	81378	96659	37008	04050	04228
87240	52716	87697	79433	16336	52862	69149
08486	10951	26832	39763	02485	71688	90936
39338	32169	03713	93510	61244	73774	01245
21188	01850	69689	49426	49128	14660	14143
13287	82531	04388	64693	11934	35051	68576
53609	04001	19648	14053	49623	10840	31915
87900	36194	31567	53506	34304	39910	79630
81641	00496	36058	75899	46620	70024	88753
19512	50277	71508	20116	79520	06269	74173

Methodological Considerations When Quantifying Attributes of Speech, Hearing, and Language Using Psychological Scaling Methods

Once the scaling method has been selected, the next step is to prepare the stimuli for scaling. Since most of the stimuli scaled by speech-language pathologists and audiologists have been auditory—that is, speech events or other acoustic signals recorded on audiotape—this discussion will emphasize the preparation of such stimuli for scaling. Most of the comments will be relevant, however, to the preparation of other types of stimuli for scaling, including videotaped ones.

Preparation of Audiotaped Stimuli for Scaling

A number of factors must be considered in preparing audiotaped stimuli for scaling, including: (1) method of assembling the tape (i.e., splicing versus dubbing), (2) ordering of the stimuli, (3) duration of the "judging interval" between stimuli, (4) selection, frequency of occurrence, and location of the standard stimuli, (5) definition and selection of stimuli, (6) equating stimuli for extraneous attributes, (7) numbering stimuli, (8) acquainting judges with the range of the target attribute present in the stimuli, and (9) determining the number of times each stimulus is to be presented. Comments relevant to each consideration are presented in the paragraphs that follow.

Method of Assembling

Two methods can be used to prepare audiotaped stimuli for scaling. The first is *splicing* together the segments of tape on which the stimuli were recorded. The second is *dubbing* the stimuli onto a master tape. The splicing method obviously cannot be used when a stimulus has to appear more than once on a master tape (as it would for pair comparisons and constant sums). The main limitation of the dubbing process is that some distortion of the signal is introduced by it. In many cases, this distortion would probably not be of sufficient magnitude to influence observers' ratings of the target attribute. While it would be unlikely to influence stuttering severity ratings, it may influence voice quality ratings.

Ordering of the Stimuli

The ordering of stimuli on the master tape should be random—that is, determined by a table of random numbers (see Appendix B). If there is a possibility of order or sequence effects (see Chapter 6) influencing the ratings, these effects could be controlled for, at least partially, by preparing several randomizations of the stimuli. Since the possibility of order and sequence effects often cannot be ruled out, it is not desirable for all members of a panel to rate a set of stimuli in the same order.

Duration of the "Judging Interval" between Stimuli

This refers to the time interval following the presentation of a stimulus during which it is rated. It must be long enough to permit the judges to make their ratings with adequate levels of validity and reliability but not so long that it will unnecessarily extend the length of the judging session. An interval duration of approximately 15 seconds appears to be adequate for rating most attributes of audiotaped speech stimuli.

Selection, Frequency of Occurrence, and Location of the Standard Stimuli

Standard stimuli serve as anchor, or reference, points on a scale. They help to reduce intrarater and interrater variability. They usually are used with the method of direct magnitude-estimation. Standard stimuli also are used occasionally with the methods of equal-appearing intervals and successive intervals.

Several decisions must be made if standard stimuli are to be used: (1) which stimulus (for direct magnitude-estimation), or which stimuli (for equal-appearing intervals and successive intervals) to select, (2) how often to present the stimulus, or stimuli, and (3) at what points during the rating session to present the stimulus, or stimuli (i.e., at the beginning only or at the beginning and periodically during the session). With direct magnitude-estimation, a stimulus is usually selected for the standard in which the amount of the attribute is at the approximate midpoint of the range (based on the judgment of the experimenter or that of a small panel of observers). Theoretically, the "location" of the standard in the range of possible values of the attribute should not influence the characteristics of the scale resulting from its use. As long as the scale is regarded as ordinal, this would probably be a safe assumption to make. However, if it is regarded as having interval or ratio properties, this assumption would be risky to make, since there is some evidence that suggests that the location of the standard used to construct a scale by the method of direct magnitude-estimation influences to some extent the spacings between points on that scale. For this reason, it would probably be most defensible to interpret direct magnitude-estimation scale values as if they had ordinal properties.

In scaling tape recorded stimuli with the method of direct magnitude-estimation, the standard stimulus usually appears two or three times (one after the other) at the beginning of the tape on which the stimuli are recorded. The standard may also appear on this tape after every third or fourth stimulus. Hence, the sequence of stimuli on a tape could be:

1. Standard Stimulus
2. Standard Stimulus
3. Standard Stimulus
4. Stimulus #1
5. Stimulus #2
6. Stimulus #3
7. Standard Stimulus
8. Stimulus #4
9. Stimulus #5
10. Stimulus #6
11. Standard Stimulus
    etc.

The more abstract or vague the target attribute, the more frequently the standard stimulus should be presented.

With the method of equal-appearing intervals and the method of successive intervals, if individual scale points are not defined, two stimuli are selected for the standard that represent the *extremes* of the range of possible values of the target attribute. It is crucial that the amounts of the target attribute present in these stimuli represent the extremes of the continuum. Otherwise, there may be an *end effect,* that is, a piling up of ratings in one or both of the extreme intervals. Both stimuli that have a value of the target attribute *equal* to that in the standard and *exceeding* that in the standard will be assigned the most extreme ratings. (Such ratings on a seven-point scale would be 1 and 7.) Standard stimuli are often not used with these methods because of the difficulty in identifying stimuli that represent the extremes of the range of possible values of the target attribute. The extremes of the scale in such cases are usually defined verbally, for example,

1 = least hypernasality and 7 = most hypernasality

or

1 = lowest stuttering severity and 7 = highest stuttering severity

When standard stimuli are used with these scaling methods, they usually are presented several times at the beginning of the stimulus tape and after every third or fourth stimulus.

Definition and Selection of Stimuli

This is not a problem in many scaling experiments because the events, or stimuli, to be rated have "natural" boundaries. (Examples of events that can be treated as such are phonemes, syllables, and words.) This can present a problem, however, when the events to be rated do not have "natural" boundaries—for example, conversational speech segments. To illustrate this point, suppose you wished to rate "before and after" therapy conversational speech segments for degree of nasality or degree of stuttering severity. How long a speech segment would be required to obtain ratings which are adequately reliable? Would 20-second segments be adequate? The answers to these questions would depend, in part, on the nature of the attribute being rated. Some attributes could be reliably rated from shorter segments than others. Nasality, for example, could probably be reliably rated from shorter segments than would be required for stuttering severity. Unfortunately, with the exception of a few attributes such as stuttering severity, there are no data in the literature that indicate the shortest segment lengths that can be expected to yield reliable ratings. The only possibly helpful observation from the literature is that in studies where the speech segments rated were 30 seconds in duration, ratings in almost all cases have been reported to be adequately reliable.

After a decision has been made concerning the duration of speech segments, it is then necessary to decide which segments of the available speech samples to rate. This obviously would be of concern only if the available samples were longer in duration than the segment length selected. There are several strategies that can be used for selecting such segments, including the following:

1. Segments are selected by the experimenter. The experimenter chooses segments that he or she feels are representative. One limitation of this strategy is that the experimenter, without being consciously aware of it, may select segments that instead of being representative would be likely to be rated in a manner consistent with his or her expectations of hypotheses. (The phenomenon of *experimenter bias* is discussed in several contexts in this book, which may be located by consulting the index.)

2. Segments are selected through the use of a random sampling procedure. The sample could be segmented, for example, into consecutive segments of the length to be rated. (A five-minute sample could be segmented into ten consecutive, 30-second segments.) These segments would be numbered consecutively, and one or more would be selected by means of a table of random numbers. This sampling strategy is more likely than the first to provide representative samples for rating.

Equating Stimuli for Extraneous Attributes

The stimuli the judges are asked to rate may possess a large number (perhaps, an infinite number) of attributes. The judges are usually instructed to attend to only one such attribute (i.e., the target attribute) when making their ratings. Two strategies have been used to *minimize* the impact of other attributes (i.e., extraneous attributes) on these ratings. The first is to instruct the judges to ignore these attributes when making their ratings, and the second is to equate the stimuli for them. Suppose you did not want judges to be influenced by disfluency level when they were rating speech segments for articulation defectiveness. If you used the first approach, you would tell them to ignore disfluency level when making their ratings. If you used the second approach, you would select speech segments in which no disfluency occurred. (If you were using a random sampling procedure for selecting such segments, you could exclude those containing instances of disfluency.)

Numbering Stimuli (or Stimulus Pairs)

Each stimulus (or stimulus pair) to be rated is usually given an identification number. If the stimuli are audiotape-recorded speech segments, a carrier phrase and number is recorded on the stimulus tape preceding each segment, for example, "sample number one." This carrier phrase-number combination performs two functions. First, it maximizes the odds that the judges will record their ratings at the appropriate places on the response sheet. Second, it alerts the judges immediately before the presentation of each stimulus, which maximizes the odds they will attend to it.

Acquainting Judges with the Range of the Target Attribute Present in the Stimuli

With equal-appearing intervals, with successive intervals, and sometimes with direct magnitude-estimation, the judges are acquainted with the range of the target attribute present in the stimuli before beginning the rating task. This may be done by presenting ten or fifteen stimuli to them that represent the range of the attribute. It also may be done by presenting all the stimuli to the judges before they begin to rate them.

Determining the Number of Times Each Stimulus Is to Be Presented

It may sometimes be necessary to present a stimulus more than once before asking judges to rate it. If the duration of individual stimuli is relatively short, such as would be the case for isolated phonemes, judges may be unable to get a sufficiently good impression of the target attribute to rate isolated vowels for nasality. You might dub each vowel on the stimulus tape three times (with a few seconds between presentations) and have judges listen to the three presentations before assigning it a nasality rating.

Considerations in Writing Instructions to Judges

One of the most important tasks associated with designing a scaling experiment is writing the instructions for the judges. The instructions they are given influence both the validity and reliability of their ratings.

The instructions given the judges in scaling experiments usually provide them with three kinds of information: (1) a description of the attribute to be rated, (2) a description of the scaling task, and (3) descriptions of attributes to be ignored. Two representative sets of instructions that include these three kinds of information are reproduced here. The first is for the method of equal-appearing intervals; the second, for the method of direct magnitude-estimation. Both were used for rating the same attribute, that is, intricacy of language usage (Sherman & Silverman, 1968).

I

You are asked to judge a series of samples of children's oral language that are presented in written form. You are to judge each sample in relation to a seven-point scale of "intricacy of language usage." Intricacy of language usage, for the purposes of this experiment, is defined as the intricacy of the arrangement of words for the purpose of conveying information. For example, consider the following four sets of words that without reference to the specific meanings, might be judged to vary with respect to intricacy of language as defined here:

(a)   two good little boys
(b)   boys in your school
(c)   boys who are orphans
(d)   really very good boys

Although each of the above sets contains four words, it is obvious that they vary with respect to type of arrangement.

Make your judgment on the basis of the whole sample. Avoid being influenced by grammatical correctness; for example, "we was" in place of the correct wording "we were." Obviously, the expressions "we was" and "we were" do not differ with respect to the intricacy of word arrangement. Also, do not give a rating based upon a judgment of the extent of vocabulary; for example, "big size" and "extensive area" are equivalent as far as the intricacy of arrangement is concerned, but they probably would not be considered equivalent if judged for the purpose of rating extent of vocabulary usage.

The scale is one of equal intervals—from 1 to 7—with 1 representing least intricacy of language usage and 7 representing most intricacy; 4 represents the midpoint between 1 and 7 with respect to intricacy, with the other numbers falling at equal distances along the scale. Do not attempt to place samples between any two of the seven points, but only at these points.

Each language sample is preceded by a number. Your task will be to record your judgment on your response sheet to the right of the identifying number of the language sample.

On the following pages there are 50 samples to be rated on a seven-point scale. The experimenter obtained these samples by requesting the children to respond to a picture stimulus. He also encouraged the children to speak by asking them questions and by making comments, as needed. These questions and comments are not included in the material you are to judge. All of the samples are in response to the same picture.

Before you record any judgments, read quickly the first 25 samples to acquaint yourself with the experimental task and to acquaint yourself with the range of samples with respect to the intricacy of language usage that you are requested to judge.

After you have acquainted yourself with the task and the range, make a judgment on every sample. If you are somewhat doubtful, make a guess as to the most suitable scale position.

II

You are asked to judge a series of samples of children's oral language that are presented in written form. You are to judge each sample for intricacy *of language usage. You are to estimate the relative intricacy of language usage of each language sample in relation to the intricacy of language usage of a standard sample that you will read before making your estimates. Your task will be to assign the number of points you believe represents the relative intricacy of language usage with reference to the standard sample.*

Intricacy of language usage, for the purposes of this experiment, is defined as the intricacy of the arrangement of words for the purpose of conveying information. For example, consider the following four sets of words that, without reference to the specific meanings, might be judged to vary with respect to intricacy of language usage as here defined:

(a) two good little boys
(b) boys in our school
(c) boys who are orphans
(d) really good little boys

Although each of the above sets contains four words, it is obvious that they vary with respect to type of arrangement of words for purpose of conveying information.

Make your judgment on the basis of the whole sample. Avoid being influenced by grammatical correctness; for example, "we was" in place of the correct wording "we were." Obviously, the expressions "we was" and "we were" do not differ with respect to the intricacy of word arrangement. Also, do not give a rating based upon a judgment of the extent of vocabulary; for example, "big size" and "extensive area" are equivalent as far as the intricacy of arrangement is concerned, but they probably would not be considered equivalent if judged for the purpose of rating extent of vocabulary.

The following sample is to be used as the standard *sample.*

> *"That's a grandpa lion and he is sitting down in a chair and he is thinking about something. And he's holding a pipe in his hand. And a little mouse is coming out of the mouse hole. Sneak up on the tiger. Cause he is gonna lay on the tiger's head. He would feel upon his head and he'd feel a mouse up on his head and try to catch him. Well, I would get out of there and crawl under the chair and go through there and run. Run away from him. I would run back under the chair and into my mousehole. He couldn't get under the chair."*

You will assign 100 *points to this sample. The point assignments you make on the succeeding samples should represent, with reference to the standard, the relative intricacy of language usage of each sample. For example, if you believe that a sample is* twice *as intricate in language usage as the standard sample, you would assign* 200 *points to it. On the other hand, if you believe that a sample is* half *as intricate in language usage as the standard, you would assign it* 50 *points.*

You may, of course, use any point assignment you choose to represent your judg-ment of the intricacy of language usage. You need not limit yourself to even frac-tions and even multiples of the 100 points assigned to the standard. You might use, for example, 85, or 65, or 20, or even 57, or 112, or 120, or 215, or any other num-ber you choose as long as it represents your judgment of the intricacy of language usage of the sample in relation to the standard sample.

On the following pages there are 50 samples to be judged in relation to the standard sample. The experimenter obtained these samples by requesting the chil-dren to respond to a picture stimulus. He also encouraged the children to speak by asking them questions and making comments, as needed. These questions and comments are not included in the material you are to judge. All of the samples are in response to the same picture.

Each experimental sample is preceded by a number. You are to record your judgments on your response sheet to the right of the identification numbers of the samples. Before you record any judgments, read quickly the first 25 samples to acquaint yourself with the experimental task. As you read think about the point assignments you would make if you were recording judgments. Now read the stan-dard sample once again; record your judgments according to the instructions that you have been given. Make a judgment on every sample. If you are somewhat doubtful about what number to assign, make a guess.

In the first set of instructions (for the method of equal-appearing intervals), the first paragraph gives a description of the attribute to be rated; the second, the attributes to be ignored; and the remaining paragraphs, a description of the scaling task. In the second set of instructions (for the method of direct magnitude-estimation), the second paragraph gives a description of the attribute to be rated; the third, the attributes to be ignored; and the remaining paragraphs, a description of the scaling task.

These sets of instructions can be modified fairly easily for rating other attributes of speech (or language) segments. Also, the equal-appearing interval instructions can be used for the method of successive intervals, with minor modifications.

Instructions can be presented to judges in oral or written form. An oral mode of pres-entation can be either tape-recorded or "live." A written mode is usually wordprocessed and photocopied. These presentation modes are often combined. The experimenter reads the instructions aloud while the judges follow along on their copies. This combined mode may be the most satisfactory one (when it is possible to use it), since some judges would prob-ably better comprehend "heard" than "read" instructions, and vice versa.

The judges usually record their ratings on a response sheet. A representative response sheet is reproduced in Figure C-1. This response sheet could be used for all the methods dis-cussed, with the exception of constant sums. For the method of pair comparisons, a 1 or 2 would be recorded in the space to the right of each identification number to designate the stimulus in each pair that possessed the greater amount of the target attribute. For the method of rank order, the number recorded to the right of a stimulus identification number would designate the rank of that stimulus in an ordering. For the methods of equal-appearing intervals and successive intervals, this number would be a numeral that designates a point

```
┌─────────────────────────────────────────────────────────┐
│                                                         │
│   Name _____     Date _____       │
│                                                         │
│       1  _____                 26  _____                 │
│       2  _____                 27  _____                 │
│       3  _____                 28  _____                 │
│       4  _____                 29  _____                 │
│       5  _____                 30  _____                 │
│       6  _____                 31  _____                 │
│       7  _____                 32  _____                 │
│       8  _____                 33  _____                 │
│       9  _____                 34  _____                 │
│      10  _____                 35  _____                 │
│      11  _____                 36  _____                 │
│      12  _____                 37  _____                 │
│      13  _____                 38  _____                 │
│      14  _____                 39  _____                 │
│      15  _____                 40  _____                 │
│      16  _____                 41  _____                 │
│      17  _____                 42  _____                 │
│      18  _____                 43  _____                 │
│      19  _____                 44  _____                 │
│      20  _____                 45  _____                 │
│      21  _____                 46  _____                 │
│      22  _____                 47  _____                 │
│      23  _____                 48  _____                 │
│      24  _____                 49  _____                 │
│      25  _____                 50  _____                 │
│                                                         │
└─────────────────────────────────────────────────────────┘
```

FIGURE C-1   A representative response sheet.

on a scale (having a finite number of points). And for the method of direct magnitude-estimation, this number would be a magnitude estimate.

To make this response sheet usable for the method of constant sums, it would be necessary to have *two* response spaces to the right of each identification number,

       A   B
  1. _____   _____

The point value assigned to the first stimulus in a pair could be recorded in the *A* space and that assigned to the second member in the *B* space.

Considerations in the Selection of a Judging Panel

All scaling methods require a panel of judges, or raters. Several considerations concerning the selection of judges for a panel will be discussed in this section, including: (1) the number to be used, (2) their characteristics, and (3) the procedure by which they are to be selected.

Number of Judges to Be Used in the Panel

If too few judges are used, the scale values for the stimuli may not be sufficiently reliable for the purposes of the experiment. If too many are used, the panel may be unnecessarily costly. The added cost here includes: (1) judges' time in performing the rating task, (2) experimenter's time in administering the task, and (3) data analysis time and expense.

There is little in the literature to assist the experimenter in deciding how many judges to use, with the possible exception of information pertaining to the magnitude of reliability coefficients reported for scaling experiments in which different numbers of judges were used (e.g., Edwards, 1957, pp. 94-95). Such information has limited usefulness, since the number of judges required to attain a specific level of reliability would be expected to vary as a function of several factors, including: (1) the degree of ambiguity of the attribute being rated, (2) the complexity of the stimuli, and (3) the extent to which the judges are trained to share a common standard. However, in almost all studies reported in which speech segments were scaled by the methods of equal-appearing intervals, successive intervals, or direct magnitude-estimation and panels of approximately fifty judges were used, the investigators concluded that the resulting scale values were adequately reliable for their purposes. Panels of fifty judges, therefore, probably would be sufficiently large for scaling attributes of speech segments for most purposes.

With the approach described, the size of the judging panel is fixed before beginning the rating task, and the reliability of the scale values is permitted to vary. An alternative approach would be to fix the minimum level of reliability desired for the scale values before beginning the rating task and to permit the size of the judging panel to vary. That is, you would gradually increase the number of judges in the panel until the scale values computed from their ratings would possess a predetermined level of reliability. One such approach, based on the principle of sequential sampling, has been described by Silverman (1968a).

Definition of the Population from Which the Panel Is to Be Selected

"Organismic" and related variables such as hearing acuity, visual acuity, intelligence, and previous exposure to the attribute being rated can systematically influence the ratings assigned by the members of a panel. A panel consisting of parents of children who stutter may tend to rate segments of disfluent speech as more abnormal than would a panel consisting of parents of children who do not stutter. Also, a panel of speech-language pathologists may tend to rate speech segments in which the speaker has a lateral lisp as more abnormal than would a panel consisting of laymen.

If it seems that a particular attribute might be rated differently by different subgroups of observers, it would be necessary for the experimenters to define the subgroup they wish to use for their panel. The characteristics of the members of this subgroup would be determined, at least, in part, by the purpose to which the ratings were to be put. Suppose an investigator wished to determine whether the speech of severe stutterers would be regarded as less defective if they paced their speech with a miniature metronome than if they spoke in their usual manner. Since the ratings of speech-language pathologists might differ from those of laymen, and since the investigator would probably be interested primarily in how laymen would react to the "metronome" as opposed to the usual speech of such stutterers, the investigator would probably be wise to limit membership in the panel to persons who have not had training in speech-language pathology.

The more heterogeneous the members of a panel are with regard to organismic variables, the greater the probable dispersion of their ratings and the lower the probable *reliability* of the scale values computed from them (for a given size panel) will be. Also, the more heterogeneous the members of a panel are with regard to such variables, the less *valid* the scale values computed from their ratings are apt to be. If a panel consisted of two or more subgroups who would tend to rate a set of stimuli differently, scale values computed from the ratings of such a panel may not correspond to how the typical member of any subgroup would rate the stimuli. They may be merely "mathematical artifacts." (For a discussion of this point in two somewhat different contexts, see Silverman, 1974.)

Selection of the Panel

The panel, strictly speaking, should consist of a random sample of persons from the defined population. Every member of this population should have an equal chance of being selected for the panel. Sometimes it is possible to have such a panel. For instance, suppose the population an investigator wished to sample for a panel consisted of speech-language pathologists who have been awarded the Certificate of Clinical Competence in Speech-Language Pathology by the American Speech-Language-Hearing Association. A reasonably complete list of such persons could be obtained from the most recent edition of the Association's Membership Directory. Each could be assigned a number, and a panel could be selected by means of a table of random numbers. Such a panel would be practical if the rating task could be mailed.

In some instances it is neither possible nor practical to sample randomly the defined population. Such a population would be adults who are not speech-language pathologists. All you can do in these instances is to try to select a panel of persons who appear to be representative of the defined population and to be cautious when generalizing from their ratings.

Modes of Stimulus Presentation

Once a scaling method has been selected, the stimuli have been prepared, the instructions have been written, and the panel has been selected, the stimuli can be presented to the panel for rating. The primary emphasis in this discussion will be on the presentation of audiotaped stimuli. Many of the comments, however, are relevant for the presentation of other types of stimuli.

A number of decisions have to be made on procedures for presenting audiotaped stimuli for scaling including the following: (1) individual versus group presentation, (2) headphones versus speakers, (3) loudness level of the stimuli, (4) physical environment, and (5) number of judging sessions.

Individual versus Group Presentation

The issue here is whether the stimuli should be presented to one member of the panel at a time or to several (possibly even the entire panel). The main advantage of group presentation is efficiency. Ordinarily it takes less time to have a set of stimuli rated using a group presentation mode than using an individual one.

The individual presentation mode has several advantages that may outweigh the efficiency advantage of the group mode. First, it ordinarily allows more control to be exerted over the presentation of the stimuli. This permits you to maximize the odds that the stimuli presented to the members of a panel will be similar. They may not be similar if a group presentation mode is used. If, for example, tape recorded stimuli are presented to a group of judges over a loudspeaker, the judges may not "hear" the same stimuli because they are sitting at different distances from the speaker. With an individual presentation mode, judges could be seated the same distance from the speaker.

A second advantage of the individual over the group presentation mode is that it permits order and sequence effects (see Chapter 6) to be minimized. The stimuli can be presented to the members of a panel in different random sequences. This would ordinarily be quite difficult to do if a group presentation mode were used.

The third advantage of the individual over the group presentation mode is that it permits the use of the sequential approach for defining the size of a panel (Silverman, 1968a). The main advantage of this approach is that it ensures that the scale values derived from the judges' ratings will possess the required level of reliability and the panel will be no larger than necessary to achieve this end.

Headphones versus Speakers

Two types of transducers can be used to present audiotape stimuli to judges: headphones and loudspeakers. The main advantage of loudspeakers is that they make it relatively easy to present a set of stimuli to more than one rater at a time. Their main disadvantage is that they permit the acoustic properties of the experimental room to interact with the stimuli. This can cause the properties of the stimuli to be distorted for at least some members of a panel. All members may not "hear" the same thing. Headphones (particularly those with a good acoustic seal) minimize the extent to which the stimuli the judges hear are distorted by the acoustical properties of the experimental room.

A second advantage of headphones over speakers is that they make the intensity level at which the stimuli are presented to the raters easier to control since the transducer-to-subject distance is constant. By the same token, headphones also make it relatively simple to compensate at least partially for differences in the hearing thresholds of judges.

Loudness Level of the Stimuli

With audiotape recorded stimuli, it is necessary to define a loudness level for presenting the stimuli to the panel. This level usually is defined by the experimenter (implicitly or explicitly) as one the judges would regard as "comfortable." While such an approach would probably be satisfactory for rating some attributes (e.g., stuttering severity), it may not be satisfactory for others—that is, those whose attributes might vary as a function of the loudness level or levels at which they were presented. For rating attributes that may be of the latter type, it would probably be a good idea to define the loudness level more precisely. One approach would be to determine each panel member's speech reception threshold (SRT) and present the stimuli a given number of decibels above this threshold.

Physical Environment

The environment in which the stimuli are rated can influence the level of reliability of the ratings. As previously indicated, the acoustical properties of the experimental room can interact with those of audiotape recorded stimuli. Such an interaction would tend to increase the dispersion of the ratings and hence reduce their reliability.

The temperature and humidity levels within the experimental room also can influence the reliability of the ratings. If the judges are uncomfortable while rating the stimuli, they may divert some of the attention they should be devoting to the stimuli to their feelings of discomfort. This could reduce the reliability of their ratings.

Number of Judging Sessions

The rating task may be administered at a single session or divided into several sessions. While it is usually most efficient to have all the stimuli rated at a single session, this may not be possible or desirable. If the rating task is relatively long (i.e., longer than one hour), it almost always is desirable to divide the task into several sessions. It would also be desirable to divide the task into several sessions if the task were relatively short but so demanding that raters would likely become fatigued before completing it. Fatigue, of course, can reduce the reliability of the judges' ratings.

Analyses of Judges' Ratings

Once the judges have rated the stimuli, the next task is to analyze their ratings to yield: (1) a scale value for each of the stimuli, (2) an estimate of the reliability of these scale values, and (3) an index of the degree of agreement among the judges in their ratings of individual stimuli. Computational procedures for these three types of analyses are presented in the references cited for the six scaling methods in the section dealing with psychological scaling methods as measuring instruments. Here a general description of each type of analysis will be presented. We will also discuss two related topics: (1) the desirability of eliminating the ratings of judges who did not appear to be following instructions, and (2) the use of multiple regression analysis for inferring the attributes of the stimuli that influenced judges' ratings.

Computation of Scale Values

A stimulus's scale value is a number that designates the amount (relative or absolute) of the attribute rated that it possesses. This number indicates the location of the stimulus on the continuum, or scale, of possible values of this attribute. If a stimulus, for example, had a scale value of 4.0 on a seven-point, equal-appearing interval scale of stuttering severity where 1 designated least possible severity and 7 designated most possible severity, its location on this continuum, or scale, would be at the midpoint.

For the methods of equal-appearing intervals and direct magnitude-estimation, either the mean or median of the ratings assigned to a stimulus can be used as its scale value. Which of these is used may not make too much difference, even though mean and median scale values for a stimulus will differ somewhat in magnitude, since both appear to order a set of stimuli in approximately the same manner (Silverman, 1967a).

For the methods of pair comparisons, constant sums, rank order, and successive intervals, the computational procedures for deriving scale values are fairly complex. The math involved is not difficult, but it is time consuming. Programs are available for some computers for computing scale values from sets of ratings yielded by these methods. If an appropriate computer program is not available, it might be worthwhile to investigate the possibility of using a spreadsheet to create one.

Estimating Reliability of Scale Values

Before a set of scale values can be interpreted, it is necessary to establish whether they are sufficiently reliable for the purpose they were intended for. If they are not sufficiently reliable for this purpose, they cannot be used to answer the question or questions they were intended to answer. Both intrasubject and intersubject differences and relationships can be obscured.

Suppose you wished to determine whether dysarthrics were less hypernasal after being fitted with some sort of palatal prosthesis. You could have "before and after" treatment speech segments from such persons rated for degree of nasality. If the ratings were not adequately reliable, you could end up concluding the treatment made no difference when, in fact, it did.

What would be the minimum acceptable level of reliability for most purposes? Unless a difference were quite large or a relationship quite strong, you would stand a good chance of failing to detect it if the reliability of your scale values were less than 0.85. A reliability coefficient of 0.90 would probably be adequate except in instances where you were attempting to detect relatively small differences or relatively weak relationships. In such instances, a reliability coefficient of at least 0.95 probably would be necessary. This level probably could be achieved by using a fairly large judging panel—that is, one with more than 50 judges.

Several approaches have been used for estimating the reliability level of a set of scale values. One such approach that can be used with any scaling method is *test-retest*. With this approach, the panel either rates the entire set of stimuli twice (usually on different days) or a randomly selected sample of the set of stimuli twice (e.g., at the beginning and at the end of the rating session). Two sets of scale values are computed from these ratings and correlated.

Suppose you wished to use the test-retest approach and the number of stimuli you were having rated were 75. You could select from these a sample of 25 by means of a table of random numbers and have them rated twice in different random orders—once at the beginning and once at the end of the rating session. The observers, then, would rate a total of 100 stimuli. Sets of scale values for the 25 stimuli could be computed from the first and second ratings, and these two sets of scale values could be correlated, possibly using a Pearson product-moment correlation coefficient (see Chapter 9). The magnitude of this coefficient would indicate whether the ratings were likely to be adequately reliable.

Another approach that can be used with any scaling method for estimating reliability is the *split-half* method. With this approach, each member of a panel is randomly assigned to one of two groups. Two sets of scale values are computed—one from the ratings of the judges in each group. These sets of scale values are correlated, usually with a Pearson product-moment correlation coefficient. The resulting correlation coefficient can be interpreted as a reliability estimate for a panel *one half* the size of the panel used. This would tend to be a conservative estimate for the entire panel. A more accurate estimate for the entire panel would be obtained by inserting the value of the Pearson product-moment correlation coefficient that was computed into the Spearman-Brown formula (Guilford, 1954, p. 391).

The main disadvantage of the split-half approach is that it is necessary to compute three sets of scale values—two of which are used solely for estimating reliability.

A third approach to estimating the reliability of scale values that can be used with the methods of equal-appearing intervals and direct magnitude-estimation utilizes the *intraclass correlation coefficient for average ratings* (Ebel, 1951). With this approach, the ratings assigned to the stimuli are subjected to an analysis of variance (see Chapter 10). An intraclass correlation coefficient is computed from the resulting mean square values, that is,

$$r_{\text{intraclass}} = 1 - \frac{MS_{AS}}{MS_A}$$

One interpretation of this coefficient (which was paraphrased from Winer, 1962) is that if the experiment were to be repeated with another random sample of the same number of judges, but with the same stimuli, the correlation between the *mean* ratings obtained from the two sets of data on the same stimuli would be approximately the value obtained for this coefficient. Because of the close correspondence between mean and median scale values, this coefficient can also be used to estimate the reliability of *median* ratings (Silverman, 1968b).

The intraclass correlation coefficient discussed here provides a reliability estimate for the average of the ratings of a *group* of judges. Sometimes it may be necessary to estimate the reliability of the ratings of the *individual* judges in a panel. Ebel (1951) provides formulas for two intraclass correlation coefficients that can be used for this purpose. One provides an estimate of the reliability of single ratings that is adjusted for systematic differences in judges' frames of reference (i.e., internal standards). It is approximately equal to the average intercorrelation between ratings given by all possible pairs of judges (Winer, 1962). This coefficient provides an estimate of how closely judges' ratings order a set of stimuli in the same manner. Suppose three judges rated five speech segments for degree of nasality by the method of direct magnitude-estimation and assigned the ratings given in Table C-1.

While the absolute ratings assigned by these judges are quite different, the five segments have been ordered by them in the same manner. For this reason, the magnitude of the intraclass correlation coefficient computed with this formula would be quite high, indicating good interjudge agreement.

Ebel's other formula provides an estimate of the reliability of the *absolute* ratings assigned by individual judges. It indicates how closely the absolute ratings assigned by indi-

TABLE C-1   Direct magnitude-estimation ratings of five speech segments by three judges for degree of nasality.

Segment	Judge #1	Judge #2	Judge #3
A	150	150	95
B	375	250	165
C	333	200	125
D	400	300	175
E	270	185	115

vidual judges agree. This formula could be used for such a purpose as estimating how well speech-language pathologists agree in their assignment of stutterers to one of the eight points on the Iowa Scale for Rating Severity of Stuttering (Darley & Spriestersbach, 1978). If it were applied to the data used to illustrate the other intraclass correlation coefficient for the ratings of individual judges, the formula would yield a coefficient that was considerably lower because of the differences in the absolute magnitudes of the judges' ratings. The magnitude of this coefficient will almost always be lower than that of the other.

One other approach that has been used for estimating the reliability of scale values utilizes the *mean Q value*. This strategy has only been used in conjunction with the method of equal-appearing intervals. The mean Q value is the mean semi-interquartile range (see Chapter 9) of the ratings assigned to each of a set of stimuli. A semi-interquartile range is computed for the ratings assigned to each stimulus in a set, and the mean of these ranges is computed.

The mean Q value is a measure of average interjudge agreement. The smaller the mean Q value, the closer the agreement of the judges in their ratings. And the closer the agreement of the judges in their ratings, the higher the reliability (or stability) of the scale values.

Information on the distribution of mean Q values for stimuli rated on a seven-point, equal-appearing interval scale has been reported (Silverman, 1967b). The relative magnitude of an obtained mean Q value can be estimated by locating it in this distribution.

Degree of Agreement among Judges in Their Ratings of Individual Stimuli

Judges do not usually assign identical ratings to stimuli. There is ordinarily some variability in their ratings. It is sometimes useful to be able to describe the degree of agreement among the judges in their ratings of specific stimuli. Such information is useful, for example, in the construction of master scales. Suppose you wished to construct an equal-appearing interval master scale of nasality. You could have a large number of speech segments from persons with cleft palates rated on a seven-point, equal-appearing interval scale of degree of nasality. You would compute from the ratings assigned to each stimulus both a scale value and a measure of dispersion, or spread (e.g., the semi-interquartile range).

Next, you would identify segments that had scale values of 1.0, 2.0, 3.0, 4.0, 5.0, 6.0, and 7.0. From the segments having scale values at each of these points, you would select the one on which the dispersion of their ratings was the smallest. These seven segments ordered on a tape would constitute a seven-point master scale of nasality.

Several measures of dispersion have been used to describe the degree of agreement among the judges in their ratings of individual stimuli, including: (1) the range, (2) the interquartile range, (3) the semi-interquartile range, and (4) the standard deviation. These measures are described in Chapter 9.

Desirability of Eliminating Judges Who Did Not Appear to Follow Instructions

There are a few judges on almost every panel whose ratings are so different from those of the others that it appears likely they failed to follow instructions. Should the ratings of such judges be thrown out? Unfortunately, this isn't an easy question to answer. It is usually quite difficult to discriminate between judges who did not follow instructions and judges who did follow instructions but reacted to the stimuli differently than the other panel members. Suppose, for example, that a judge who was instructed to rate a set of stimuli by the method of equal-appearing intervals assigned 1s, 4s, and 7s to the stimuli. While it is likely that he or she failed to follow instructions, it is possible that all the stimuli fell at one of these points on his or her internally generated scale.

If the ratings of only a small proportion of the members of a panel are questionable, the scale values would probably not be influenced very much by including them. There would be no need in such a case to throw them out. If, on the other hand, a relatively high percentage of the members of a panel assigned ratings in a manner that suggested they were not following instructions, it would be important to determine whether this was the case. If it were established that they were not following instructions, it would be justifiable to throw out their ratings.

Use of Multiple Regression for Inferring Characteristics of the Stimuli That Influenced Judges' Ratings

A speech-language pathologist or audiologist may on occasion wish to answer a question such as the following:

1. What aspects of a stutterer's communicative behavior are apt to influence observers' judgments of his or her stuttering severity?
2. What aspects of the communicative behavior of an esophageal speaker are apt to influence observers' judgments of the "acceptability" of his or her speech?

Obviously many aspects of communicative behavior could influence observer judgments such as these. A procedure will be outlined in this section that can be helpful in identifying relevant aspects. This procedure utilizes multiple regression analysis (see Chapter 9). Representative studies from the speech-language pathology literature in which it has been used include those of Jordan (1960) and Shriner and Sherman (1967).

The procedure can be summarized briefly as follows:

1. A set of stimuli is rated by one of the scaling methods for the attribute the investigator wishes to study. This attribute for the first question would be stuttering severity and for the second question would be acceptability of speech. A scale value is computed from these ratings for each of the stimuli in the set. (These scale values serve as the *dependent variable* in the multiple regression analysis.)

2. Aspects of the stimuli that the investigator feels may have influenced the observers' ratings are measured. One such aspect relevant to the first question would be stuttering frequency; to the second question, speaking rate. (These measures serve as the *independent variables* in the multiple regression analysis.

3. A coefficient of multiple correlation (see Chapter 9) is computed between the dependent variable (i.e., the scale values) and the composite of the independent variables (i.e., the measures of the aspects of the stimuli the investigator felt may have influenced the observers' ratings). A multiple regression equation (see Chapter 9) is also computed. It is used for predicting the dependent variable from the independent variables.

4. Independent variables that do not appear to be related to the dependent variable are eliminated. Such variables are unlikely to have influenced the observers' ratings. The basic strategy here is to identify the independent variable that is least related to the observers' ratings and eliminate it. The coefficient of multiple correlation then is recomputed without this variable. If this coefficient is not significantly lower than the original one, the independent variable that is least related to the observers' ratings is identified and eliminated from among the remaining ones. The coefficient of multiple correlation is then recomputed. If it is not significantly (in a statistical sense) lower than the original one, the identification and elimination process is continued until the point is reached where a statistically significant difference exists between a multiple correlation coefficient computed on a reduced set of independent variables and the original multiple correlation coefficient. The independent variables remaining at this point are *hypothesized* to have influenced the observers' ratings. They are not, of course, the only independent variables that could have influenced the observers' ratings. There may have been other aspects of the stimuli which, if measured, would have been found to correlate with the observers' ratings.

A p p e n d i x **D**

Representative Regulations Governing the Use of Human Subjects

Nuremberg Code (1946)*

Note: The Nuremberg Code, which was one of the first attempts to regulate human experimentation, consists of ten points that delimit permissible experimentation on human subjects. It was motivated by abuses of such experimentation that occurred in Nazi Germany during World War II.

1. The voluntary consent of the human subject is absolutely essential. This means that the persons involved should have the capacity to give legal consent; should be situated as to be able to exercise free power of choice, without the intervention of any element of force, fraud, deceit, duress, over-reaching, or other ulterior form of constraint or coercion, and should have sufficient knowledge and comprehension of the elements of the subject matter involved as to enable him to make an understanding and enlightened decision. This latter element requires that before the acceptance of an affirmative decision by the experimental subject there should be made known to him the nature, duration, and purpose of the experiment; the method and means by which it is to be conducted; all inconveniences and hazards reasonably to be expected; and the effects upon his health or person which may possibly come from his participation in the experiment.

The duty and responsibility for ascertaining the quality of the consent rests upon each individual who initiates, directs, or engages in the experiment. It is a personal duty and responsibility which may not be delegated to another with impunity.

---

*Reprinted from "Permissible medical experiments" (no date) in *Trials of War Criminals before the Nuremberg Military Tribunals under Control Council Law No. 10: Nuremberg 1946 to April 1949.* Washington, DC: U.S. Government Printing Office.

2. The experiment should be such as to yield fruitful results for the good of society, unprocurable by other methods or means of study, and not random and unnecessary in nature.

3. The experiment should be designed and based on the results of animal experimentation and a knowledge of the natural history of the disease or other problem under study that the anticipated result will justify the performance of the experiment.

4. The experiment should be so conducted to avoid all unnecessary physical and mental suffering and injury.

5. No experiment should be conducted where there is an *a priori* reason to believe that death or disabling injury will occur; except, perhaps, where the experimental physicians also serve as subjects.

6. The degree of risk to be taken should never exceed that determined by the humanitarian importance of the problem to be solved by the experiment.

7. Proper preparations should be made and adequate facilities provided to protect the experimental subject against even remote possibilities of injury, disability, or death.

8. The experiment should be conducted only by scientifically qualified persons. The highest degree of skill and care should be required through all stages of the experiment of those who conduct or engage in the experiment.

9. During the course of the experiment the human subject should be at liberty to bring the experiment to an end if he has reached the physical or mental state where continuation of the experiment seems to him to be impossible.

10. During the course of the experiment the scientist in charge must be prepared to terminate the experiment at any stage, if he has probable cause to believe, in the exercise of good faith, superior skill and careful judgment required of him that a continuation of the experiment is likely to result in injury, disability, or the death of the experimental subject.

*Declaration of Helsinki (1964)**

Note: This document has replaced the Nuremberg Code to some extent. The recommendations contained in it for conducting experiments using human subjects has been adopted by the World Medical Association. It represents one of the first attempts by the international scientific community to regulate human experimentation. Although its emphasis is medical, most of the recommendations are applicable to research in speech-language pathology and audiology. To increase its relevancy to our field, I have substituted the word "clinician" for the words "doctor" and "physician;" the word "patient" for "sick person;" and the words "he and she" for "he."

Introduction

It is the mission of the clinician to safeguard the health of the people. His or her knowledge and conscience are dedicated to the fulfillment of this mission. . . .

Because it is essential that the results of laboratory experiments be applied to human

*Reproduced with permission of *The World Medical Journal*.

beings to further scientific knowledge and to help suffering humanity, the World Health Association has prepared the following recommendations as a guide to each clinician involved in clinical research. It must be stressed that the standards as drafted are only a guide to clinicians all over the world. They are not relieved from criminal, civil and ethical responsibilities under the laws of their own country.

In the field of clinical research a fundamental distinction must be recognized between clinical research in which the aim is essentially therapeutic for the patient and clinical research, the essential object of which is purely scientific and without therapeutic value to the person subjected to the research.

I. Basic Principles

1. Clinical research must conform to the moral and scientific principles that justify such research and should be based on . . . experiments or other scientifically established facts.
2. Clinical research should be conducted only by scientifically qualified persons. . .
3. Clinical research cannot legitimately be carried out unless the importance of the objective is in proportion to the inherent risk to the subject.
4. Every clinical research project should be preceded by careful assessment of inherent risks in comparison to foreseeable benefits to the subject or to others.
5. Special caution should be exercised by the clinician in performing clinical research in which the personality of the subject is liable to be altered by drugs or experimental procedure.

II. Clinical Research Combined with Professional Care

1. In the treatment of a patient, the clinician must be free to use a new therapeutic measure, if in his or her judgment it offers hope. . .

   If at all possible, consistent with patient psychology, the clinician should obtain the patient's freely given consent after the patient has been given a full explanation. In case of legal incapacity, consent should also be procured from the legal guardian; in the case of physical incapacity the permission of the legal guardian replaces that of the patient.
2. The clinician can combine clinical research with professional care, the objective being the acquisition of new clinical knowledge, only to the extent that clinical research is justified by its therapeutic value for the patient.

III. Non-Therapeutic Clinical Research

1. In the purely scientific application of clinical research carried out on a human being, it is the duty of the clinician to remain the protector of the life and health of that person on whom clinical research is being carried out.
2. The nature, the purpose and the risk of clinical research must be explained to the subject by the clinician.
3a. Clinical research on a human being cannot be undertaken without his or her free consent after he or she has been informed; if he or she is legally incompetent, the consent of the legal guardian should be procured.

3b. The subject of clinical research should be in such a mental, physical and legal state to be able to exercise fully his or her power of choice.

3c. Consent should, as a rule, be obtained in writing. However, the responsibility for clinical research always remains with the research worker; it never falls on the subject, even after consent is obtained.

4a. The investigator must respect the right of each individual to safeguard his personal integrity, especially if the subject is in a dependent relationship to the investigator.

4b. At any time during the course of clinical research the subject or his or her guardian should be free to withdraw permission for research to be continued.

The investigator or the investigating team should discontinue the research if in his, her, or their judgment, it may, if continued, be harmful to the individual.

Glossary

Many of the terms relevant to statistics and research design that were used in this book are briefly defined here. For definitions of other terms or for more complete definitions of those defined, consult the index. For a glossary of symbols used in Appendix A, see p. 296. Words in capital letters are defined elsewhere in the glossary.

Alpha Level   See LEVEL OF CONFIDENCE.

Answerable Question   A question that can be answered by observations that can be made and that implicitly or explicitly (preferably the latter) specifies the observation or observations necessary to answer it.

Applied Research   RESEARCH that implicitly or explicitly is intended to increase our understanding of how to prevent the development of, or modify behaviors contributing to, communicative disorders.

Attributes of Events   Measurable or verbally describable properties of EVENTS.

"Before and After" Design   Research design in which measures are made before and after the administration of a TREATMENT (e.g., a therapy program).

Bivariate Distribution   A DISTRIBUTION in which the observations are assigned to categories on the basis of two of their ATTRIBUTES.

Causality   Assumption of the SCIENTIFIC METHOD that every event has a cause.

Chance   See RANDOM FLUCTUATION.

Clinician-Investigator   A speech-language pathologist or audiologist who functions as both a clinician and a clinical investigator.

Confidence Interval   An INFERENTIAL STATISTIC for estimating POPULATION values of DESCRIPTIVE STATISTICS and differences between such statistics.

Constant Sums   A PSYCHOLOGICAL SCALING METHOD.

Correlation Coefficient   An INDEX OF ASSOCIATION.

Criterion Measure   A measure of an ATTRIBUTE of an EVENT.

Cubic Relationship   A NONLINEAR RELATIONSHIP between VARIABLES (see Figure 6-6).

Curvilinear Relationship   A NONLINEAR RELATIONSHIP between VARIABLES (see Figure 6-5).

Data   Symbolic representations (numerical or verbal descriptions) of ATTRIBUTES of EVENTS. See QUANTITATIVE and QUALITATIVE DATA.

Degrees of Freedom   This value for a set of DATA designates the DISTRIBUTION (row and/or column) in the table that contains the critical value of the statistic for testing the NULL HYPOTHESIS.

Dependent Measures   Sets of measures made on the same subjects or on matched groups of subjects.

Dependent Variable   A VARIABLE whose value one seeks to determine.

Descriptive Statistics   Indices that describe an ATTRIBUTE of a set of measures. See MEASURES OF ASSOCIATION, CENTRAL TENDENCY, and VARIABILITY.

df   Abbreviation for DEGREES OF FREEDOM.

Direct Magnitude-Estimation   A PSYCHOLOGICAL SCALING METHOD.

Distribution   A set of categories to which measures are assigned. See BIVARIATE, MULTIVARIATE, and UNIVARIATE DISTRIBUTIONS.

End Effect   A piling up of ratings in one or both of the extreme intervals when the method of EQUAL-APPEARING INTERVALS is used.

Equal-Appearing Intervals   A PSYCHOLOGICAL SCALING METHOD.

Event   A phenomenon that occurs in a certain place during a particular interval of time.

Experimental Condition   A set of circumstances under which observations are made.

Experimenter Bias   The impact of an experimenter's expectations and beliefs on his or her observations.

Extensional Definition   Pointing to or exhibiting in some way the actual objects, phenomena, and so on that the term you wish to define refers to.

Face Validity   Refers to a test or observational procedure intuitively appearing to be valid for the purpose intended.

Generality   The extent to which the persons or events observed are representative of those in the POPULATION to which a question refers.

Hypothesis   A tentative theory adopted to explain certain observations.

Independent Measures   Sets of measures made on different groups of persons.

Independent Variable   A VARIABLE whose values are known.

Index of Association   See MEASURES OF ASSOCIATION.

Index of Central Tendency   See MEASURES OF CENTRAL TENDENCY.

Index of Variability   See MEASURES OF VARIABILITY.

Inferential Statistics   Indices that allow one to answer certain kinds of questions about a set of data that go beyond analyses that were made of it. See SIGNIFICANCE TESTS and CONFIDENCE INTERVALS.

Interval Scale   A measurement SCALE in which NUMERALS designate points on a continuum that have equal amounts of the ATTRIBUTE being measured between them.

Laboratory Setting   An artificial controlled environment in which observations are made.

Level of Confidence   States how small the PROBABILITY of a NULL HYPOTHESIS being true has to be before it is rejected. See SIGNIFICANCE TESTS.

Linear Relationship   When two VARIABLES are linearly related, an increase (or decrease) in the magnitude of one is associated with a proportional increase (or decrease) in the value of the other. The points in a SCATTERGRAM for two VARI-ABLES that are linearly related lie on a straight line.

Logarithmic Scale A measurement SCALE in which NUMERALS designate points on a continuum that have unequal, but known, mathematically defined amounts of the ATTRIBUTE being measured between them.

Mean An INDEX OF CENTRAL TENDENCY that is the arithmetic average of a set of measures.

Measurement The assignment of NUMERALS to ATTRIBUTES of EVENTS according to rules.

Measurement Error Various forms of RANDOM and SYSTEMATIC ERROR that influence the reliability of observations.

Measures of Association Indices used to describe the strength and direction of the relationships between sets of measures.

Measures of Central Tendency Indices that designate the "average," "typical," or most frequently occurring NUMERAL in a set of numerals. See MEAN, MEDIAN, and MODE.

Measures of Variability Indices that designate the spread, dispersion, homogeneity, or variability of a set of NUMERALS.

Median An INDEX OF CENTRAL TENDENCY; it is the measure at the midpoint of a set of measures when they are ordered from lowest to highest (or from highest to lowest).

Mode An INDEX OF CENTRAL TENDENCY; it is the most frequently occurring measure in a set of measures.

Multivariate Distribution A DISTRIBUTION in which observations are assigned to categories on the basis of two or more of their attributes.

N Abbreviation for number of subjects.

Negative Relationship A relationship between two VARIABLES in which individuals who tend to score highly on one tend to have relatively low scores on the other, and vice versa (see Figure 6-4).

Nominal Scale A measurement SCALE in which NUMERALS merely designate, or label, categories.

Nonlinear Relationship When two VARIABLES are not linearly related, an increase (or decrease) in the magnitude of one is not associated with a proportional increase (or decrease) in the magnitude of the other. The points on a SCATTERGRAM for the two VARIABLES would not lie on a straight line.

Nonrandom Sample A SAMPLE that is not generated by a RANDOM SAMPLING METHOD.

Normal Distribution A symmetrical, bell-shaped curve in which certain relationships hold regarding its height at specified distances from its center (see Figure 9-1).

Null Hypothesis The hypothesis tested by a SIGNIFICANCE TEST. It states that observed differences or relationships are due to CHANCE, or RANDOM FLUCTUATION.

Numerals Number symbols; their meanings are determined by the rules used to assign them.

One-Tailed Test A SIGNIFICANCE TEST intended to detect a difference between measures (e.g., MEANS) in one direction only.

Order Effect   A phenomenon that systematically improves or impairs a subject's performance on a series of tasks (e.g., learning or fatigue).

Ordinal Scale   A MEASUREMENT SCALE in which NUMERALS designate locations in a rank order.

Organismic Variables   Properties, or ATTRIBUTES, of the individual. Examples are sex, chronological age, and educational level.

Paired Comparisons   A PSYCHOLOGICAL SCALING METHOD.

Placebo Effect   Changes produced by placebo—that is, therapeutic procedures that are objectively without specific activity for the condition being treated.

Population   The group of persons to whom a research question refers.

Positive Relationship   A relationship between two VARIABLES in which individuals who tend to score highly on one also tend to score highly on the other and vice versa.

Probability   The likelihood of the occurrence of an EVENT.

Psychological Scaling Methods   Techniques for MEASURING, or quantifying, ATTRIBUTES of EVENTS through the use of observer judgments.

Pure Research   Research that implicitly or explicitly is intended to increase our understanding of the etiology of communicative disorders.

Qualitative Data (or Concepts)   Verbal descriptions of ATTRIBUTES of EVENTS.

Quantitative Data (or Concepts)   Numerical descriptions of ATTRIBUTES of EVENTS.

Random Error   A form of error present to some degree in all MEASUREMENT processes that does not bias the data resulting from such processes.

Random Fluctuation   Unpredictable variation in measures of ATTRIBUTES of EVENTS.

Random Sample   A SAMPLE selected by a random sampling process—for example, a table of random numbers (see Appendix B).

Ratio Scale   A MEASUREMENT SCALE in which NUMERALS designate points on a continuum that both have equal amounts of an ATTRIBUTE between them and are related to an absolute zero.

Reliability   This refers to the repeatability of the observations used to answer a question.

Replication   Repetition of a study or observational procedure used to answer a question or questions.

Representativeness   Refers to the extent to which the ATTRIBUTES of the persons or EVENTS in a SAMPLE are similar to those in the POPULATION from which the sample was selected.

Research   This refers to the process underlying the asking and answering of questions. See APPLIED RESEARCH and PURE RESEARCH.

Research Hypothesis   The HYPOTHESIS an investigator seeks to test.

Sample   Part of a POPULATION.

Scale   A succession or progression of steps or degrees, or a graduated series of categories.

Scaling Method   See PSYCHOLOGICAL SCALING METHOD.

Scattergram   A two-dimensional graphical display used for assessing the relationship between two variables (see Figures 6-2 through 6-7).

Scientific Method   A set of rules for asking and answering questions.

Sequence Effect   Occurs when a subject's performance on a task is enhanced or impaired by his or her having performed a particular task prior to it.

Significance Tests   INFERENTIAL STATISTICS used to estimate the PROBABILITY that observed differences and relationships between DESCRIPTIVE STATISTICS resulted from RANDOM FLUCTUATION.

Statistical Inference   Statistical techniques that provide information needed to generalize beyond a set of DATA or SAMPLE of subjects. See CONFIDENCE INTERVALS and SIGNIFICANCE TESTS.

Statistically Significant Result   A finding is regarded as statistically significant if the NULL HYPOTHESIS is rejected.

Statistics   Numerical procedures for analyzing, organizing, and summarizing QUANTI- TATIVE DATA. See DESCRIPTIVE STATISTICS and INFERENTIAL STATISTICS.

Subject Bias   Results from subjects responding to experimental conditions in the manner in which they feel the experimenter either would like them to respond or expects them to respond.

Successive Intervals   A PSYCHOLOGICAL SCALING METHOD.

Systematic Error   A form of error that can be present in a MEASUREMENT process that can bias the DATA resulting from that process.

Systematic Observation   A process that permits individual ATTRIBUTES of EVENTS to be described with adequate levels of VALIDITY and RELIABILITY.

Treatment   An experimental condition under which subjects are observed.

Two-Tailed Test   A SIGNIFICANCE TEST intended to detect a difference between mea- sures (e.g., MEANS) in either direction.

Type I Error   Rejection of the NULL HYPOTHESIS when it should not have been rejected—that is, when the observed difference or relationship really was the result of RANDOM FLUCTUATION.

Type II Error   Failure to reject the NULL HYPOTHESIS when it should have been rejected.

Univariate Distribution   A DISTRIBUTION in which observations are assigned to cate- gories on the basis of one of their ATTRIBUTES.

Validity   The appropriateness of observations for answering a question they are used to answer.

Variable   A quantity that can assume more than one value. See DEPENDENT VARI- ABLE and INDEPENDENT VARIABLE.

References

Agnew, N.M., & Pyke, S.W. (1975). *The Science Game*. Englewood Cliffs, NJ: Prentice-Hall.

Albright, R.G. (1988). *A Basic Guide to Online Information Systems for Health Care Professionals*. Arlington, VA: Information Resources Press.

Anderson, N.B. (1991). Understanding cultural diversity. *American Journal of Speech-Language Pathology*, 1(1), 9–10.

Anderson, N.B. (1992). Understanding cultural diversity. *American Journal of Speech-Language Pathology*, 1(2), 11–12.

Anderson, P., & Fenichel, E. (1989). *Serving Culturally Diverse Families of Infants and Toddlers with Disabilities*. Washington, DC: National Center for Clinical Infant Programs.

Angle, E. (1907). *Malocclusion of the Teeth* (Seventh Edition). Philadelphia: S.S. White Dental Manufacturing Company.

Applebaum, P.S., Lidz, C.W., & Meisel, A. (1987). *Informed Consent: Legal Theory and Clinical Practice*. New York: Oxford University Press.

Attanasio, J.S. (1986). Therapy and research: Response to Siegel and Spradlin (1985). *Journal of Speech and Hearing Disorders*, 51, 378.

Baer, D.M., Wolf, M.M., & Risley, T.R. (1968). Some current dimensions in applied behavior analysis. *Journal of Applied Behavior Analysis*, 1, 91–97.

Barber, T.X. (1976). *Pitfalls in Human Research*. New York: Pergamon Press.

Barlow, D.H., & Hayes, S.C. (1979). Alternating treatments design: One strategy for comparing the effects of two treatments on a single subject. *Journal of Applied Behavior Analysis*, 12 (2), 199–210.

Barlow, D.H., & Hersen, M. (1973). Single-case experimental designs: Uses in applied clinical research. *Archives of General Psychiatry*, 29, 319–325.

Barlow, D.H., & Hersen, M. (1984). *Single Case Experimental Designs: Strategies for Studying Behavior Change* (Second Edition). New York: Pergamon Press.

Basilevsky, A. (1994). *Statistical Factor Analysis and Related Methods*. New York: Wiley.

Bat-Chava, Y. (1993). Antecedents of self-esteem in deaf people: A meta-analytic review. *Rehabilitation Psychology*, 38(4), 221–234.

Battle, D.E. (1993). *Communication Disorders in Multicultural Populations*. Boston: Andover Medical Publishers.

Bauer, D.G. (1995). *The "How To" Grants Manual: Successful Grantseeking Techniques for Obtaining Public and Private Grants* (Third Edition). Phoenix, AZ: Oryx Press.

Beasley, D.S., & Manning, J.I. (1973). Experimenter bias and speech pathologists' evaluation of children's language skills. *Journal of Communication Disorders*, 6, 93–101.

Bebout, L., & Arthur, B. (1992). Cross-cultural attitudes toward speech disorders. *Journal of Speech and Hearing Research*, 35, 45–52.

Bench, R.J. (1989). Science and theory in communication disorders: A response to Siegel and Ingham (1987). *Journal of Speech and Hearing Disorders*, 54, 296–298.

Berkman, R.I. (1990). *Find It Fast*. New York: Harper & Row.

Berry, R.C., & Silverman, F.H. (1972). Equality of intervals on the Lewis-Sherman scale of stuttering severity. *Journal of Speech and Hearing Research*, 15, 185–188.

Berry, W.R., Darley, F.L., Aronson, A.E., & Goldstein, N.P. (1974). Dysarthria in Wilson's disease. *Journal of Speech and Hearing Research*, 17, 160–183.

Best, J.W., & Kahn, J.V. (1989). *Research in Education* (Sixth Edition). Englewood Cliffs, NJ: Prentice-Hall.

Bird, J., Bishop, D.V.M., & Freeman, N.H. (1995). Phonological awareness and literacy development in children with expressive phonological impairments. *Journal of Speech and Hearing Research*, 38, 446–462.

Birnbrauer, J.S., Peterson, C.R., & Solnick, J.V. (1974). Design and interpretation of studies of single subjects. *American Journal of Mental Deficiency*, 79, 191–203.

Bloodstein, O. (1987). *A Handbook on Stuttering*. Chicago: National Easter Seal Society for Crippled Children and Adults.

Bloom, C.M., & Silverman, F.H. (1973). Do all stutterers adapt? *Journal of Speech and Hearing Research*, 16, 518–521.

Bogartz, R.S. (1994). *An Introduction to the Analysis of Variance*. Westport, CT: Praeger.

Booth, V. (1993). *Communicating in Science : Writing a Scientific Paper and Speaking at Scientific Meetings* (Second Edition). New York: Cambridge University Press.

Borgman, C.L., Moghdam, D., & Corbett, P.K. (1984). *Effective Online Searching*. New York: Marcel Dekker.

Bridgman, P.W. (1927). *The Logic of Modern Physics*. New York: The Macmillan Company.

Briggs, J., & Peat, F.D. (1989). *Turbulent Mirrors: An Illustrated Guide to Chaos Theory and the Science of Wholeness*. New York: Harper & Row.

Bromley, D.B. (1986). *The Case-study Method in Psychology and Related Disciplines*. New York: John Wiley & Sons.

Brookshire, R.H. (1983). Subject description and generality of results in experiments with aphasic adults. *Journal of Speech and Hearing Disorders*, 48, 342–346.

Buckley, W., (Ed.) (1968). *Modern Systems Research for the Behavioral Scientist*. Chicago: Aldine Publishing Company.

Bush, S.G. (1974). Should the history of science be rated X? *Science*, 183, 1164–1172.

Campbell, C.R., & Jackson, S.T. (1995). Transparency of one-handed Amer-Ind hand signals to nonfamiliar viewers. *Journal of Speech and Hearing Research*, 38, 1284–1289.

Campbell, D.T. (1963). From description to experimentation: Interpreting trends as quasi-experiments. In C.W. Harris (Ed.), *Problems in Measuring Change* (pp. 212–242). Madison: University of Wisconsin Press.

Campbell, D.T., & Stanley, J.C. (1966). *Experimental and Quasi-Experimental Designs for Research*. Chicago: Rand McNally.

Campbell, S.K. (1974), *Flaws and Fallacies in Statistical Thinking*. Englewood Cliffs, NJ: Prentice-Hall.

Carlson, M. (1995). *Winning Grants Step by Step: Support Centers of America's Complete Workbook for Planning, Developing, and Writing Successful Proposals*. San Francisco: Jossey-Bass Publishers.

Caruso, A.J., Chodzko-Zajko, W.J., Bidinger, D.A., & Sommers, R.K. (1994). Adults who stutter: Responses to cognitive stress. *Journal of Speech and Hearing Research*, 37, 746–754.

Catlett, C. (1989). Constructing a competitive proposal. *Asha*, 31 (2), 70–72.

Chadwick, B.A., Bahr, H.M., & Albrecht, S.L. (1984).

Social Science Research Methods. Englewood Cliffs, NJ: Prentice-Hall.

Cheng, L. (1989). Service delivery to Asian/Pacific LEP children: A cross-cultural framework. *Topics in Language Disorders*, 9(3), 1–14.

Clark, J.G., & Stemple, J.C. (1982), Assessment of three modes of alaryngeal speech with a synthetic sentence identification (SSI) task in varying message-to-completion ratios. *Journal of Speech and Hearing Research*, 25, 333–338.

Code, C., & Ball, M. (Eds.) (1984). *Instrumentation in Speech-Language Pathology*. San Diego: College-Hill.

Cohen, S.H., & Reese, H.W. (1994). *Life-span Developmental Psychology : Methodological Contributions*. Hillsdale, NJ : Lawrence Erlbaum Associates.

Cole, E. (1989). E. pluribus pluribus: Multicultural imperatives for the 1990s and beyond. *Asha*, 31(9), 66–70.

Cole, L. (1986). The social responsibility of the researcher. *Concerns for Minority Groups in Communication Disorders. ASHA Reports*, 16, 93–98.

Comrey, A.L., & Lee, H.B. (1992). *A First Course in Factor Analysis* (Second Edition). Hillsdale, NJ: Lawrence Erlbaum Associates.

Connell, P.J., & Thompson, C.K. (1986). Flexibility of single-subject experimental designs. Part III: Using flexibility to design or modify experiments. *Journal of Speech and Hearing Disorders*, 51, 204–214.

Cook, T.D., & Campbell, D.T. (1979). *Quasi-experimentation*. Boston: Houghton Mifflin.

Costello, J.M. (1979). Clinicians and researchers: A necessary dichotomy? *Journal of the National Student Speech and Hearing Association*, 7, 6–26.

Cudahy, E. (1988). *Introduction to Instrumentation in Speech and Hearing*. Baltimore: Williams and Wilkins.

Culatta, R.A. (1984). Why articles don't get published in Asha. *Asha*, 26 (3), 25–27.

Curtis, J.F., & Schultz, M.C. (1986). *Basic Laboratory Instrumentation for Speech and Hearing*. Boston: Little, Brown.

Cuvo, A.J. (1979). Multiple-baseline design in instruc-

tional research: Pitfalls of measurement and procedural advantages. *American Journal of Mental Deficiency*, 84, 219–228.

Darley, F.L., & Spriestersbach, D.C. (1978). *Diagnostic Methods in Speech Pathology* (Second Edition). New York: Harper and Row, Publishers.

Davidson, P.O., & Costello, C.G.N. (1969). *N=1: Experimental Studies of Single Cases*. New York: Van Nostrand Reinhold.

Davison, M.L. (1992). *Multidimensional Scaling* (Second Edition). Malabar, FL: Krieger Publishing Company.

Day, R.A. (1992). *Scientific English : A Guide for Scientists and Other Professionals*. Phoenix, AZ: Oryx Press.

Day, R.A. (1994). *How to Write & Publish a Scientific Paper* (Fourth Edition). Phoenix, AZ : Oryx Press.

Decker, L.E. (1993). *Grantseeking*. Charlottesville, VA: Community Collaborators.

Decker, T.N. (1989). *Instrumentation: An Introduction for Students in Speech and Hearing Sciences*. White Plains, NY: Longman.

De Krom, G. (1994). Consistency and reliability of voice quality ratings for different types of speech fragments. *Journal of Speech and Hearing Research*, 37, 985–1000.

De Krom, G. (1995). Some spectral correlates of pathological breathy and rough voice quality for different types of vowel fragments. *Journal of Speech and Hearing Research*, 38, 794–811.

Dowell, R.C, Martin, L.F.A., Tong, Y.C., Clark, G.M., Seligman, P.M., & Patrick, J.F. (1982). A 12-consonant confusion study of a multiple-channel cochlear implant patient. *Journal of Speech and Hearing Research*, 25, 509–516.

Dubno, J.R., Lee, F.-S., Klein, A.J., Matthews, L.J., & Lam, C.F. (1995). Confidence limits for maximum word-recognition scores. *Journal of Speech and Hearing Research*, 38, 490–502.

Duffy, J.R., Watt, J., & Duffy, R.J. (1981). Path analysis: A strategy for investigating multivariate causal relationships in communication disorders. *Journal of Speech and Hearing Research*, 24, 474–490.

Dukes, W.F. (1965). N=1. *Psychological Bulletin*, 64, 74–79.

Durlak, J.A. (1995). Understanding meta-analysis. In L. Grimm & P. Yarnold (Eds.), *Reading and Understanding Multivariate Statistics* (pp. 319–352). Washington, DC: American Psychological Association.

Ebel, R. (1951). Estimation of the reliability of ratings. *Psychometrika*, 16, 407–424.

Edgar, E., & Billingsley, F. (1974). Believability when N=1. *Psychological Record*, 24, 147–160.

Edgington, E.S. (1967). Statistical inference from N=1 experiments. *Journal of Psychology*, 65, 195–199.

Edgington, E.S. (1972). N=1 experiments: Hypothesis testing. *Canadian Psychology*, 13, 121–135.

Edgington, E.S. (1984). Statistics and single case analysis. In M. Hersen, R.M. Eisler, & P.M. Miller (Eds.), *Progress in Behavior Modification* (Volume 16). Orlando: Academic Press.

Edwards, A.L. (1957). *Techniques of Attitude Scale Construction*. New York: Appleton-Century-Crofts.

Edwards, A.L. (1985). *Multiple Regression and the Analysis of Variance and Covariance* (Second Edition). New York: W.H. Freeman.

Einstein, A., & Infeld, L. (1938). *The Evolution of Physics*. New York: Simon and Schuster.

Elbert, M., Shelton, R.L., & Arndt, W.B. (1967). A task for evaluation of articulation change: I. Development of methodology. *Journal of Speech and Hearing Research*, 10, 281–288.

Elliott, L. (1986). Discrimination and response bias for CV syllables differing in voice onset time among children and adults. *Journal of the Acoustical Society of America*, 80, 1250–1255.

Elliott, L., & Hammer, M.A. (1993). Fine-grained auditory discrimination: Factor structure. *Journal of Speech and Hearing Research*, 36, 396–409.

Erickson, J., & Iglesias, A. (1986). Assessment of communication disorders in non-English proficient children. In O. Taylor (Ed.), *Nature of Communication Disorders in Culturally and Linguistically Diverse Populations* (pp. 181–218). San Diego: College-Hill.

Everitt, B.S. (1993). *Cluster Analysis* (Third Edition). New York: Halsted Press.

Ezekiel, M., & Fox, K.A. (1963). *Methods of Correlation and Regression Analysis* (Third Edition). New York: John Wiley & Sons.

Fain, M. (1990). Opportunities for service in third world countries. *Asha*, 32(5), 45–46.

Feigl, H. (1953). The scientific outlook: Naturalism and humanism. In H. Feigl & M. Brodbeck (Eds.), *Readings in the Philosophy of Science* (pp. 8–18). New York: Appleton-Century-Crofts.

Felsenfeld, S., Broen, P.A., & McGue, M. (1994). A 28-year follow-up of adults with a history of moderate phonological disorder: Educational and occupational results. *Journal of Speech and Hearing Research*, 37, 1341–1353.

Ferguson, G.A. (1989). *Statistical Analysis in Psychology and Education* (Sixth Edition). New York: McGraw-Hill.

Fey, M.E., Cleave, P.L., Ravida, A.I., Long, S.H., Dejmal, A.E., & Easton, D.L. (1994). Effects of grammatical facilitation on the phonological performance of children with speech and language impairments. *Journal of Speech and Hearing Research*, 37, 594–607.

Final regulations amending basic HHS policy for the protection of human research subjects (1981). *Federal Register*, 46, 8366–8392.

Finn, P., & Glow, M. (1990). Clinical implications from Meyers (1989) on preschool stutterers and their conversational partners: Too much ado about null. *Journal of Speech and Hearing Disorders*, 55, 172–173.

Finn, P., & Ingham, R.J. (1994). Stutterers' self-ratings of how natural speech sounds and feels. *Journal of Speech and Hearing Research*, 37, 326–340.

Fisher, R.A. (1960). *The Design of Experiments* (Seventh Edition). New York: Hafner.

Fitz-Gibbon, C.T. (1986). In defence of randomized controlled trials, with suggestions about the possible use of meta-analysis. *British Journal of Disorders of Communication*, 21, 117–124.

Freund, P. (Ed.) (1970). *Experimentation with Human Subjects*. New York: George Braziller.

Fried, C. (1974). *Medical Experimentation: Personal Integrity and Social Policy*. New York: American Elsevier.

Gardner, M.J., & Altman, D.G. (1990). Confidence—and clinical importance in research findings. *British Journal of Psychiatry*, 156, 472–474.

Gelatt, J.P. (1989). Obtaining grant funding: Ten steps to success. *Asha*, 31 (2), 67–69.

Girolametto L., & Tannock, R. (1994). Correlates of directiveness in the interactions of fathers and mothers of children with developmental delays. *Journal of Speech and Hearing Research*, 37, 1178–1192.

Gitlin, L.N. (1996). *Successful Grant Writing*. New York: Springer Publishing Company.

Glass, G.V., McGaw, B., & Smith, M.L. (1981). *Meta-analysis in Social Research*. Beverly Hills, CA: Sage Publications.

Glass, G.V., Wilson, V.L., & Gottman, J.M. (1975). *Design and Analysis of Time-series Experiments*. Boulder, CO: Colorado Associated University Press.

Golenpaul, D. (Ed.) (1973). *Information Please Almanac, Atlas, and Yearbook 1974*. New York: Simon and Schuster.

Gorenflo, C.W., Gorenflo, D.W., & Santer, S.A. (1994). Effects of synthetic voice output on attitudes toward the augmented communicator. *Journal of Speech and Hearing Research*, 37, 64–68.

Gosling, C.G., Knight, N.H., & McKenney, L.S. (1989). *Search PsycINFO*. Washington, DC: American Psychological Association.

Gostin, L. (1991). Ethical principles for the conduct of human subject research: Population-based research and ethics. *Law, Medicine & Health Care*, 19(3–4), 191–201.

Gottman, J.M. (1973). N-of-one and N-of-two research in psychotherapy. *Psychological Bulletin*, 80, 93–105.

Gottman, J.M. (1981). *Time-Series Analysis*. Cambridge: Cambridge University Press.

Gottman, J.M., & Glass, G.V. (1978). Analysis of interrupted time-series experiments. In T.R. Kratochwill (Ed.), *Single Subject Research—Strategies for Evaluating Change* (pp. 197–236). New York: Academic Press.

Gottman, J.M., & Notarius, C. (1978). Sequential analysis of observational data using Markov chains. In T.R. Kratochwill (Ed.), *Single Subject Research—Strategies for Evaluating Change* (pp. 237–285). New York: Academic Press.

Green, P.E., Carmone, Jr., J., & Smith, S.M. (1989). *Multidimensional Scaling: Concepts and Applications*. Boston: Allyn & Bacon.

Greenwald, A. (1975). Consequences of prejudice against the null hypothesis. *Psychological Bulletin*, 82, 1–20.

Greenwald, M.K., Ryan, M.K., & Mulvihill, J.E. (Eds.) (1982). *Human Subject Research: A Handbook for Institutional Review Boards*. New York: Planum Press.

Grodin, M.A., & Glantz, L.H. (1994). *Children as Research Subjects: Science, Ethics, and Law*. New York: Oxford University Press.

Grose, J.H., Hall III, J.W., Gibbs, C. (1993). Temporal analysis in children. *Journal of Speech and Hearing Research*, 36, 351–356.

Grose, J.H., Poth, E.A., & Peters, R.W. (1994). Masking level differences for tones and speech in elderly listeners with relatively normal audiograms. *Journal of Speech and Hearing Research*, 37, 422–428.

Guidelines for nonsexist language in journals of ASHA. (1979). *Asha*, 21, 973–978.

Guilford, J.P. (1954). *Psychometric Methods*. New York: McGraw-Hill.

Gutierrez-Clellen, V.F., & Hofstetter, R. (1994). Syntactic complexity in Spanish narratives: A developmental study. *Journal of Speech and Hearing Research*, 37, 645–654.

Hall, M. (1988). *Getting Funded: A Complete Guide to Proposal Writing*. Portland, OR: Continuing Education Publications.

Hall, N.E., Yamashita, T.S., & Aram, D.M. (1993). Relationship between language and fluency in children with developmental language disorders. *Journal of Speech and Hearing Research*, 36, 568–579.

Hammer, C.S. (1994). Working with families of Chamorro and Carolinian children. *American Journal of Speech-Language Pathology*, 3(3), 5–12.

Hamre, C.E. (1972). Research and clinical practice: A unifying model. *Asha*, 14, 542–545.

Harris, R.J. (1994). *ANOVA : An Analysis of Variance Primer*. Itasca, IL: F.E. Peacock Publishers.

Hart, M.K., & Hart, R.F. (1989). *Quantitative Methods for Quality and Productivity Improvement*. Milwaukee, WI : ASQC Quality Press.

Hays, W.L. (1973). *Statistics for the Social Sciences*. New York: Holt, Rinehart and Winston.

Head, H. (1926). *Aphasia and Kindred Disorders of Speech*. New York: Cambridge University Press.

Head, H. (1963). *Aphasia and Kindred Disorders of Speech*, Vol. 1. New York: Hafner.

Hedges, L.V., & Olkin, I. (1985). *Statistical Methods for Meta-analysis*. New York: Academic Press.

Hempel, C.G. (1952). *Fundamentals of Concept Formation in Empirical Science*. Chicago: University of Chicago Press.

Henerson, M.E., Morris, L.L., & Fitz-Gibbon, C.T. (1987). *How to Measure Attitudes*. Beverly Hills, CA: Sage Publications.

Hillenbrand, J., & Gayvert, R.T. (1993). Vowel classification based on fundamental frequency and formant frequencies. *Journal of Speech and Hearing Research*, 36, 694–700.

Hinds, P.S., Scandrett-Hibden, S., & McAulay, L.S. (1990). Further assessment of a method to estimate reliability and validity of qualitative research findings. *Journal of Advanced Nursing*, 15 (4), 430–435.

Holland, A.L., Greenhouse, J.B., Fromm, D., & Swingell, C.S. (1989). Predictors of language restitution following stroke: A multivariate analysis. *Journal of Speech and Hearing Research*, 32, 332–338.

Holtzman, W.H. (1963). Statistical models for the study of change in the single case. In C.W. Harris (Ed.), *Problems in Measuring Change* (pp. 199–211). Madison: University of Wisconsin Press.

Horner, R.D., & Baer, D.M. (1978). Multiple-probe technique: A variation of the multiple baseline. *Journal of Applied Behavior Analysis*, 11 (1), 189–196.

How to be sure you don't get funded (1989). *Asha*, 31(2), 76.

Howard, D. (1986). Beyond randomised controlled trials: The case for effective case studies of the effects of treatment in aphasia. *British Journal of Disorders of Communication*, 21, 89–102.

Hsu, L.M. (1989). Random sampling, randomization, and equivalence of contrasted groups in psychotherapy outcome research. *Journal of Consulting and Clinical Psychology*, 57, 131–137.

Humes, L.E., Watson, B.U., Christensen, L.A., Cokely, C.G., Halling, D.C., & Lee, L. (1994). Factors associated with individual differences in clinical measures of speech recognition among the elderly. *Journal of Speech and Hearing Research*, 37, 465–474.

Hunter, J.E. (1990). *Methods of Meta-Analysis*. Beverly Hills, CA: Sage Publications.

Hunter, J.E., & Schmidt, F.L. (1990). *Meta-analysis: Correcting Error and Bias in Research Findings*. Beverly Hills, CA: Sage Publications.

Ingham, R.J., & Siegel, G.M. (1989). On statements and overstatements: A response to Bench (1989). *Journal of Speech and Hearing Disorders*, 54, 298–299.

Jansen-Wilde, M.L., Duchan, J.F., & Higginbotham, D.J. (1995). Successful use of facilitated communication with an oral child. *Journal of Speech and Hearing Research*, 38, 658–676.

Jerger, J. (1960). Bekesy audiometry in analysis of auditory disorders. *Journal of Speech and Hearing Research*, 3, 275–287.

Jerger, J. (1962). Scientific writing can be readable. *Asha*, 4, 101–104.

Jerger, J. (1963a). Viewpoint. *Journal of Speech and Hearing Research*, 6, 203–206.

Jerger, J. (1963b). Who is qualified to do research? *Journal of Speech and Hearing Research*, 6, 301.

Jerger, J. (1964a). More on "Who is qualified to do research." *Journal of Speech and Hearing Research*, 7, 4–6.

Jerger, J. (1964b). Subject-oriented research. *Journal of Speech and Hearing Research*, 7, 207–208.

Johnson, W. (1946). *People in Quandaries*. New York: Harper and Row.

Johnson, W., & Associates (1959). *The Onset of Stuttering*. Minneapolis: University of Minnesota Press.

Johnson, W., Darley, F.L., & Spricstersbach, D.C. (1963). *Diagnostic Methods in Speech Pathology.* New York: Harper and Row.

Jordan, E.P. (1960). Articulation test measures and listener ratings of articulation defectiveness. *Journal of Speech and Hearing Research,* 3, 303–319.

Journals in Communication Sciences and Disorders (1991). Rockville, MD: American Speech-Language-Hearing Association.

Kaiser, A.P., & Hester, P.P. (1994). Generalized effects of enhanced milieu teaching. *Journal of Speech and Hearing Research,* 37, 1320–1340.

Karlsen, E.A., Mikhail, H.H., Norris, C.W., & Hassanein, R.S. (1992). Comparison of responses to air, water, and closed-loop caloric irrigators. *Journal of Speech and Hearing Research,* 35, 186–191.

Kaufman, L., & Rousseeuw, P.J. (1990). *Finding Groups in Data: An Introduction to Cluster Analysis.* New York: Wiley.

Kazdin, A.E. (1981). External validity and single case experimentation: Issues and limitations. *Analysis and Intervention in Developmental Disabilities,* 1, 133–143.

Kazdin, A.E. (1982a). Single-case experimental designs in clinical research and practice. In A.E. Kazdin & A.H. Tuma (Eds.), *Single-case Research Designs* (pp. 33–47). San Francisco: Jossey-Bass.

Kazdin, A.E. (1982b). *Single-Case Research Designs: Methods for Clinical and Applied Settings.* London: Oxford University Press.

Kearns, K.P. (1986). Flexibility of single-subject experimental designs. Part II: Design selection and arrangement of experimental phases. *Journal of Speech and Hearing Disorders,* 51, 204–214.

Kelly, D.J., & McReynolds, L.V. (1987). The role of research in the clinic. Paper presented at the 1987 annual meeting of the American Speech-Language-Hearing Association, New Orleans.

Kempster G.B., Kistler, D.J., & Hillenbrand, J. (1991). Multidimensional scaling analysis of dysphonia for two speaker groups. *Journal of Speech and Hearing Research,* 34, 534–543.

Kendall, P.C. (1981). Assessing generalization and the single subject strategies. *Behavior Modification,* 5 (3), 307–319.

Kimball, A.W. (1957). Errors of the third kind in statistical consulting. *Journal of the American Statistical Association,* 52, 133–142.

Kline, P. (1994). *An Easy Guide to Factor Analysis.* New York: Routledge.

Korzybski, A. (1958). *Science and Sanity: An Introduction to Non-Aristotelian Systems and General Semantics.* Lakeville, CT: Institute of General Semantics.

Kratochwill, T.R. (Ed.) (1978). *Single Subject Research.* New York: Academic Press.

Kratochwill, T.R., & Brody, G.H. (1978). Single subject designs—A perspective on the controversy over employing statistical inference and implications for research and training in behavior modification. *Behavior Modification,* 2 (3), 291–307.

Kratochwill, T.R., & Levin, J.R. (1980). On the applicability of various data analysis procedures to the simultaneous and alternating treatment designs in behavior therapy research. *Behavioral Assessment,* 2, 353–360.

Kratochwill, T.R., & Levin, J.R. (1992). *Single-Case Research Design and Analysis: New Directions for Psychology and Education.* Hillsdale, NJ: Lawrence Erlbaum Associates.

Kreiman, J., Gerratt, B.R., Kenpster, G.B., Erman, A., & Berke, G.S. (1993). Perceptual evaluation of voice quality: Review, tutorial, and a framework for future research. *Journal of Speech and Hearing Research,* 36, 21–40.

Kreiman, J., Gerratt, B.R., Precoda, K., & Berke, G.S. (1992). Individual differences in voice quality perception. *Journal of Speech and Hearing Research,* 35, 512–520.

Kuehn, D.P., & Moon, J.B. (1994). Levator veli palatini muscle activity in relation to intraoral air pressure variations. *Journal of Speech and Hearing Research,* 37, 1260–1270.

Kunh, T.S. (1962). *The Structure of Scientific Revolutions.* Chicago: University of Chicago Press.

Ladimer, I. (1970). Protection and compensation for injury in human studies. In P.A. Freund (Ed.), *Experimentation with Human Subjects.* New York: George Braziller.

Lahey, M. (1992). Linguistic and cultural diversity: Further problems for determining who shall be called language disordered. *Journal of Speech and Hearing Research*, 35, 638–639.

Laird, N.M., & Mosteller, F. (1990). Some statistical methods for combining experimental results. *International Journal of Technology Assessment in Health Care*, 6 (1), 5–30.

Langmore, S.E., & Lehman, M.E. (1994). Physiologic deficits in the orofacial system underlying dysarthria in amyotrophic lateral sclerosis. *Journal of Speech and Hearing Research*, 37, 28–37.

Lawson, C. (1995). Research participation as a contract. *Ethics & Behavior*, 5(3), 205–215.

Lee, A. (1989). A socio-cultural framework for the assessment of Chinese children with special needs. *Topics in Language Disorders*, 9(3), 38–44.

Leitenberg, H. (1973). The use of single case methodology in psychotherapy research. *Journal of Abnormal Psychology*, 82, 87–101.

Leonard, L.B., McGregor, K.K., & Allen, G.D. (1992). Grammatical morphology and speech perception in children with specific language impairment. *Journal of Speech and Hearing Research*, 35, 1076–1085.

Levin, J.R., Marascuilo, L.A., & Hubert, L.J. (1978). N = Nonparametric randomization tests. In T.R. Kratochwill (Ed.), *Single Subject Research—Strategies for Evaluating Change* (pp. 167–196). New York: Academic Press.

Levine, G. (1991). *A Guide to SPSS for Analysis of Variance*. Hillsdale, NJ : Lawrence Erlbaum Associates.

Lewis, D., & Sherman, D. (1951). Measuring the severity of stuttering. *Journal of Speech and Hearing Disorders*, 16, 320–326.

Lieber, R.L. (1990). Statistical significance and statistical power in hypothesis testing. *Journal of Orthopedic Research*, 8 (2), 304–309.

Liles, B.Z., Duffy, R.J., Merritt, D.D., & Purcell, S.L. (1995). Measurement of narrative discourse ability in children with language disorders. *Journal of Speech and Hearing Research*, 38, 415–425.

Lindquist, E.F. (1953). *Design and Analysis of Experiments in Psychology and Education*. Boston: Houghton Mifflin.

Linville, S.E. (1992). Glotal gap configurations in two age groups of women. *Journal of Speech and Hearing Research*, 35, 1209–1215.

Locke, L.F. (1993). *Proposals That Work*. Newbury Park, CA: Sage Publications.

Logemann, J.A., Gibbons, P., Rademaker, A.W., Pauloski, B.R., Kahrilas, P.J., Bacon, M., Bowman, J., & McCracken, E. (1994). Mechanisms of recovery of swallow after supraglottic laryngectomy. *Journal of Speech and Hearing Research*, 37, 965–974.

Lore, J.I., & Gutter, F.J. (1968). The embryogeny of an NIH research grant. *Asha*, 10, 7–9.

Lucas, R.A. (1992). *The Grants World Inside Out*. Urbana: University of Illinois Press.

MacMillan, N., Goldberg, R., & Braida, L. (1988). Resolution for speech sounds: Basic sensitivity and context memory on vowel and consonant continua. *Journal of the Acoustical Society of America*, 84, 1262–1280.

MacRae, J.H. (1995). Temporary and permanent threshold shift caused by hearing aid use. *Journal of Speech and Hearing Research*, 38, 949–959.

Maestas, A.G., & Erickson, J.G. (1992). Mexican immigrant mother's beliefs about disability. *American Journal of Speech-Language Pathology*, 1(4), 5–10.

Maré, M.J., Dreschler, W.A., & Verschuure, H. (1992). The effects of input-output configuration in syllabic compression on speech perception. *Journal of Speech and Hearing Research*, 35, 675–685.

Martin, D., Fitch, J., & Wolfe, V. (1995). Pathologic voice type and acoustic prediction of severity. *Journal of Speech and Hearing Research*, 38, 765–771.

Martin, R., & Haroldson, S.K. (1992). Stuttering and speech naturalness: Audio and audiovisual judgments. *Journal of Speech and Hearing Research*, 35, 521–528.

Martinez, A., Bedore, L.M., & Ludwig, J.L. (1994). On cultural sensitivity in assessing cross-cultural attitudes: Comments on Bebout and Arthur (1992).

Journal of Speech and Hearing Research, 37, 341–342.

Matsuda, M. (1989). Working with Asian parents: Some communication strategies. *Topics in Language Disorders*, 9(3), 45–53.

Matt, G.E. (1989). Decision rules for effect sizes in meta-analysis: A review and reanalysis of psychotherapy outcome studies. *Psychological Bulletin*, 105, 106–115.

Mayberry, R.I. (1993). First-language acquisition after childhood differs from second-language acquisition: The case of American Sign Language. *Journal of Speech and Hearing Research*, 36, 1258–1270.

McCall, G.J., & Simmons, J.L. (1969). *Issues in Participant Observation: A Text and Reader.* Reading, MA: Addison-Wesley.

McClean, M.D., Levandowski, D.R., & Cord, M.T. (1994). Intersyllabic movement timing in the fluent speech of stutterers with different disfluency levels. *Journal of Speech and Hearing Research*, 37, 1060–1066.

McCullough, J.P. (1984). Single case investigative research and its relevance for the nonoperant clinician. *Psychotherapy*, 21, 382–388.

McLeod, S., Hand, L., Rosenthal, J.B., & Hayes, B. (1994). The effect of sampling condition on children's productions of consonant clusters. *Journal of Speech and Hearing Research*, 37, 868–882.

McPherson, D.L., & Thatcher, J.W. (1977). *Instrumentation in the Hearing Sciences.* New York: Grune and Stratton.

McReynolds, L.V., & Kearns, K.P. (1983). *Single-subject Experimental Designs in Communicative Disorders.* Baltimore: University Park Press.

McReynolds, L.V., & Thompson, C.K. (1986). Flexibility of single-subject experimental designs. Part I: Review of the basics of single-subject designs. *Journal of Speech and Hearing Disorders*, 51, 194–203.

Meitus, I.J., Ringel, R.L., House, A.S., & Hotchkiss, J.C. (1973). Clinical bias in evaluating speech proficiency. *British Journal of Disorders of Communication*, 8, 146–151.

Merriam, S.B. (1988). *Case Study Research in Education: A Qualitative Approach.* San Francisco: Jossey-Bass.

Meslin, E.M. (1990). Protecting human subjects from harm through improved risk judgments. *IRB· A Review of Human Subject Research*, 12 (1), 7–10.

Metz, D.E., & Folkins, J.W. (1985). Protection of human subjects in speech and hearing research. *Asha*, 27 (3), 25–29.

Meyers, S.C. (1990). Tempest in a t-test: A reply to Finn and Glow. *Journal of Speech and Hearing Disorders*, 55, 173–174.

Moore, M.V. (1969). Pathological writing. *Asha*, 11, 535–538.

Mower, D.E. (1969). Evaluating speech therapy through precision recording. *Journal of Speech and Hearing Disorders*, 34, 329–344.

Mulligan, M., Carpenter, J., Riddel, J., Delaney, M.K., Badger, G., Krusinski, P., & Tandan, R. (1994). Intelligibility and acoustic characteristics of speech in amyotrophic lateral sclerosis (ALS). *Journal of Speech and Hearing Research*, 37, 496–503.

Murray, G.D. (1989). Confidence intervals. *Nuclear Medicine Communications*, 10 (6), 387–388.

National Institutes of Health (1993a). *Guidelines for the Conduct of Research Involving Human Subjects at the National Institutes of Health.* Bethesda, MD: National Institutes of Health.

National Institutes of Health (1993b). *Preparing a Research Grant Application to the National Institutes of Health : Selected Articles.* Bethesda, MD: National Institutes of Health.

Nellum-Davis, P. (1993). Clinical practice issues. In D.E. Battle (Ed.), *Communication Disorders in Multicultural Populations* (pp. 306–316). Boston: Andover Medical Publishers.

Ogden, T.E., & Goldberg, I.A. (1995). *Research Proposals : A Guide to Success* (Second Edition). New York: Raven Press.

Olswang, L.B. (1990). Treatment efficacy research: A path to quality assurance. *Asha*, 32 (1), 45–47.

Orne, M.T. (1969). Demand characteristics and the concept of quasi-controls. In R. Rosenthal & R.L.

Rosnow (Eds.), *Artifacts in Behavioral Research* (pp. 143–179). New York: Academic Press.

Orque, M., Block, L., & Monroy, L. (1983). *Ethnic Nursing Care: A Multicultural Approach*. St. Louis, MO: C. V. Mosby.

Osgood, C.E., Suci, G.J., & Tannenbaum, P.H. (1957). *The Measurement of Meaning*. Urbana: University of Illinois Press.

Panush, R. (1989). The limits of science in communication disorders: A reply to Siegel. *Journal of Speech and Hearing, Disorders*, 54, 301–302.

Pap, A. (1949). *Elements of Analytic Philosophy*. New York: The Macmillan Company.

Pap, A. (1953). Does science have metaphysical presuppositions? In H. Feigl & M. Brodbeck (Eds.), *Readings in the Philosophy of Science* (pp. 21–33). New York: Appleton-Century-Crofts.

Parsonson, B.S., & Baer, D.M. (1978). The analysis and presentation of graphic data. In T.R. Kratochwill (Ed.), *Single Subject Research—Strategies for Evaluating Change* (pp. 101–166). New York: Academic Press.

Patton, M.Q. (1990). *Qualitative Evaluation and Research Methods*. Newbury Park, CA: Sage.

Peach, R.K. (1992). Factors underlying neuropsychological test performance in chronic severe traumatic brain injury. *Journal of Speech and Hearing Research*, 35, 810–818.

Penner, M.J., & Bilger, R.C. (1989). Adaptation and the masking of tinnitus. *Journal of Speech and Hearing Research*, 32, 339–346.

Penslar, R.L. (1993). *Protecting Human Research Subjects: Institutional Review Board Guidebook* (Second Edition). Bethesda, MD: U.S. Dept. of Health and Human Services, Public Health Service, National Institutes of Health, Office of Extramural Research, Office for Protection from Research Risks.

Perkins, W.H. (1986). Functions and malfunctions of theories in therapies. *Asha*, 28 (2), 31–33.

Perlman, A.L., Grayhack, J.P., & Booth, B.M. (1992). The relationship of vallecular residue to oral involvement, reduced hyoid elevation, and epiglottic function. *Journal of Speech and Hearing Research*, 35, 734–741.

Petitti, D.B. (1994). *Meta-Analysis, Decision Analysis, and Cost-Effectiveness Analysis*. New York: Oxford University Press.

Pfaffenberger, B. (1990). *Democratizing Information: Online Databases and the Rise of End-User Searching*. Boston: G. K. Hall.

Pitt, M.A., & Samuel, A.G. (1993). An empirical and meta-analytic evaluation of the phoneme identification task. *Journal of Experimental Psychology: Human Perception & Performance*, 19(4), 699–725.

PlusNet2 Medline System: End-user Introduction (1990). New York: CD Plus.

Polanyi, M. (1967). *The Tacit Dimension*. Garden City, NY: Doubleday Anchor Books.

Porch, B. (1971). Multidimensional scoring in aphasia testing. *Journal of Speech and Hearing Research*, 14, 776–792.

Porter, R.E., & Samovar, L.A. (1976). Communicating interculturally. In L.A. Samovar & R.W. Porter (Eds.), *Intercultural Education: A Reader*. Belmont, CA: Wadsworth.

Prather, E.M. (1960). Scaling defectiveness of articulation by direct magnitude-estimation. *Journal of Speech and Hearing Research*, 3, 380–392.

Preparing a Research Grant Application to the National Institutes of Health (1989). Bethesda, MD: National Institutes of Health.

Pring, T.R. (1986). Evaluating the effects of speech therapy for aphasics: Developing the single case methodology. *British Journal of Disorders of Communication*, 21, 103–115.

Prutting, C.A., Mentis, M., & Nelson, P. (1989). Critique of Siegel: The limits of "The Limits of Science in Communication Disorders." *Journal of Speech and Hearing Disorders*, 54, 299–300.

The Publication Process: A Guide for Authors (1991). Rockville, MD: American Speech-Language-Hearing Association.

Publications Manual for the American Psychological Association (Fourth Edition). (1994). Washington, DC: American Psychological Association.

Purtilo, R., & Cassel, C.K. (1981). *Ethical Dimensions in the Health Professions*. Philadelphia: W. B. Saunders.

Radil-Weiss, T. (1983). Men in extreme conditions: Some medical and psychological aspects of the Auschwitz Concentration Camp. *Psychiatry*, 46, 259–268.

Reif-Lehrer, L. (1995). *Grant Application Writer's Handbook*. Boston: Jones & Bartlett Publishers.

Reiner, B.J., & Ludlow, C.L. (1979a). *MEDLINE Users Manual and Thesaurus for Specialists in Communicative Disorders*, Vol. I (Users Manual NIH 79-1997). Bethesda, MD: U.S. Department of Health Services, Public Health Service, National Institutes of Health.

Reiner, B.J., & Ludlow, C.L. (1979b). *MEDLINE Users Manual and Thesaurus for Specialists in Communicative Disorders*, Vol. II (Thesaurus NIH 79-1998). Bethesda, MD: U.S. Department of Health Services, Public Health Service, National Institutes of Health.

Reiner, B.J., & Ludlow, C.L. (1981). Using MEDLINE for literature retrieval in the communicative disorders. *Asha*, 23, 655–662.

Revusky, S.H. (1967). Some statistical treatments compatible with individual organism methodology. *Journal of Experimental Analysis of Behavior*, 10, 319–330.

Rickels, K., Schweizer, E., & Case, W.G. (1988). The uncontrolled case report: A double-edged sword. *Journal of Nervous and Mental Diseases*, 176 (1), 50–52.

Ries, J.B. (1995). *Applying for Research Funding*. Thousand Oaks, CA: Sage Publications.

Ringel, R.L. (1972). The clinician and the researcher: An artificial dichotomy. *Asha*, 14, 351–353.

Ringel, R.L., Tachtman, L.E., & Prutting, C.A. (1984). The science in human communication sciences. *Asha*, 26 (12), 33–36.

Roark, R.M., Dowling, E.M., DeGrote, R.D., Watson, B.C., & Schaefer, S.D. (1995). Time-frequency analyses of thyroarytenoid myoelectric activity in normal and spasmodic dysphonia subjects. *Journal of Speech and Hearing Research*, 38, 289–303.

Robey, R.R. (1994). The efficacy of treatment for aphasic persons: A meta-analysis. *Brain & Language*, 47, 582–608.

Rochon, J. (1990). A statistical model for the "N-of-1" study. *Journal of Clinical Epidemiology*, 43, 499–508.

Rosenthal, R. (1976). *Experimenter Effects in Behavioral Research*. New York: Halsted Press.

Rosenthal, R. (1978). Combining results of independent studies. *Psychological Bulletin*, 85, 185–193.

Rosenthal, R., & Rosnow, R.L. (1969). *Artifacts in Behavioral Research*. New York: Academic Press.

Rosenthal, R., & Rosnow, R.L. (1985). *Contrast Analysis : Focused Comparisons in the Analysis of Variance*. New York: Cambridge University Press.

Rosnow, R.L. (1990). Teaching research ethics through role-play and discussion. *Teaching of Psychology*, 17(3) 179–181.

Rosnow, R.L., Rotheram-Borus, M.J., Ceci, S.J., & Blanck, P.D. (1993). The Institutional Review Board as a mirror of scientific and ethical standards. *American Psychologist*, 48(7), 821–826.

Roth, C.R., Aronson, A.E., & Davis, L.J., Jr. (1989). Clinical studies in psychogenic stuttering of adult onset. *Journal of Speech and Hearing Disorders*, 54, 634–646.

Rusch, F.R., & Kazdin, A.E. (1981). Toward a methodology of withdrawal designs for the assessment of response maintenance. *Journal of Applied Behavior Analysis*, 14 (2), 131–140.

Schiavetti, N., Martin, R.R., Haroldson, S.K., & Metz, D.E. (1994). Psychophysical analysis of audiovisual judgments of speech naturalness of nonstutterers and stutterers. *Journal of Speech and Hearing Research*, 37, 46–52.

Schober-Peterson, D., & Johnson, C.J. (1989). Conversational topics of 4-year-olds. *Journal of Speech and Hearing Research*, 32, 857–870.

Schuell, H., Jenkins, J., & Jimenez-Pabon, E. (1964). *Aphasia in Adults*. New York: Harper and Row.

Schultz, M.C., Roberts, W.H., & Yairi, E. (1972). The clinician and the researcher: Comments. *Asha*, 14, 539–541.

Schumacher, D. (1992). *Get Funded*. Newbury Park, CA: Sage Publications.

Schwartz, S.M. (1992). *A Guide to NIH Grant Programs*. New York: Oxford University Press.

Scott, D.M. (1995). June 8th memorandum to program

chairpersons about multicultural affairs. Rockville, MD: Office of Multicultural Affairs, American Speech-Language-Hearing Association.

Screen, R.M., & Anderson, N.B. (1994). *Multicultural Perspectives in Communication Disorders*. San Diego, CA: Singular Publishing Group.

Seymour, H.N. (1992). The invisible children: A reply to Lahey's perspective. *Journal of Speech and Hearing Research*, 35, 640–641.

Seymour, H.N., & Seymour, C.M. (1981). Black English and Standard American English contrasts in consonantal development of four- and five-year-old children. *Journal of Speech and Hearing Disorders*, 46, 274–280.

Shapiro, A.K. (1964). Factors contributing to the placebo effect: Implications for psychotherapy. *American Journal of Psychotherapy*, 18 (Supplement 1), 73–88.

Shelton, R.L., Paesani, A., McClelland, K.D., & Bradfield, S.S. (1975). Panendoscope feedback in the study of voluntary velopharyngeal movements. *Journal of Speech and Hearing Disorders*, 40, 232–244.

Sherman, D., & Silverman, F.H. (1968). Three psychological methods applied to language development. *Journal of Speech and Hearing Research*, 11, 837–841.

Shipley, K.G. (Ed.) (1982). *A Style Manual for Writers in Communicative Disorders*. Tucson, AZ: Communication Skill Builders.

Shriberg, L.D. (1993). Four new speech and prosody-voice measures for genetics research and other studies in developmental phonological disorders. *Journal of Speech and Hearing Research*, 36, 105–140.

Shriberg, L.D., & Kwiatkowski, J. (1982). Phonological disorders III: A procedure for assessing severity of involvement. *Journal of Speech and Hearing Disorders*, 47, 256–270.

Shriberg, L.D., Kwiatkowski, J., & Gruber, F.A. (1994). Developmental phonological disorders II: Short-term speech-sound normalization. *Journal of Speech and Hearing Research*, 37, 1127–1150.

Shriner, T.H., & Sherman, D. (1976). An equation for assessing language development. *Journal of Speech and Hearing Research*, 10, 41–48.

Sidman, M. (1960). *Tactics of Scientific Research*. New York: Basic Books.

Siegel, G.M. (1988). Science and communication disorders: A reply to Bloodstein. *Journal of Speech and Hearing Disorders*, 53, 348–349.

Siegel, G.M., & Ingham, R.J. (1987). Theory and science in communication disorders. *Journal of Speech and Hearing Disorders*, 52, 99–104.

Siegel, G.M., & Spradlin, J.E. (1985). Therapy and research. *Journal of Speech and Hearing Disorders*, 50, 226–230.

Siegel, S. (1956). *Nonparametric Statistics for the Behavioral Sciences*. New York: McGraw-Hill.

Siegel, S. (1988). *Nonparametric Statistics for the Behavioral Sciences* (Second Edition). New York: McGraw-Hill.

Silverman, E.-M. (1972). Generality of disfluency data collected from preschoolers. *Journal of Speech and Hearing Research*, 5, 84–92.

Silverman, F.H. (1967a). Correspondence between mean and median scale values for sets of stimuli scaled by the method of equal-appearing intervals. *Perceptual and Motor Skills*, 25, 727–728.

Silverman, F.H. (1967b). Interpretation of mean Q values for sets of stimuli rated on a seven-point equal-appearing interval scale. *Perceptual and Motor Skills*, 24, 842 (1967).

Silverman, F.H. (1968a). An approach to determining the number of judges needed for scaling experiments. *Perceptual and Motor Skills*, 17, 1333–1334.

Silverman, F.H. (1968b). Intraclass correlation coefficient as an index of reliability of median scale values for sets of stimuli rated by equal-appearing intervals. *Perceptual and Motor Skills*, 26, 878.

Silverman, F.H. (1974). The Porch Index of Communicative Ability (PICA): A psychometric problem and its solution. *Journal of Speech and Hearing Disorders*, 39, 225–226.

Silverman, F.H. (1977a). A bibliography of literature relevant to nonspeech communication modes for the speechless. *Ohio Journal of Speech and Hearing*, 12, 83–102.

Silverman, F.H. (1977b). Criteria for assessing therapy outcome in speech pathology and audiology. *Journal of Speech and Hearing Research*, 20, 5–20.

Silverman, F.H. (1984). *Speech-Language Pathology and Audiology: An Introduction.* Columbus, Ohio: Merrill.

Silverman, F.H. (1987). *Microcomputers in Speech-Language Pathology and Audiology.* Englewood Cliffs, NJ: Prentice-Hall.

Silverman, F.H. (1988). The "Monster" Study. *Journal of Fluency Disorders*, 13, 225–231.

Silverman, F.H. (1992). *Legal-Ethical Considerations, Restrictions, and Obligations for Clinicians who Treat Communicative Disorders* (Second Edition). Springfield, IL: Charles C. Thomas.

Silverman, F.H. (1995a). *Communication for the Speechless* (Third Edition). Needham Heights, MA: Allyn & Bacon.

Silverman, F.H. (1995b). *Speech, Language, and Hearing Disorders.* Needham Heights, MA: Allyn & Bacon.

Silverman, F.H. (1996). *Stuttering and Other Fluency Disorders* (Second Edition). Needham Heights, MA: Allyn & Bacon.

Silverman, F.H. (1997). *Computer Applications for Augmenting the Management of Speech, Language, and Hearing Disorders.* Needham Heights, MA: Allyn & Bacon.

Silverman, F.H., & Johnston, R.G. (1975). Direct interval-estimation: A ratio scaling method. *Perceptual and Motor Skills*, 41, 464–466.

Silverman, F.H., & Klees, J. (1989). Adolescents' attitudes toward peers who wear visible hearing aids. *Journal of Communication Disorders*, 22, 147–150.

Silverman, F.H., & Paulus, P.G. (1989). Peer reactions to teenagers who substitute /w/ for /r/. *Language, Speech, and Hearing Services in Schools*, 20, 219–221.

Silverman, F.H., & Trotter, W.D. (1973). Impact of pacing speech with a miniature electronic metronome upon the manner in which a stutterer is perceived. *Behavior Therapy*, 4, 414–419.

Silverman, F.H., & Williams, D.E. (1973). Use of revision by elementary-school stutterers and nonstutterers during oral reading. *Journal of Speech and Hearing Research*, 16, 584–585.

Simes, J. (1990). Meta-analysis: Its importance in cost-effectiveness studies. *Medical Journal of Australia*, 153 (Supplement), 13–16.

Snider, J.G., & Osgood, C.E., (Eds.) (1968). *Semantic Differential Technique: A Sourcebook.* Chicago: Aldine Publishing Company.

Snow, D. (1994). Phrase-final syllable lengthening and intonation in early child speech. *Journal of Speech and Hearing Research*, 37, 831–840.

Sparks, R.D. (1989). Matching ideas and funds. *Asha*, 31 (2), 77, 99.

Spradley, J.P. (1979). *The Ethnographic Interview.* New York: Holt, Rinehart, and Winston.

Stagray, J.R., Downs, D., & Sommers, R.K. (1992). Contributions of the fundamental, resolved harmonics, and unresolved harmonics in tone-phoneme identification. *Journal of Speech and Hearing Research*, 35, 1406–1409.

Stanley, B. (1985). Toward "applicable" single-case research. *Bulletin of the British Psychological Society*, 38, 33–36.

Sternberg, R.J. (1993). *The Psychologist's Companion: A Guide to Scientific Writing for Students and Researchers* (Third Edition). New York: Cambridge University Press.

Stevens, S.S. (1951). Mathematics, measurement, and psychophysics. In S.S. Stevens (Ed.), *Handbook of Experimental Psychology* (pp. 1–49). New York: John Wiley and Sons.

Stewart, C.J., & Cash, W.B. (1988). *Interviewing: Principles and Practices.* Dubuque, IA: William C. Brown.

Stout, M.B. (1962). *Basic Electrical Measurements* (Second Edition). Englewood Cliffs, NJ: Prentice Hall.

Strain, P.S., & Shores, R.E. (1979). Additional comments on multiple baseline designs in instructional research. *American Journal of Mental Deficiency*, 84, 229–234.

Strohmetz, D.B., & Skleder, A.A. (1992). The use of role-play in teaching research ethics: A validation study. *Teaching of Psychology*, 19(2), 106–108.

Stutt-L for researchers, clinicians (1990). *Asha*, 32 (2), 12.

Sue, S. (1983). Ethnic minority issues in psychology: A reexamination. *American Psychologist*, 38(5), 583–592.

Summers, R.R. (1987). Research and training programs of the National Institute of Neurological and Communicative Disorders and Stroke. In H.J. Oyer (Ed.), *Administration of Programs in Speech-Language Pathology and Audiology*. Englewood Cliffs, NJ: Prentice-Hall.

Sussman, J.E. (1993a). Auditory processing in children's speech perception: Results of selective adaptation and discrimination tasks. *Journal of Speech and Hearing Research*, 36, 380–395.

Sussman, J.E. (1993b). Perception of formant transition cues to place of articulation in children with language impairment. *Journal of Speech and Hearing Research*, 36, 1286–1299.

Sutor, D.C., & White, D.B. (1992). *Nonparametric Statistics*. Reading, MA: Addison-Wesley.

Swanson, L.A., Leonard, L.B., & Grandour, J. (1992). Vowel duration in mothers' speech to young children. *Journal of Speech and Hearing Research*, 35, 617–625.

Takahashi, G.A., & Bacon, S.P. (1992). Modulation detection, nodulation masking, and speech understanding in noise in the elderly. *Journal of Speech and Hearing Research*, 35, 1410–1421.

Talbott, R.E. (1969). Bacteriology of earphone contamination. *Journal of Speech and Hearing Research*, 12, 326–329.

Tawney, J.W., & Gast, D.L. (1984). *Single Subject Research in Special Education*. Columbus, OH: Charles C. Merrill.

Taylor, O.L. (1986). *Treatment of Communicative Disorders in Culturally and Linguistically Diverse Populations*. Boston: College Hill.

Taylor, O.L. (1992). Clinical practice as a social occasion: An ethnographic model. In L. Cole & V. Deal (Eds.), *Communication Disorders in Multicultural Populations*. Rockville, MD: American Speech-Language-Hearing Association.

Terrell, B.Y., & Hale, J.E. (1992). Serving a multicultural population: Different learning styles. *American Journal of Speech-Language Pathology*, 1(2), 5–8.

Thal, D.J., & Tobias, S. (1992). Communicative gestures in children with delayed onset of oral expressive vocabulary. *Journal of Speech and Hearing Research*, 35, 1281–1289.

Thompson, R.A. (1990). Behavioral research involving children: A developmental perspective on risk. *IRB: A Review of Human Subject Research*, 12 (2), 1–6.

Tomes, L., & Shelton, R.L. (1989). Children's categorization of consonants by manner and place characteristics. *Journal of Speech and Hearing Research*, 32, 432–438.

Trotter, W.D., & Kools, J.A. (1955). Listener adaptation to the severity of stuttering. *Journal of Speech and Hearing Disorders*, 29, 385–387.

Van Ijzendoorn, M.H., Dijkstra, J., & Bus, A.G. (1995). Attachment, intelligence, and language: A meta-analysis. *Social Development*, 4(2), 115–128.

Van Kleeck, A. (1994). Potential cultural bias in training parents as conversational partners with their children who have delays in language development. *American Journal of Speech-Language Pathology*, 3(1), 67–78.

Van Riper, C. (1958). Experiments in stuttering therapy. In J. Eisenson (Ed.), *Stuttering: A Symposium* (pp. 273–390). New York: Harper and Row.

Van Riper, C. (1982). *The Nature of Stuttering* (Second Edition). Englewood Cliffs, NJ: Prentice-Hall.

Vekovius, G.T. (1995). Managed care 101. *Asha*, 37(9), 44–47.

Villarruel, F., Mathy-Laikko, P., Ratcliff, A., & Yoder, D. (1987). *Alternative and Augmentative Communication Bibliography*. Madison, WI: Trace Research & Development Center, University of Wisconsin.

Viswanath, N.S., & Neel, A.T. (1995). Part-word repetitions by persons who stutter: Fragment types and their articulatory processes. *Journal of Speech and Hearing Research*, 38, 740–750.

Wachter, K.W., & Straf, M.E. (Eds.) (1990). *The Future of Meta-analysis*. New York: Russell Sage Foundation.

Walden, B.E., Busacco, D.A., & Montgomery,

A.A. (1993). Benefit from visual cues in auditory-visual speech recognition by middle-aged and elderly persons. *Journal of Speech and Hearing Research*, 36, 431–436.

Washington, J.A., & Craig, H.K. (1994). Dialectal forms during discourse of poor, urban, African American preschoolers. *Journal of Speech and Hearing Research*, 37, 816–823.

Watson, P.J. & Workman, E.A. (1981). The non-concurrent multiple baseline across-individuals design: An extension of the traditional multiple baseline design. *Journal of Behavior Therapy and Experimental Psychiatry*, 12 (3), 257–259.

Wayman, I., Lynch, E., & Hanson, M. (1990). Home-based early childhood services: Cultural sensitivity in a family systems approach. *Topics in Early Childhood Special Education*, 10(4), 56–75.

Weston, A.D., & Shriberg, L.D. (1992). Contextual and linguistic correlates of intelligibility in children with developmental phonological disorders. *Journal of Speech and Hearing Research*, 35, 1316–1332.

Whitaker, V.B., Dill, C.A., & Whitaker, R., Jr. (1990). Experimenter behavior: Influences on research outcomes? *Insight*, 15 (4), 18–19.

White, B.C. (1994). *Competence to Consent*. Washington, DC: Georgetown University Press.

Whorf, B.E. (1956). *Language, Thought, and Reality*. Cambridge, MA: Cambridge Technology Press of MIT.

Wilkinson, L. (1988). *SYSTAT: The System for Statistics*. Evanston, IL: SYSTAT, Inc.

Williams, D.E. (1968). Stuttering therapy: An overview. In H. H. Gregory (Ed.), *Learning Theory and Stuttering Therapy* (pp. 52–66). Evanston, IL: Northwestern University Press.

Wilson, B.U., & Miller, T.K. (1993). Auditory perception, phonological processing, and reading ability/disability. *Journal of Speech and Hearing Research*, 36, 850–863.

Winer, B.J. (1962). *Statistical Principles in Experimental Design*. New York: McGraw-Hill.

Winer, B.J. (1991). *Statistical Principles in Experimental Design* (Third Edition). New York: McGraw-Hill.

Wit, J., Maassen, B., Gabreëls, F.J.M., & Thoonen, G. (1993). Maximum performance tests in children with developmental spastic dysarthria. *Journal of Speech and Hearing Research*, 36, 452–459.

Wolery, M., & Harris, S.R. (1982). Interpreting results of single-subject research designs. *Physical Therapy*, 62 (4), 445–452.

Yairi, E. (1974). A sudden onset of high-pitched voice associated with unilateral vocal fold paralysis: A case report. *Journal of Speech and Hearing Disorders*, 39, 373–375.

Yin, R.K. (1984). *Case Study Research: Design and Methods*. Beverly Hills, CA: Sage Publications.

Young, F.W. (1987). *Multidimensional Scaling—History, Theory, and Applications*. Hillsdale, NJ: Lawrence Erlbaum Associates.

Zaidel, E., Aboitiz, F., Clarke, J., Kaiser, D., & Matteson, R. (1995). Sex differences in interhemispheric relations for language. In F. Kitterle (Ed.), *Hemispheric Communication: Mechanisms and Models* (pp. 85–175). Hillsdale, NJ: Lawrence Erlbaum Associates.

Author Index

Subject Index